Pharmacovigilance:
A Practical Approach

Pharmacovigilance: A Practical Approach

THAO DOAN, MD
Senior Medical Director
Safety Science
Pharmacovigilance and Patient Safety
AbbVie
North Chicago, Illinois, United States

CHERYL RENZ, MS, MD
Senior Medical Director
Safety Science
Pharmacovigilance and Patient Safety
AbbVie
North Chicago, Illinois, United States

MONDIRA BHATTACHARYA, MD
Former Senior Medical Director
Safety Science
Pharmacovigilance and Patient Safety
AbbVie
North Chicago, Illinois, United States

FABIO LIEVANO, MD
Vice President
Safety Science
Pharmacovigilance and Patient Safety
AbbVie
North Chicago, Illinois, United States

LINDA SCARAZZINI, MD
Vice President
Pharmacovigilance and Patient Safety
AbbVie
North Chicago, Illinois, United States

ELSEVIER

ELSEVIER

3251 Riverport Lane
St. Louis, Missouri 63043

PHARMACOVIGILANCE: A PRACTICAL APPROACH   ISBN: 978-0-323-58116-5

Content Strategist: Kayla Wolfe
Content Development Manager: Christine McElvenny
Content Development Specialist: Jennifer Horigan
Publishing Services Manager: Shereen Jameel
Project Manager: Nadhiya Sekar
Designer: Gopalakrishnan Venkatraman

Printed in United States of America

Last digit is the print number: 9 8 7 6 5 4 3 2 1

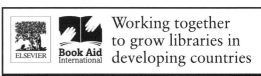

List of Contributors

Jabeen Ahmad, BSc (Hons)
Regional Director
Affiliate Vigilance Excellence
Pharmacovigilance and Patient Safety
AbbVie
Maidenhead, United Kingdom

Hans Peter Bacher, MD, PhD
Mature Products
Global Medical Affairs
AbbVie
North Chicago, IL, United States

Mondira Bhattacharya, MD
Former Senior Medical Director
Safety Science
Pharmacovigilance and Patient Safety
AbbVie
North Chicago, IL, United States

Deepa H. Chand, MD, MHSA
Associate Medical Director
Safety Science
Pharmacovigilance and Patient Safety
AbbVie
North Chicago, IL, United States

Monali Desai, MD, MPH
Senior Medical Director
Pharmacovigilance and Patient Safety
AbbVie
North Chicago, IL, United States

Thao Doan, MD
Senior Medical Director
Safety Science
Pharmacovigilance and Patient Safety
AbbVie
North Chicago, IL, United States

James Duhig, PhD
Director
Safety Science
Pharmacovigilance and Patient Safety
AbbVie
North Chicago, IL, United States

Vicki Edwards, BPharm (Hons)
Vice President
Pharmacovigilance Excellence
Pharmacovigilance and Patient Safety
AbbVie
Maidenhead, United Kingdom

Jawed Fareed, PhD, DSc, FAHA
Professor of Pathology and Pharmacology
Director of Hemostasis and Thrombosis
Research Laboratories
Division Director Cardiovascular Institute,
Vascular Biology
Chair, Institutional Animal Care and
Usage Committee
Loyola University Medical Center
Maywood, IL, United States

Carl Fischer, PhD
Senior Advisor
Center for Device and Radiological Health
U.S. Food & Drug Administration
Silver Spring, MD, United States

Cheryl Foit, BS
Director
Project Management
Pharmacovigilance and Patient Safety
AbbVie
North Chicago, IL, United States

Suzanne Pauline Green, MD, MBChB, FFPM
Former Medical Director
Safety Science
Pharmacovigilance and Patient Safety
AbbVie
Maidenhead, United Kingdom

Barbara A. Hendrickson, MD
Senior Medical Director
Safety Science
Pharmacovigilance and Patient Safety
AbbVie
North Chicago, IL, United States

Robert Hogan, PhD
President
Terminologix LLC
Antigo, WI, United States

Syed S. Islam, MBBS, MPH, MSPH, Dr.PH
Senior Medical Director
Epidemiology
Pharmacovigilance and Patient Safety
AbbVie
North Chicago, IL, United States

Calvin Johnson, BSc (Hons), MSc (PhV)
Director
Affiliate Vigilance Excellence
Pharmacovigilance and Patient Safety
AbbVie
Maidenhead, United Kingdom

Jeremy D. Jokinen, PhD, MS
Senior Director
Safety Science
Pharmacovigilance and Patient Safety
AbbVie
North Chicago, IL, United States

Ryan Kilpatrick, PhD
Senior Director
Epidemiology
Pharmacovigilance and Patient Safety
AbbVie
North Chicago, IL, United States

Karolyn Kracht, MS
Associate Director
Safety Science
Pharmacovigilance and Patient Safety
AbbVie
North Chicago, IL, United States

Gweneth Levy, MD
Medical Director
Safety Science
Pharmacovigilance and Patient Safety
AbbVie
North Chicago, IL, United States

Fabio Lievano, MD
Vice President
Safety Science
Pharmacovigilance and Patient Safety
AbbVie
North Chicago, IL, United States

Murray Malin, MD, MBA
Senior Medical Director
Medical Quality Assurance
AbbVie
North Chicago, IL, United States

Anthony G. Oladipo, PharmD, MPH, BCPS
Senior Director
Safety Science
Pharmacoviligance and Patient Safety
AbbVie
North Chicago, IL, United States

Denise M. Oleske, PhD
Director
Epidemiology
Pharmacovigilance and Patient Safety
AbbVie
North Chicago, IL, United States

Meenal Patwardhan, MD, MHSA
Senior Medical Director
Safety Science
Pharmacovigilance and Patient Safety
AbbVie
North Chicago, IL, United States

James M. Pauff, MD, PhD
Associate Medical Director
Oncology Clinical Development
AbbVie
North Chicago, IL, United States

Ariel Ramirez Porcalla, MD, MPH
Medical Director
Safety Science
Pharmacovigilance and Patient Safety
AbbVie
North Chicago, IL, United States

Radhika M. Rao, MD, MPH
Medical Director
Pharmacovigilance Operations
Pharmacovigilance and Patient Safety
AbbVie
North Chicago, IL, United States

Nicholas Rees, MBBS, BSc
Medical Director
Pharmacovigilance Excellence
Pharmacovigilance and Patient Safety
AbbVie
Maidenhead, United Kingdom

Cheryl Renz, MS, MD
Senior Medical Director
Safety Science
Pharmacovigilance and Patient Safety
AbbVie
North Chicago, IL, United States

Adrienne M. Rothstein, PharmD
Associate Director
Safety Science
Pharmacovigilance and Patient Safety
AbbVie
North Chicago, IL, United States

Linda Scarazzini, MD
Vice President
Pharmacovigilance and Patient Safety
AbbVie
North Chicago, IL, United States

Charles Schubert, MD, MPH
Senior Medical Director
Safety Science
Pharmacovigilance and Patient Safety
AbbVie
North Chicago, IL, United States

Sundeep Sethi, MD, MBA
Vice President
Pharmacovigilance Operations
Pharmacovigilance and Patient Safety
AbbVie
North Chicago, IL, United States

Arsalan Shabbir, MD, PhD
Former Associate Medical Director
Global Medical Affairs
AbbVie
North Chicago, IL, United States

Melissa M. Truffa, BSPharm
Director
Safety Science
Pharmacovigilance and Patient Safety
Abbvie
North Chicago, IL, United States

Jerzy Edward Tyczynski, PhD
Senior Director
Epidemiology
Pharmacovigilance and Patient Safety
AbbVie
North Chicago, IL, United States

Marietta Vazquez, MD, FAAP
Associate Professor Pediatrics
Infectious Diseases
Pediatrics
Yale University School of Medicine
New Haven, CT, United States

Verghese Mathew, MD, FACC, FSCAI
Chair in Cardiology
Director, Division of Cardiology
Professor of Medicine
Loyola University Medical Center
Maywood, IL, United States

Acknowledgments

We would like to thank our families, friends, and colleagues for their insights, support, and encouragement in this endeavor to make an impact on the future of medical safety and pharmacovigilance.

We appreciate the following reviewers for their thoughtful comments: Ronda Goldfein, Sherrie Gallas, Katherine Hiegel, Paul J. Lee, Jianzhong Liu, Jennifer Manski, Gregory Pawell, Pam Puttfarcken, Jorge Ng Zheng, Sudhir Penugonda, Diane Schommer, and Susanna Sit.

We also acknowledge the help of Christopher Sinclair and David Sternala with the artwork in several chapters.

We wish to thank Dawn Dvorak, Shannon Gacke, Jennifer Koeller, Mary Locicero, Rosalind Munoz, Pam Spezialetti, and Adrienne Towles for their assistance.

The authors acknowledge and thank their patients whose lived experiences have contributed to the science of pharmacovigilance.

Finally, we appreciate the support from Elsevier, with special thanks to Kayla Wolfe, Nadhiya Sekar, and Jennifer Horrigan.

Introduction

After 20 years of protecting patients through pharmacovigilance, Dr. Linda Scarazzini and Dr. Fabio Lievano are acutely aware of the need for concise and accessible resources on drug safety.

Pharmacovigilance plays a lifesaving role in the practice of medicine, yet there is no definitive sourcebook on the topic. Current textbooks are dense in black-and-white text, lack graphics, and are updated infrequently.

With *Pharmacovigilance: A Practical Approach*, Dr. Linda Scarazzini and Dr. Fabio Lievano provide comprehensive, easy-to-read, and up-to-date information on the principles and practice of pharmacovigilance. This book focuses on the evolving regulatory landscape, case studies, and current and future use of digital technologies.

Topics include
- The Regulatory Environment
- Safety Data and Real-World Evidence
- Special Topics and Special Populations
- The Next Frontier: the Future of Safety Science

Besides having timely information with graphics and pragmatic applications, the text is engaging and easy to read.

Pharmacovigilance: A Practical Approach is an essential resource for clinical researchers and healthcare students and professionals. This book can form the basis for undergraduate, graduate, and professional level courses.

Contents

CHAPTER 1

Does Regulation Drive Science or Does Science Drive Regulation?

JABEEN AHMAD, BSC (HONS) • CALVIN JOHNSON, BSC (HONS), MSC (PHV) •
VICKI EDWARDS, BPHARM (HONS) • NICHOLAS REES, MBBS, BSC

INTRODUCTION

The pharmaceutical industry is highly regulated to protect both the patients taking medicines and the industry making them. No one wants to see a repeat of the serious drug-related disasters of the past that have shaped the current regulatory environment. However, we live in a fast-moving world of technology and innovative science where agility is key to ground-breaking new medicines for patients. Regulations can take a long time to develop and implement; changes are not easily made. They also have a reputation for being bureaucratic and static while innovation races past. Regulators ideally should balance the need for appropriate controls to ensure medicines have the best possible benefit-risk profile while allowing innovation to drive the development of new medicines.

Historically, regulations related to pharmacovigilance (PV) were developed only in response to an event and were fairly rudimentary in scope and application. Several key events, however, have triggered the evolution of PV regulations since the beginning of the 20th century. Over time, these regulations have become increasingly comprehensive and thoughtful.

IMPORTANT EVENTS IN PHARMACOVIGILANCE

The most significant events in the history of PV regulation are depicted in Fig. 1.1. At the end of the 19th century, large-scale production of vaccines for the prevention of diphtheria and smallpox promised to save lives and potentially eradicate these terrible diseases in the US. However, there were no government controls in place for biological products at the time. Consequently, safety issues occurred; for example, vaccine products derived from the blood of a horse contaminated with tetanus were given to patients and resulted in several deaths. This led to the Biologics Control Act of 1902[1] that required manufacturers to apply for a license to produce and sell biological products. In addition clear product labeling was required and significant sanctions were introduced if requirements were not met—true regulation was born!

In the 1930s, liquid sulfanilamide was introduced in the US as an additional formulation to the established capsules and tablet formulations available to treat streptococcal infections. The elixir was formulated using diethylene glycol as a solvent. More than 100 adults and children died after taking the elixir. Investigations showed diethylene glycol to be the cause of the deaths. This national disaster led to the Food, Drug and Cosmetics Act of 1938[1] that required the food and drug administration (FDA) to monitor the safety of new drugs. This act, although significantly modified, is still the basis of regulation in the US today.

Probably the most significant event that has shaped PV was the thalidomide disaster of the early 1960s.[2] Thalidomide was a drug developed as a mild sedative and marketed as being safe for adults and children. It was also observed to be effective in alleviating morning sickness and was used extensively by pregnant women "off label", meaning the drug was not labeled to treat morning sickness. The drug was first marketed in Germany in 1957 and was available in 43 countries, although it was never approved by the FDA. The drug was available over the counter. In 1961 the true horror of the effects of thalidomide began to unfold. Reports of phocomelia; a very rare birth defect that results in shortened, deformed, or absent limbs, were received in distressingly large numbers. The drug was eventually withdrawn in 1962 when it became clear that the birth defect was caused by thalidomide. It is estimated that

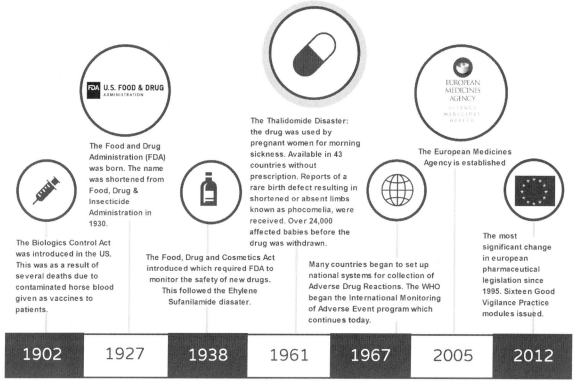

The Food and Drug Administration (FDA) was born. The name was shortened from Food, Drug & Insecticide Administration in 1930.

The Thalidomide Disaster: the drug was used by pregnant women for morning sickness. Available in 43 countries without prescription. Reports of a rare birth defect resulting in shortened or absent limbs known as phocomelia, were received. Over 24,000 affected babies before the drug was withdrawn.

The European Medicines Agency is established

The Biologics Control Act was introduced in the US. This was as a result of several deaths due to contaminated horse blood given as vaccines to patients.

The Food, Drug and Cosmetics Act introduced which required FDA to monitor the safety of new drugs. This followed the Ehylene Sufanilamide diasater.

Many countries began to set up national systems for collection of Adverse Drug Reactions. The WHO began the International Monitoring of Adverse Event program which continues today.

The most significant change in european pharmaceutical legislation since 1995. Sixteen Good Vigilance Practice modules issued.

| 1902 | 1927 | 1938 | 1961 | 1967 | 2005 | 2012 |

FIG. 1.1 Important events in pharmacovigilance.

BOX 1.1
The Trigger for Global PV

The thalidomide disaster triggered global regulations requiring evaluation of both efficacy and safety of new medicines.

BOX 1.2
Thalidomide Use Today

Thalidomide is available today for the treatment of several devastating medical conditions, such as leprosy and multiple myeloma, due to risk minimization measures being implemented.

24,000 affected babies were born worldwide, with a significantly large number of miscarriages and stillbirths in women also attributable to thalidomide. The disaster resulted in significant changes globally to the regulation of medicines, requiring more rigorous clinical trial testing and the need to demonstrate both the efficacy and the safety of new medicines. Much of what occurs today in PV is rooted in the lessons learned from thalidomide (Box 1.1).

Interestingly, the drug is still used today because it was found to be effective in a complication of leprosy and multiple myeloma.[3] In addition to the lessons learned from the birth defects, the continued use of thalidomide has been made possible for diseases where the benefit-risk balance is determined to be positive (Box 1.2). This has provided the opportunity to develop strategies and methodologies for risk minimization (see chapter 13). When thalidomide was reintroduced into the market, it came with one of the first comprehensive Pregnancy Prevention Programs. The program provides educational information for both prescribers and patients on the risks of using thalidomide and the importance of avoiding pregnancy while receiving the drug. The supply of the drug is also carefully controlled. Dispensing pharmacies must register with the program and understand the limited circumstances under which the drug can be dispensed. Female patients of childbearing age must agree to use contraception and a negative pregnancy test result must be provided before each month's supply of drug is issued. Pharmacies are required to maintain accurate records of treatment. Although the program has been very successful, it has not completely prevented further babies from being born with the devastating birth defects.

Worldwide there was a unified desire to never let another thalidomide tragedy happen again. Countries began to set up national systems for the collection of adverse drug reaction reports. In 1967 the World Health Organization (WHO) received their mandate to start a research project on the International Monitoring of Adverse Drug Reaction Reports; this work continues today.[4] In 1968 the UK regulatory authority introduced the Medicines Act that governs the control of medicines for human use and veterinary use, including the manufacture and supply of medicines. This act remains the foundation of UK legislation today. The importance of PV took hold across the world but responses continued to be reactive.

IMPORTANT PHARMACOVIGILANCE ORGANIZATIONS

The creation of the most influential PV organizations throughout the world is described in Fig. 1.2.[5–11] Some of these groups were developed as non-profit, non-governmental organizations whose aim was to set international harmonized PV principles and standards.

Two main organizations, supported by a number of non-profit industry trade organizations, are credited with creating the foundation of modern PV: the Council for International Organizations of Medical Sciences (CIOMS) and the International Council for Harmonisation (ICH).

CIOMS was established in 1949. Based in Switzerland, the mission of CIOMS was to advance public health through guidance on health research, including ethics, medicine development, and safety. Through its different expert advisory working groups, CIOMS has set many of the global standards and thinking around key PV topics. The CIOMS-1 form[12] is one of the best known examples of CIOMS work and it sets the international standard for exchange of safety information between organizations, regulators, and countries (Box 1.3).

ICH was formed by regulators in the United States, Europe, and Japan in the 1990s. By this time, some countries had developed national PV regulation aimed at protecting patient safety and public health. However, as each country's regulations were developed in isolation, the results were sometimes contradictory or duplicative. The

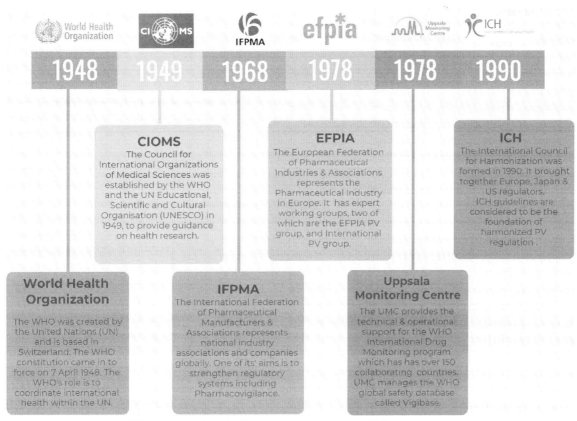

FIG. 1.2 Timeline of influential pharmacovigilance (PV) organizations.

mission of ICH is to achieve greater harmonization worldwide to ensure that safe, effective, and high-quality medicines are developed and registered in the most resource-efficient manner. The ICH guidelines are recognized internationally as a neutral international standard for the safety, quality, and efficacy of medicines and they continue to be influential today (Box 1.3).

In Japan the Pharmaceuticals and Medical Devices Agency (PMDA) was established in 2004. Its creation consolidated existing bureaus for Adverse Drug Reactions. The PMDA is responsible for the review of new drug applications and postmarketing safety activities. PDMA works closely with the Ministry of Health, Labour and Welfare (MHLW) in Japan.[13]

A significant event for PV in Europe was the establishment of the European Medicines Agency (EMA) in 2005.[14] The mission of EMA is to foster scientific excellence in the evaluation and supervision of medicines for the benefit of public and animal health in the European Union. The EMA supervised medicines in 28 countries of the European Union (known as the member states) and in the countries (Norway, Liechtenstein, and Iceland) that are part of the European Economic Area (EEA) (Box 1.4).[15] Together, the EMA, FDA, and MHLW regulators have played a significant role in shaping PV legislation today.

IMPORTANT REGULATORY AUTHORITIES AND REGIONS

Most countries in the world now have a regulatory authority whose aim is to protect public health. Fig. 1.3 shows important global regulatory authorities and countries which have regional multi-country PV

frameworks. Significant progress has been made since 1990 to establish national PV systems, especially in low- to middle-income countries, by the WHO International Drug Monitoring program[16] and the Uppsala Monitoring Centre. More than 150 countries have now joined the WHO program, representing over 90% of the world's population.[17]

Similar to the EMA model, regional PV frameworks (in which more than one country adopts the same PV regulations) have begun developing throughout the world. Although the intention of regional frameworks is to harmonize regulation across countries, this does not always happen. When countries transpose regional regulation into their national laws, often additional requirements are added or requirements are removed. To date, none of the regional PV frameworks operate like the European Union, which has legal authority over all the countries it operates in. Of note, however, a multi-country regulatory agency is being planned for the continent of Africa; 54 countries![18]

THE WORLD OF REGULATORY SCIENCE

In recent years, regulators have moved from a reactive to a proactive approach to regulating medicines. In the past, legislation was put in place in response to an event; typically, it was narrowly focused and inclined to be inflexible. New legislation therefore has tended not to take into account advances in science and medicine, innovative technologies, or changes in societal behaviors and needs.

Currently, EMA and FDA are aligned on the definition of regulatory science as the science of developing new tools, standards, and approaches to assess the safety, efficacy, quality, and performance of medicinal products. Regulatory science informs decision-making throughout the life cycle of a medicine and can encompass basic and applied medicinal science and social sciences.[19,20] Today patients and the public want more information about medicines and sooner; this is driving the need for regulatory transparency and timely information sharing. Patients also want to participate in decision-making in the choice of their treatments and to have a voice in the development of new medicines.

Societal expectations have strongly influenced current regulations. In 2010, the EMA updated the existing directive on medicinal products for human use. This update was implemented in 2012 by practical guidelines known as the Good Pharmacovigilance Practice Modules or EU GVPs[21] (Box 1.5). The aim of this legislation was to reduce the number of adverse drug related reactions in Europe through a wide range of measures. This includes better data collection on medicines and their

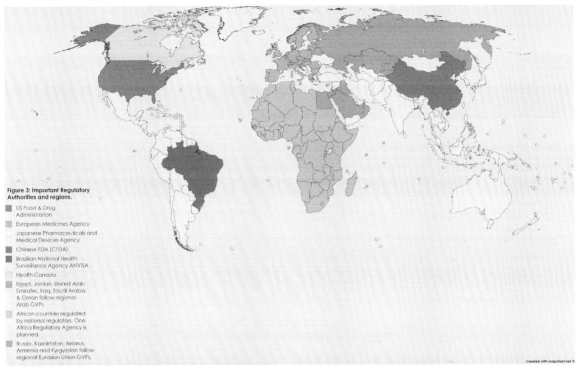

Figure 3: Important Regulatory Authorities and regions.

- US Food & Drug Administration
- European Medicines Agency
- Japanese Pharmaceuticals and Medical Devices Agency
- Chinese FDA (CFDA)
- Brazilian National Health Surveillance Agency ANVISA
- Health Canada
- Egypt, Jordan, United Arab Emirates, Iraq, Saudi Arabia & Oman follow regional Arab GVPs
- African countries regulated by national regulators. One Africa Regulatory Agency is planned.
- Russia, Kazakhstan, Belarus, Armenia and Kyrgyzstan follow regional Eurasian Union GVPs.

Created with mapchart.net ®

FIG. 1.3 Important global regulatory authorities and regional frameworks.

BOX 1.5
EMA Good Vigilance Practice Modules

The EU good pharmacovigilance practices (GVPs)

- Module I   PV systems and their quality systems
- Module II   PV system master file (PSMF)
- Module III   PV inspections
- Module IV   PV audits
- Module V   Risk management systems
- Module VI   Management and reporting of adverse reactions to medicinal products
- Module VII   Periodic safety update report (PSUR)
- Module VIII   Postauthorization safety studies (PASS)
- Module IX   Signal management
- Module X   Additional monitoring
- Module XV   Safety communication
- Module XVI   Risk minimization measures: Selection of tools and effectiveness indicators

---

safety, rapid assessment of safety issues, and empowerment of patients. This regulatory change has had a significant impact on global PV requirements and represents the current best practices. A number of countries and regions have since developed regulation that closely resembles the EU GVPs. Regional framework heavily influenced by EU GVPs are the Arab GVPs and the Eurasian GVPs. The Arab GVPs were developed by the Arab League organization[22] and have been adopted fully or partially by Egypt, Iraq, Jordan, Kuwait, Oman, Tunisia, and Saudi Arabia. The Eurasian Economic Commission[23] developed the Eurasian GVPs or EAEU GVPs (referred to in Fig. 1.3), which cover the Eurasian region of Russia, Belarus, Kazakhstan, Armenia, and Kyrgyzstan.

Fig. 1.4 shows a high-level comparison of the FDA and EMA PV requirements. Although there are a few differences, notably the requirement of a Qualified Person for Pharmacovigilance (QPPV)[24] in every company marketing medicines in Europe and a PV System Master File (PSMF),[25] the overall general approach to drug safety is very similar.

EMA PHARMACOVIGILANCE RISK ASSESSMENT COMMITTEE

A significant component of the EU GVPs intended to promote a more proactive safety approach and to strengthen transparency and communication was the establishment of the Pharmacovigilance Risk Assessment Committee (PRAC).[26] PRAC is responsible for assessing and monitoring the safety of human

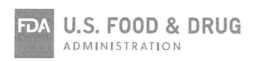

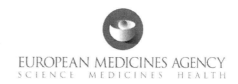

FDA		EMA
Responsible for protecting public health by ensuring the safety, efficacy and security of human and animal drugs, biologics and medical devices	**AIMS**	To foster scientific excellence in the evaluation and supervision of medicines, for the benefit of public and animal health
325 million people	**Population**	500 million people
FDA is a centralized agency that oversees drug and veterinary safety in one country. AE reporting system is FAERS and vaccines system is VAERs.	**Structure**	EMA is a de-centralized agency of the European Union. EMA protects public and animal health in 28 member states. Has one adverse event database Eudravigilance
All serious and unexpected, global and national adverse drug reactions to be reported within 15 calendar days	**Adverse Event Reporting**	All serious global and national adverse drug reactions to be reported within 15 calendar days. Non serious EU ADRs in 90 days.
No requirement for a Qualified Person for Pharmacovigilance	**Qualified Person**	Companies with EU marketing approval must have a QPPV residing in the EU, who has global oversight of the PV system
No requirement for a PSMF	**Pharmacovigilance Master File**	PSMF required. This is a detailed description of the global PV system including resources, database, programs and vendors
The Risk Evaluation & Mitigation Strategy or REMS is a strategy to manage a known or potentially serious drug related risk to enable patients to have continued access	**Risk Management**	The EU RMP is a written document that outlines a products' risks, the post-marketing surveillance plan and risk minimization activites to manage risk.
Known as Periodic Adverse Drug Experience Report (PADERS) or Periodic Adverse Experience Reports (PAERS). Require narrative information on all expected events	**Periodic Reports**	Known as Periodic Benefit Risk Update reports (PBRER). Summary of data relevent to benefits and risks of product including clinical studies

FIG. 1.4 Comparison between the US and EU pharmacovigilance regulations. (Sources: FDA & EMA websites November 06, 2017.)

medicines and for reviewing and assessing all aspects of risk management (Box 1.6).

Specifically, the PRAC reviews:
- Product referrals for safety reasons;
- Safety signal assessment and prioritization;
- Risk management plans, both pre- and post-authorization;
- Periodic Safety Update Reports;
- Post authorization Safety Studies (PASS);
- Renewals of marketing authorizations.

Each PRAC member is chosen on the basis of the strength of their expertise in PV and risk assessment of medicines. Although the meetings themselves are

> **BOX 1.6**
> **Pharmacovigilance Risk Assessment Committee**
>
> The mandate of the EMA PRAC:
> - All aspects of risk management of medicines including detection, assessment, minimization, and communication of a medicine's benefit and risk.
> - The design and approval of postauthorization safety studies.
> - Input into the risk-based programme for routine PV inspections. Recommendations on the need for inspections "for cause", meaning unannounced PV inspections of companies triggered by specific safety concerns.
>
> The PRAC committee is composed of
> - Six independent scientific experts
> - One health care professional
> - One patient organization representative
> - One member and one alternate member nominated by each member state and the EEA countries Norway and Iceland.

not public, the agendas and minutes are publically available on the EMA website.[26] Additionally, companies referred to as Marketing Authorisation Holders (MAHs) receive an advanced notification of products or new signals that will be discussed in each meeting.

PRAC may invite companies to participate in meetings by way of a Scientific Advisory Group meeting, where experts on the topic under discussion are also invited or, in more formal circumstances, at an Oral Hearing when there is a complex or controversial issue under discussion.

Trade associations such as the European Federation of Pharmaceutical Industries and Associations (EFPIA) view PRAC as a positive and effective part of the European medicine legislation. However, PRAC is not the ultimate decision-maker; rather, it makes recommendations to the Committee for Medicinal Products for Human Use (CHMP) who then provides an opinion to the European Commission, which is the ultimate decision-maker. On occasion, the CHMP will not agree with or will reverse PRAC's recommendation. The transparency of PRAC activities have had unanticipated and in some respects unintended consequences for the industry. The publically available agendas and minutes are keenly read by regulatory authorities outside Europe. In consequence, companies have seen an increase in questions from non-European authorities related to the issues under discussion. These questions may have a slightly different focus but are commonly seeking information related to the relevance of the issue to the population of the requesting country. In addition, global regulatory authorities now want to receive the outcomes of assessment at the same time as PRAC and want assurance that any action taken with respect to European licenses will be simultaneously taken with non-European licenses.

NEW WAVE OF GLOBAL PHARMACOVIGILANCE REGULATION

In the past, the most sophisticated and developed drug safety regulation was isolated to the ICH regions: the United States, Europe, and Japan. In recent years, other regions have moved from no or rudimentary legislation to adoption of robust and complex requirements. Although both commendable and understandable, if the requirements are not harmonized with existing global standards, this does put an increased burden on industry. In response, the industry is monitoring the evolving legislation to promote international harmonization. The recent wave of legislation in emerging markets is leading to a second wave of harmonization efforts. However situations are very different in resource-constrained countries, and decisions need to be made by these regulatory authorities as to where is best to focus limited resource. Therefore the focus of industry advocacy efforts should be to promote "right-sized" PV systems that are harmonized where possible. For example, aligning with complex PV frameworks, such as the EMA GVPs, may not be the answer for countries with limited resources. Instead, regulators in emerging markets may decide to focus on the reporting, collection and monitoring of local adverse reactions.

THE EU QPPV

Since 1995, European legislation has required the appointment of a Qualified Person for Pharmacovigilance (QPPV). A QPPV (Box 1.7) is required for any MAH with a marketed product in any country within the EEA.[24] The QPPV must reside in a European country and act as the single point of contact for the EMA and any national competent authority on a 24 hour basis. The main duties of the QPPV are to maintain oversight of the global PV system including drug safety profiles and emerging safety concerns, to influence the performance of the quality system for PV to improve compliance, and to provide input into regulatory action such as updates of product information with healthcare professionals and patients.[25]

Although the QPPV role is a European requirement, the QPPV is required to have oversight of the *global* PV system; therefore, the EU QPPV in a global company should be authorized to have oversight of global PV matters. The QPPV assumes both individual and company responsibility for compliance with regulation; thus, the QPPV can be individually prosecuted for a company's failings.

THE RISE OF THE NATIONAL QPPV

Some EU countries have a requirement for the appointment of a national QPPV; an individual at the national level who is responsible for PV in that country. For example, France, Germany, Italy, and Spain have this requirement. The national QPPV must reside in the specific country so that they are able to speak in the local language and understand country-specific nuances.

Many non-European countries have begun to adopt the requirement for a national QPPV. The requirements to fulfil the national QPPV role varies from country to country. In some instances, the requirement is as simple as providing the national regulatory agency with contact details for the responsible person. In comparison, some countries require specific training for the role. In Ghana, the QPPV must attend mandatory QPPV training provided by the Ghanaian regulatory authority.[27] For Arab countries who follow the Arab Good Vigilance Practice Guidelines[22], the training and education of the QPPV is exactly the same as extensive EU requirements.

One of the challenges of the national QPPV concept is the requirement for the individual to reside in the local country. In emerging countries, there is a dearth of PV expertise and companies may struggle to find a

suitably qualified candidate. Also, products are marketed in countries where companies may not have a local office and therefore do not have any local staff resident in the country to become the QPPV. This often results in the company contracting a third party to meet the local QPPV requirement. When a third party fulfils the role, it remains the responsibility of the company to have oversight of the national QPPV.

In the case of third-party vendors fulfilling the QPPV requirement, a good understanding of the role and the importance of PV is required. The importance of embedding the local QPPV role within the global organization of a company has led to the development of in-house national QPPV training by companies.

The Pharmacovigilance System Master File

The Pharmacovigilance System Master File (PSMF) is a mandatory requirement in Europe, as described in EU GVP Module II.[25] The PSMF is a dynamic document which describes the global PV system of the MAH in a prescribed format, with a focus on how the system affects products authorized in Europe. It includes how all departments within a company interact with PV and if any tasks have been delegated to third parties.

The PSMF is maintained and updated at frequent intervals by MAHs. It contains contact details and the resume of the EU QPPV plus a summary of the PV organizational structure including the physical site(s) where specific safety information is handled (such as data entry of adverse events into the global database, signal detection, and safety analysis). The PSMF documents the sources of safety data, including clinical trials and marketed drug data collection programs.

The purpose of the PSMF is to provide the EMA and EU competent authorities with an overview of a company's PV system. It is used by EU regulators in a risk-based manner when selecting companies for PV inspection.

Some non-European regulators still use the Detailed Description of the PV System (DDPS) (referred to in superseded EU PV legislation), meaning that MAHs must maintain both document formats. To complicate matters, other countries have duplicated the EU PSMF requirements and have added extra requirements. For example, countries following the Arab GVPs accept the EU PSMF but also require an additional document referred to as the Pharmacovigilance System Sub-File, which focuses on the national PV system. More recently, the Eurasian Economic Union has requested a separate Eurasian Union PSMF. This is clearly an area that lacks harmonization.

Is Regulatory Guidance Just Guidance?

In addition to regulations stated in law, regulatory guidance linked to PV activities can exist in different forms. This includes formal published guidance, question and answer documents, letters to MAHs, written correspondence between the MAH and the regulatory authority, and verbal guidance given during conferences and symposia. Additional detail provided in published guidance enables clarity in interpretation of the legal obligations. There is a hierarchy associated with guidance. For example, in Europe the EU GVP guidance[28] is at the top of this hierarchy, so any deviation from it should be carefully considered. When it comes to the assessment of compliance with the EU guidance through regulatory inspections, a critical finding is defined as

A deficiency in pharmacovigilance systems, practices or processes that adversely affects the rights, safety or well-being of patients or that poses a potential risk to public health or that represents a serious violation of applicable legislation and guidelines.[29]

This is in contrast to the more pragmatic approach of the formal FDA Guidance for Industry that states that that guidance contains nonbinding recommendations and includes the following statement:

This guidance represents the current thinking of the Food and Drug Administration (FDA or Agency) on this topic. It does not establish any rights for any person and is not binding on FDA or the public. You can use an alternative approach if it satisfies the requirements of the applicable statutes and regulations. To discuss an alternative approach, contact the FDA office responsible for this guidance as listed on the title page.[30]

Collaborative partnership among MAHs, regulatory agencies, and patients will facilitate evolution of thoughtful and practical PV regulations, which is critical for advancing benefit-risk monitoring of medicines and their use in the real world.

How can Industry Influence Regulation?

Even as recently as 10 years ago the pace of change in regulations was relatively slow. More recently, there has been an unprecedented explosion of new global PV legislation.

The pharmaceutical industry has undertaken efforts to "speak with one voice" via trade associations (see Fig. 1.1) such as the International Federation of Pharmaceutical Manufacturers and Associations (IFPMA), EFPIA (European Union), and the Pharmaceutical Research and Manufacturers of America (PhRMA, United States). When new legislation is issued as a draft for public consultation, the industry and trade associations can proactively identify any potential divergence from existing international requirements and promote alignment with neutral international standards (such as ICH or CIOMS) or influence the addition of new requirements.

Regulators such as EMA and FDA hold regular public meetings with all stakeholders who have an interest in PV (for example, industry trade associations, academia, and patient associations) and are willing to meet with the industry. Industries have been successful in driving meaningful change through these interactions.

Enforcement of Pharmacovigilance Regulations

Similar to other industries, regulatory authorities who define PV regulations need to have an effective mechanism in place to monitor and enforce compliance to the requirements (Box 1.8). There are slightly different approaches taken globally, but the key to achieve the greatest degree of compliance is linked to the effectiveness of the following strategies:

1. *Setting the standards*
   If requirements are sufficiently detailed and are clear and proportionate to the local environment and needs, there is a greater likelihood of compliance being achieved for the majority of companies that strive to comply.
2. *Performing inspections*
   This is the main approach to assess compliance. Regulatory inspectors visit MAHs to assess the systems, personnel, and procedures in place to determine the degree of compliance. Any deficiencies are graded into three categories: critical, major and minor. A report is usually provided, to which the company must respond and commit to taking action to address any deficiency. Adequacy of these actions can be assessed on re-inspection of the MAH at a future date. If the finding is significant some

---

BOX 1.8
Pharmacovigilance Enforcement

Pharmacovigilance regulation enforcement strategies:
1. Setting standards: publishing clear and detailed PV regulations proportionate to the country need.
2. Performing inspections of marketing authorization holders.
3. Education and advisory tools: through conferences, written guides, and engagement with trade associations.
4. Warning letters published in the public domain.
5. Enforcement actions: legal process such as product withdrawal and financial penalties.

regulatory authorities require written evidence of completion of the action. There is a harmonized approach to inspections in the EU that is coordinated by the EMA;[31] however, there is no international harmonization for PV inspections. A risk-based approach is commonly adopted to determine which companies are inspected and how frequently they are inspected. This may include gathering information from other parts of the regulatory agency that monitor quality and timeliness of safety information submitted by a company.

3. *Educating and advising*
   Regulatory authorities engage and educate stakeholders through trade association meetings or conferences to enhance understanding and practical application of the requirements, which in turn increases the likelihood of compliance. Additional methods include publishing guidance such as the Medicines and Healthcare products Regulatory Agency's (MHRA) Good Pharmacovigilance Practice guide (the "Purple" guide) and publishing inspection metrics.[32,33]

4. *Warnings*
   Warning letters and making information public where there is significant and/or persistent noncompliance provides an opportunity for the recipient to rectify the noncompliance before formal legal action is taken. It also acts as either a deterrent to others or a means of educating and adds further clarity to the authorities' expectations. Two examples of these letters are the used in the United Kingdom and the FDA 483 warning letters.[32,34]

5. *Enforcement action*
   Regulators can take legal action for the most serious and persistent contravention of PV regulations. For example, in the EU, financial penalties can be imposed for the infringement of PV obligations. This can be up to 5% of the company's European sales, in the preceding business year, which is a significant deterrent.[35]

CONCLUSIONS

In recent years, regulators and This is resulting in newer regulations are more focused on proactive safety measures. There is emphasis on earlier signal detection capabilities and risk proportionate approaches to decision-making. This is resulting in earlier provision of relevant safety information to prescribers and patients. Robust and comprehensive PV legislation is in place in countries with mature PV systems, which include education and enforcement processes. Risk

assessment of medicines has become much more transparent and dynamic. Leading regulatory agencies are hugely influential globally and information made public from these agencies can lead to a global focus on safety issues. However the breadth and complexity of PV frameworks in well-resourced countries, may not be the right approach for resource-limited regulators. A "right-size" PV approach is advised to newer regulators, with harmonization of PV legislation where possible. Early identification of safety issues via more recent sources of safety information such as social media is a priority for regulators and the industry alike.

Regulators are working hard to keep up with new technologies such as robotic automation and artificial intelligence, and with innovation in drug development and delivery. However, the rate of change is very fast. Therefore the answer to whether regulation drives science or whether science drives regulation is that science and technology appear to be driving regulation in our rapidly moving digital environment.

REFERENCES

1. US Food and Drug Administration. http://wwwfda.gov. AboutFDA/WhatWedo/History; 2017.
2. Thalidomide Society. www.thalidomidesociety.org; 2017.
3. Greenstone G. Special feature: the revival of thalidomide: from tragedy to therapy. *BC Med J*. 2011;53(5):203−233.
4. World Health Organization. http://www.who.int/medicines/areas/quality_safety/safety_efficacy/advdrugreactions/en/; 2017.
5. World Health Organization. http://www.who.int/about/en/; 2017.
6. Council for international Organizations of Medical Sciences. https://cioms.ch/about/; 2017.
7. International Federation of Pharmaceutical Manufacturers & Associations. https://www.ifpma.org/who-we-are/ifpma-in-brief/; 2017.
8. European Federation of Pharmaceutical Industries and Associations. https://www.efpia.eu/about-us/; 2017.
9. Uppsala Monitoring Centre. https://www.who-umc.org/global-pharmacovigilance/who-programme/; 2017.
10. The International Council for Harmonization of Technical Requirements for Pharmaceuticals for Human Use. http://www.ich.org/home.html; 2017.
11. The International Society of Pharmacovigilance. http://isoponline.org/; 2017.
12. CIOMS-1. Form: https://cioms.ch/wp-content/uploads/2017/05/cioms-form1.pdf; 2017.
13. The Pharmaceutical and Medical Devices Agency. https://www.pmda.go.jp/english/; 2017.
14. European Medicines Agency. http://www.ema.europa.eu/ema/index.jsp?curl=pages/about_us/general/general_content_000091.jsp; 2017.

15. European Economic Area. http://www.europarl.europa.eu/atyourservice/en/displayFtu.html?ftuId=FTU_6.5.3.html; 2017.

16. Olsson S, Pal SN, Dodoo A. Pharmacovigilance in resource-limited countries. *Expert Rev Clin Pharmacol*. 2015;8(4):449−460.

17. UMC. https://www.who-umc.org/vigibase/vigibase/; 2017.

18. Website: *African Medicines Regulatory Harmonisation (AMRH) NEPAD*; 2017. www.nepad.org.

19. EMA. *European Medicines Agency Process for Engaging in External Regulatory Sciences and Process Improvement Activities for Public and Animal Health*. 2017. EMA/573402/2017.

20. FDA. *Office of the Chief Scientist: Advancing Regulatory Science for Public Health*. Oct. 2010.

21. *EMA Good Vigilance Practices*; 2017. http://www.ema.europa.eu/ema/index.jsp?curl=pages/regulation/document_listing/document_listing_000345.jsp.

22. *The League of Arab Common States; Guideline on Good Pharmacovigilance Practices (GVP) for Arab Countries, Version 2*. December 2014.

23. The Eurasian Economic Commission. *Rules of Good Pharmacovigilance Practice (GV) of Eurasian Economic Union, Decision No. 87*. November 3, 2016.

24. EU Guideline on Good Pharmacovigilance Practices Module I: Pharmacovigilance Systems and Their Quality Systems, June 25, 2012. EMA/541760/2011.

25. *EU Guideline on Good Pharmacovigilance Practices Module II: Pharmacovigilance System Master File*. March 28, 2017. EMA/816573/2011 Revision 2.

26. EMA Pharmacovigilance Risk Assessment Committee (PRAC). http://www.ema.europa.eu/ema/index.jsp?curl=pages/about_us/general/general_content_000537.jsp; 2017.

27. *Ghana Food and Drugs Authority Guidelines for Qualified Person for Pharmacovigilance*. March 1, 2013. FDA/SMC/SMD/GL-QPP/2013/03, Version 2.

28. *EMA GVP Modules*; 2017. http://www.ema.europa.eu/ema/index.jsp?curl=pages/regulation/document_listing/document_listing_000345.jsp.

29. EMA. *Union Procedure on the Preparation, Conduct and Reporting on EU Pharmacovigilance Inspections*. March 21, 2014. EMA/INS/PhV/192230/2014.

30. *FDA Providing Postmarketing Periodic Safety Reports in the ICH E2C (R2) Format (Periodic Benefit Risk-Benefit Evaluation Report) Guidance for Industry, CDER, CBER*. November 2016.

31. *EMA Coordination of Pharmacovigilance Inspections*; 2017. http://www.ema.europa.eu/ema/index.jsp?curl=pages/regulation/general/general_content_000160.jsp&mid=WC0b01ac058002708a.

32. *MHRA Good Pharmacovigilance Practice (GPvP)*; November 11, 2017. https://www.gov.uk/guidance/good-pharmacovigilance-practice-gpvp#history.

33. *MHRA Good Pharmacovigilance Practice Guide*. 1st ed. London: Pharmaceutical Press; 2008.

34. US FDA 4-1- Warning Letters. In: *https://www.fda.gov/ICECI/ComplianceManuals/RegulatoryProceduresManual/ucm176870.htm#SUB4-1-1*; 2017.

35. *EU Commission Regulation (EC) Concerning Financial Penalties for Infringement of Certain Obligations on Connection with Marketing Authorisations Granted under Regulation (EC) No 726/2004 of the European Parliament and of the Council, No 658/2007*. June 14, 2017.

CHAPTER 2

Signal Management and Methods of Signal Detection

MELISSA M. TRUFFA, BS PHARM • ADRIENNE M. ROTHSTEIN, PHARMD • CHERYL FOIT, BS • JEREMY D. JOKINEN, PHD, MS

INTRODUCTION

Understanding both the benefits and the risks of medicines is essential to prescribers and patients. This understanding is based on the idea of collecting data (adverse events), weighing the importance of the data, processing the information, and providing insight into the safety profile that can result in informed decisions by prescribers and patients about the treatment of their diseases and medical conditions. These activities are the cornerstone of the science of pharmacovigilance (PV) and start with an adverse event report (Box 2.1).

An adverse event is any untoward medical occurrence associated with the use of a drug in humans, whether or not considered related. Not all adverse events are necessarily risks, but determining which ones are risks and which ones are not is critical to understand the safety profiles of drugs, biologics, or vaccines.

The science and activities related to the detection, assessment, understanding, and minimization of adverse events or any other drug-related problems are referred to as PV. The key aspects of PV are the detection of new safety signals and the further characterization of new patterns for recognized signals (e.g., risk factors, severity, and outcome). PV utilizes data gathered from multiple sources such as clinical trials, spontaneous individual case reports, scientific literature, observational studies, and electronic medical records. Examples of how adverse event data are gathered from different sources are provided in the following. The MedWatch form to report to the US Food and Drug Administration (FDA) is shown in Fig. 2.1. There are also mobile applications (apps) for reporting adverse events directly to regulatory authorities (see Fig. 2.2).

Adverse events from clinical trials can be submitted directly to the sponsor of the clinical trial or to a regulatory authority for a government-funded study.

Large safety databases of adverse events provide a rich source of data for PV activities for interested stakeholders such as global regulatory authorities, pharmaceutical companies, and researchers. The FDA Adverse Events Reporting System (FAERS) and the EudraVigilance database are two such large safety databases. The FAERS public dashboard allows users to visualize and search safety data in the FAERS database. Fig. 2.3A shows screenshots of the FAERS dashboard, with an example of an overview for acetaminophen (see Fig. 2.3B).

The EudraVigilance database is the European information system of adverse events for medicines that are authorized or being studied in clinical trials in the European Economic Area. The EudraVigilance system also has a public dashboard. Sample views of this data are shown for ACTOS in Fig. 2.4A and 2.4B.

SIGNALS (BOX 2.2)

Detection of safety signals is a key aspect of PV but what is a signal? There are many definitions for a signal. For the purposes of PV, there are two commonly

---

BOX 2.1
Pharmacovigilance

- Pharmacovigilance is the science of identifying, assessing, and minimizing the risk of adverse events within a population.
- Clinical trials, case reports, studies, and medical records are data sources used in PV practices.
- Data is collected via submissions to regulatory authorities, mobile applications, and from clinical trial submissions
- Public data is housed in FAERS (FDA) and EudraVigilance (EU).

Reset Form

U.S. Department of Health and Human Services

MEDWATCH

The FDA Safety Information and
Adverse Event Reporting Program

For VOLUNTARY reporting of
adverse events, product problems and
product use errors

Page 1 of 3

Form Approved: OMB No. 0910-0291. Expires: 9/30/2018
See PRA statement on reverse

FDA USE ONLY

Triage unit
sequence #

FDA Rec. Date

PLEASE TYPE OR USE BLACK INK

Note: For date prompts of "dd-mmm-yyyy" please use 2-digit day, 3-letter month abbreviation, and 4-digit year; for example, 01-Jul-2015.

A. PATIENT INFORMATION

1. Patient Identifier
2. Age ☐ Year(s) ☐ Month(s) ☐ Week(s) ☐ Days(s) or Date of Birth (e.g., 08 Feb 1925)
3. Sex ☐ Female ☐ Male
4. Weight ☐ lb ☐ kg

In Confidence __ __ - __ __ __ - __ __ __ __

5.a. Ethnicity (Check single best answer)
☐ Hispanic/Latino
☐ Not Hispanic/Latino

5.b. Race (Check all that apply)
☐ Asian ☐ American Indian or Alaskan Native
☐ Black or African American ☐ White
☐ Native Hawaiian or Other Pacific Islander

B. ADVERSE EVENT, PRODUCT PROBLEM

1. Check all that apply
☐ Adverse Event ☐ Product Problem (e.g., defects/malfunctions)
☐ Product Use Error ☐ Problem with Different Manufacturer of Same Medicine

2. Outcome Attributed to Adverse Event (Check all that apply)
☐ Death Include date (dd-mmm-yyyy): __ __ - __ __ __ - __ __ __ __
☐ Life-threatening
☐ Hospitalization – initial or prolonged
☐ Disability or Permanent Damage
☐ Congenital Anomaly/Birth Defects
☐ Other Serious (Important Medical Events)
☐ Required Intervention to Prevent Permanent Impairment/Damage (Devices)

3. Date of Event (dd-mmm-yyyy) __ __ - __ __ __ - __ __ __ __
4. Date of this Report (dd-mmm-yyyy) __ __ - __ __ __ - __ __ __ __

5. Describe Event, Problem or Product Use Error

(Continue on page 3)

6. Relevant Tests/Laboratory Data, Including Dates

(Continue on page 3)

7. Other Relevant History, Including Preexisting Medical Conditions (e.g., allergies, pregnancy, smoking and alcohol use, liver/kidney problems, etc.)

(Continue on page 3)

C. PRODUCT AVAILABILITY

2. Product Available for Evaluation? (Do not send product to FDA)
☐ Yes ☐ No ☐ Returned to Manufacturer on (dd-mmm-yyyy) __ __ - __ __ __ - __ __ __ __

D. SUSPECT PRODUCTS

1. Name, Manufacturer/Compounder, Strength (from product label)

#1 – Name and Strength	#1 – NDC # or Unique ID
#1 – Manufacturer/Compounder	#1 – Lot #
#2 – Name and Strength	#2 – NDC # or Unique ID
#2 – Manufacturer/Compounder	#2 – Lot #

---

3. Dose or Amount | Frequency | Route
#1
#2

4. Dates of Use (From/To for each) (If unknown, give duration, or best estimate) (dd-mmm-yyyy)
#1
#2

5. Diagnosis or Reason for Use (Indication)
#1
#2

6. Is the Product Compounded?
#1 ☐ Yes ☐ No
#2 ☐ Yes ☐ No

7. Is the Product Over-the-Counter?
#1 ☐ Yes ☐ No
#2 ☐ Yes ☐ No

8. Expiration Date (dd-mmm-yyyy)
#1 __ __ - __ __ __ - __ __ __ __ #2 __ __ - __ __ __ - __ __ __ __

9. Event Abated After Use Stopped or Dose Reduced?
#1 ☐ Yes ☐ No ☐ Doesn't apply
#2 ☐ Yes ☐ No ☐ Doesn't apply

10. Event Reappeared After Reintroduction?
#1 ☐ Yes ☐ No ☐ Doesn't apply
#2 ☐ Yes ☐ No ☐ Doesn't apply

E. SUSPECT MEDICAL DEVICE

1. Brand Name

2. Common Device Name | 2b. Procode

3. Manufacturer Name, City and State

4. Model #
Catalog #
Serial #

Lot #
Expiration Date (dd-mmm-yyyy) __ __ - __ __ __ - __ __ __ __
Unique Identifier (UDI) #

5. Operator of Device
☐ Health Professional
☐ Lay User/Patient
☐ Other

6. If Implanted, Give Date (dd-mmm-yyyy) __ __ - __ __ __ - __ __ __ __
7. If Explanted, Give Date (dd-mmm-yyyy) __ __ - __ __ __ - __ __ __ __

8. Is this a single-use device that was reprocessed and reused on a patient? ☐ Yes ☐ No

9. If Yes to Item 8, Enter Name and Address of Reprocessor

F. OTHER (CONCOMITANT) MEDICAL PRODUCTS

Product names and therapy dates (Exclude treatment of event)

(Continue on page 3)

G. REPORTER (See confidentiality section on back)

1. Name and Address

Last Name:	First Name:
Address:	
City:	State/Province/Region:
Country:	ZIP/Postal Code:
Phone #:	Email:

2. Health Professional? ☐ Yes ☐ No
3. Occupation
4. Also Reported to: ☐ Manufacturer/Compounder ☐ User Facility ☐ Distributor/Importer

5. If you do NOT want your identity disclosed to the manufacturer, please mark this box: ☐

FORM FDA 3500 (10/15) Submission of a report does not constitute an admission that medical personnel or the product caused or contributed to the event.

FIG. 2.1 The US Food and Drug Administration MedWatch form. (Data from: https://www.fda.gov/downloads/AboutFDA/ReportsManualsForms/Forms/UCM163919.pdf.)

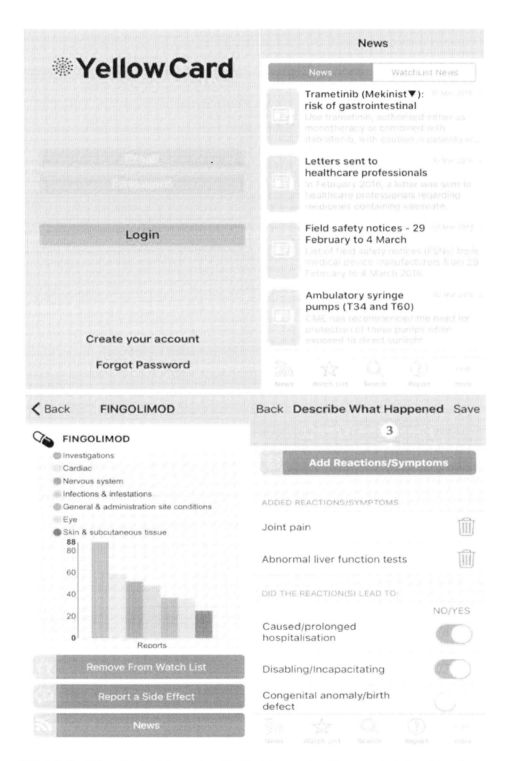

FIG. 2.2 The Yellow Card mobile app from the Medicines and Healthcare products Regulatory Agency.

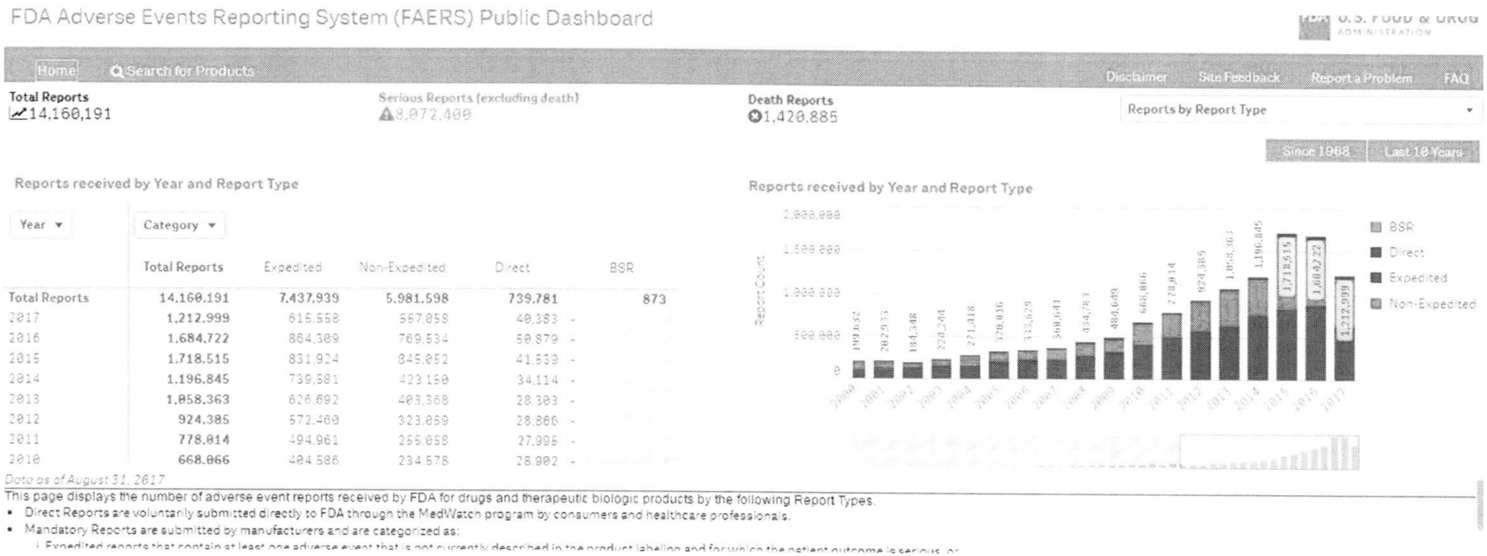

FIG. 2.3A The FDA Adverse Events Reporting System public dashboard. (Data from: https://www.fda.gov/Drugs/GuidanceCompliance RegulatoryInformation/Surveillance/AdverseDrugEffects/ucm070093.htm **(data as of 31 August 2017)**.)

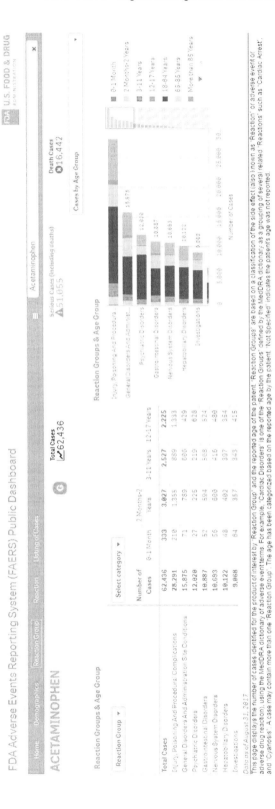

FIG. 2.3B The FDA Adverse Events Reporting System public dashboard—acetaminophen overview. (Data from: https://fis.fda.gov/sense/app/777e9f4d-0cf8-448e-8068-f564c31baa25/sheet/7a47a261-d58b-4203-a8aa-6d3021737452/state/analysis **(data as of 31 August 2017)**.)

B

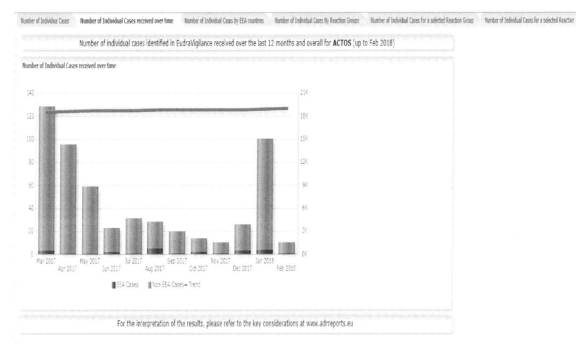

A

FIG. 2.4A EudraVigilance system public dashboard: individual cases received over time, ACTOS example (February 2018). (https://bi.ema.europa.eu/analyticsSOAP/saw.dll?PortalPages)

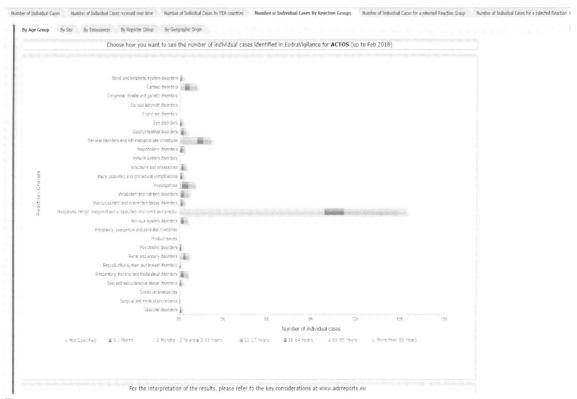

B

FIG. 2.4B EudraVigilance system public dashboard: individual cases by reaction groups and age groups, ACTOS example (February 2018). (https://bi.ema.europa.eu/analyticsSOAP/saw.dll?PortalPages)

recognized definitions: one from the International Council for Harmonisation of Technical Requirements for Pharmaceuticals for Human Use (ICH) and another from the World Health Organization (WHO).

A signal, as defined by the ICH,[1] is information arising from one or multiple sources, including observations and experiments, which suggests a new potentially causal association or a new aspect of a known association between an intervention and an event or a set of related events, either adverse or beneficial, that is judged to be of sufficient likelihood to justify verificatory action.

The WHO[2] defines a signal as "Reported information on a possible causal relationship between an adverse event and a drug, the relationship being previously unknown or incompletely documented. Usually more than a single case report is required to generate a signal depending on the seriousness of the event and the quality of the information."

A critical activity of how signals are managed is the weighing of the available evidence to look for an association between the drug and the reported adverse event. This is done by utilizing an EIQ framework (see Fig. 2.5) that considers the following factors:

- *EVIDENCE* of association between the drug and adverse event
- clinical *IMPACT* (seriousness and severity)
- *QUANTITATIVE* assessment of available data (reporting frequency, disproportionality scores).

These factors outline a framework of questions to be considered when evaluating available evidence from data sources, such as clinical trials, scientific literature, and spontaneous reports for potential signals.

- What is the temporal relationship between drug exposure and the adverse event?

- Is the association biologically plausible?
- Is there a possible class effect?
- Are the adverse events commonly considered to be drug induced (e.g., anaphylaxis, Stevens-Johnson syndrome, and acute drug-induced liver injury)?
- Are there alternative causes or etiologies for the adverse event?

The signal management process includes four key steps: signal detection, signal validation, signal assessment, and any resulting actions to address or mitigate a risk (see Fig. 2.6).

The process of signal management includes both quantitative and qualitative aspects. Intuitive assessment through the integration and weighing of different sources of data by individual safety scientists provides a qualitative aspect (see Fig. 2.7). Safety scientists also use clinical judgement to assess the medical importance of safety issues, which complements the quantitative signal detection methodology.

SIGNAL DETECTION

Signal detection during ongoing clinical trials relies on integrative insight and qualitative rather than quantitative assessments, particularly in the early stages of drug development. There may be limited human data to inform on a safety issue and doses being studied, especially in Phase 1 studies. It is possible that there are no other marketed drug products in the same class and that there is limited information in the published literature about ongoing studies for related products. When a potential signal is detected from clinical trial sources, a safety scientist must integrate data from preclinical studies, timing of the adverse event relative to study drug exposure, knowledge of the study population's comorbid conditions and concomitant medications, and information from the published literature on related products. The safety scientist preliminarily weighs available evidence to determine if a reported adverse event is indicative of a signal.

Signal detection involves systematic examination of data, sometimes referred to as data mining, which provides quantitative assessments regarding the safety of medicinal products particularly in the postmarketing setting.[3] Large-scale databases that continually accumulate adverse event information are maintained by healthcare companies and regulatory authorities globally. These databases serve as valuable resources to ensure public health; however, the volume of information contained therein can make meaningful use of these data challenging.[4] As a result, methods for mining these databases for safety signals have been a topic of regulatory, academic, and industry research for more than

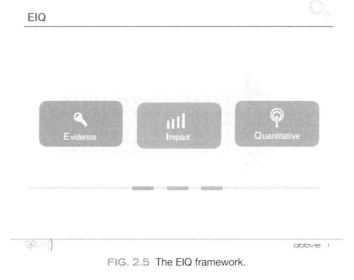

FIG. 2.5 The EIQ framework.

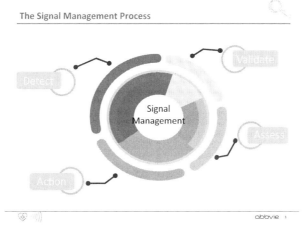

FIG. 2.6 The Signal management process (Box 2.3).

- Signal management involves both a quantitative and qualitative factor analysis
- Signal detection in clinical trials relies on qualitative data
  - Multifactorial analysis
- Signal detection in postmarketing uses quantitative data mining
  - Disproportionality analysis compares the observed proportion of an adverse event for a specific drug to its expected proportion within a given set of data
  - Disproportionality stems from the observed proportion being greater than the expected
  - If sufficiently large, it is a signal of disproportionate reporting
  - Frequency-based analysis counts the occurrence of an event for a drug during a specified time period
  - Expected value is constructed from previous time frames to monitor sufficiently different values from the evaluated time period

Qualitative – Intuitive

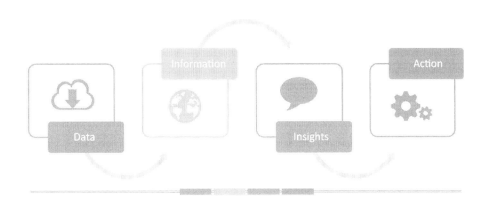

FIG. 2.7 Qualitative—intuitive aspects.

20 years.[5−7] Signal detection describes a series of analytical approaches intended to identify changes in the pattern of incoming data. The analyses can be described very generally as a comparison of expected value to some observed value. What differentiates methods is the specification of what is "expected" and how the comparison to what is observed is conducted.

The most common approach to mine PV databases is the use of disproportionality measures.[7,8] Disproportionality measures are a series of methods that compare an observed proportion, the occurrence of a specific adverse event associated with a drug of interest (e.g., aspirin and nausea), to the expected proportion, defined as the occurrence of the specific adverse event in all other data contained in the database (e.g., nausea for all other drugs). If the proportion of the drug of interest is greater than the proportion measured in the remainder of the database, then there is evidence of disproportionality. If the disproportionality is sufficiently large, the result is a signal of disproportionate reporting. There are numerous methods to compute disproportionalities, such as proportional reporting ratio, Empirical Bayes Geometric Mean, and reporting odds ratio, that are described in various publications.[8−10]

The size or composition of the database may not lend itself to analysis by disproportionality or the safety scientist may have interest in analyses that answer questions different from disproportion. If so, alternatives to disproportionalities, such as frequency-based analyses, are used.[11−13] In frequency-based analyses the observed value is usually a count of occurrence of some adverse event for a given drug at a specified time period. The expected value is constructed from the time periods prior to the current time period—the counts observed over time leading up to the current time period. If the current time period counts are sufficiently different from the previous time periods, a signal is identified. Regardless of the signal detection method employed, if a signal is identified, the information must be further examined.

SIGNAL VALIDATION
Signal validation is the preliminary evaluation of data after a signal has been identified in order to determine if a further comprehensive assessment should be undertaken. This step considers if there is sufficient evidence (e.g., index case, rare serious unexpected event,

rechallenge information, biological plausibility, and similar event with others in the class) based on a preliminary look at the data. The preliminary data can demonstrate the existence of a new potential causal association between a product and an adverse event, or a new aspect of an already known association, which therefore justifies a further comprehensive assessment.

SIGNAL ASSESSMENT

Safety scientists use medical and clinical expertise to critically assess validated signals for a potential association. Data are compiled and analyzed from a variety of available sources, depending on a product's life cycle. Potential data sources include clinical trials; postmarketing (spontaneous data) from individual case reports; literature and, if available, observational studies; and electronic medical records. Other considerations at this stage include exposure data (including the number of patients using the product, the patient population, and the setting), the epidemiology of the medical event of interest in the population of use, and the prevalence or incidence rates from the literature or calculated from clinical trial data (Box 2.4).

It is imperative to develop a case definition of the medical event of interest before assessing cases to ensure consistent objective evaluation of the data. The case definition defines the medical concept of interest and determines which individual cases to include or exclude during the medical assessment. An example of a case definition is the one developed by a working group for the diagnosis of acute pancreatitis, which utilizes signs and symptoms and laboratory and other diagnostic criteria.[14] This example stipulates that the diagnosis of acute pancreatitis requires two of the following three features:

1. abdominal pain consistent with acute pancreatitis (acute onset of a persistent, severe, epigastric pain often radiating to the back),
2. serum lipase activity (or amylase activity) at least three times greater than the upper limit of normal,
3. characteristic findings of acute pancreatitis on contrast-enhanced computed tomography (CECT) and, less commonly, on magnetic resonance imaging or transabdominal ultrasonography.

The authors note that if abdominal pain suggests strongly that acute pancreatitis is present, but the serum amylase and/or lipase activity is less than three times the upper limit of normal, as may be the case with delayed presentation, imaging will be required to confirm the diagnosis. If the diagnosis of acute pancreatitis is established by abdominal pain and by increases in the serum pancreatic enzyme activities, a CECT is not usually required for diagnosis in the emergency room or on admission to the hospital.

Each case is read and reviewed to determine the importance of the case and to apply the case definition. Is it out of scope, biologically implausible, missing critical information for medical assessment, or confounded by prior medical history, comorbid disease state(s), or concomitant medications? Is there an alternative etiology for the event? Most importantly, are there nonconfounded cases in a reasonable time frame to support a causal relationship?

Safety scientists summarize the results of their analysis and determine next steps based on the strength of the evidence. Following this assessment, signals are either refuted or confirmed. If a signal is refuted, the recommendation is to continue to monitor through standard surveillance activities. If a signal is confirmed, safety scientists must determine if the event represents a new risk or a change to a known risk and further categorize the risk as an important identified risk or an important potential risk. Of note, not every confirmed signal will be categorized as a risk.

The assessment of a confirmed signal for determination of risk should consider

- the strength of the signal (e.g., probability that the drug contributed to the adverse event),
- whether or not the signal or some aspect/characteristic of it is new,
- the clinical importance (e.g., severity of event and outcome),
- the potential for high impact to patient safety,

BOX 2.4
Signal Assessment

- Signal assessment is multifaceted with multiple data sources
  - Source data include exposure data, clinical trial/postmarketing data, literature, observational studies, medical records, and epidemiology of population of interest
- Case definition captures the medical concept of interest for case categorization
- Safety scientists determine the strength of potential risk
- Signal confirmation requires determination if event is a new risk or change to a known risk
  - Important potential risk
  - Important identified risk
- Designated medical event is a drug-related serious event that requires further evaluation

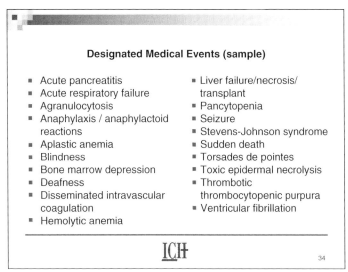

Designated Medical Events (sample)

- Acute pancreatitis
- Acute respiratory failure
- Agranulocytosis
- Anaphylaxis / anaphylactoid reactions
- Aplastic anemia
- Blindness
- Bone marrow depression
- Deafness
- Disseminated intravascular coagulation
- Hemolytic anemia

- Liver failure/necrosis/transplant
- Pancytopenia
- Seizure
- Stevens-Johnson syndrome
- Sudden death
- Torsades de pointes
- Toxic epidermal necrolysis
- Thrombotic thrombocytopenic purpura
- Ventricular fibrillation

ICH

34

FIG. 2.8 Designated medical events (sample). (Data from: http://www.ich.org/fileadmin/Public_Web_Site/Training/GCG_-_Endorsed_Training_Events/ASEAN_MedDRA_March_2010/Day_3/Regulatory_Perspective_SBrajovic.pdf.)

- the potential need for preventative measures to be implemented.

A designated medical event (DME) is an event that is inherently serious and often drug-related and is of critical importance to evaluate further. Serious events such as drug-induced liver injury or QT prolongation/torsades de pointes, if shown to be associated with the use of a drug, can critically impact the continuation of a drug development program or real-world use of the drug and should be assessed immediately. Given the severity and seriousness of these events, they are a priority for a safety scientist to validate the signal and conduct a signal assessment, as warranted. See Fig. 2.8 for some examples of DMEs.

DETERMINING BENEFIT/RISK (BOX 2.5)

The safety scientist should assess and summarize the public health impact of the newly identified risk or an update to a known risk. The safety scientist should consider the impact to the established benefit-risk profile, patient population affected, available alternative therapies, and circumstances of use. Possible next steps and recommendations for action are

- change in reference safety information,
- initiate or revise risk minimization strategies (see Chapter 13),
- conduct additional studies or surveillance activities,
- communicate new safety information to prescribers and patients.

The description of signal management and methods as described earlier has largely focused on traditional (Box 2.6) methods of obtaining safety information, i.e., case reports from clinical trials and spontaneous sources. However, the number, type, and size of data available are continually evolving. In order to capture events that are occurring in the real world in a timely manner, novel sources of adverse event data will need

---

BOX 2.5
Determining Benefit/Risk

Assess and summarize the impact of newly identified risk or update to a known risk with regard to
- benefit-risk profile
- patient population affected
- alternative therapies
- circumstances of use

BOX 2.6
Novel Data Sources

- Integrate new data into signal management process
- Social media listening is a new technological platform for signal detection and management
- Signal detection is evolving based on technology and the continuous improvement of signal detection approach

to be integrated into the signal management processes (see Box 2.6). For example, data could be obtained by reviewing photos of skin adverse events, videos of seizures, and audio files of respiratory events, certain neurologic events, and even patient or caregiver testimonials. As data sources expand, there will be a need for new approaches to store and analyze these data. Additionally, alternatives to data collection are needed for patients in developing countries who have increasing access to medications but are limited in opportunities to provide adverse event information.

For more technologically enabled patients, personal devices may be used to capture health data, such as blood pressure, heart rate, weight, and blood glucose levels. Similarly, patients may have implanted devices (such as pacemakers and insulin pumps) integrated. If data from wearable or implanted devices were compiled and evaluated on a periodic basis, perhaps an unforeseen risk could be identified and investigated sooner in a vulnerable population, such as patients with diabetes or congestive heart failure.

Another new source of information, on a larger scale, is social media. Patients have found a voice on social media and want other patients (and possibly physicians, regulatory authorities, and pharmaceutical companies) to know how their diseases, conditions, and therapies affect them. Safety scientists will need to develop best practices for social media listening and evaluation of data from popular search engines and social media platforms.

These new and evolving challenges represent an opportunity for a dramatically expanded role for signal detection and management. Two important aspects are technology (better analytical and visualization tools) and the continuous improvement of our approach and methodology to signal detection. The future is very promising. PV as a scientific field needs to fully understand critical datamining decision factors that can be augmented by more advanced machine learning algorithms, which allow our mining to "learn" over time and subsequently become better at identifying signals and processing large amounts of data.

The future of signal detection involves ever-changing data sources, analyses, and agglomeration of information. Health records and electronic claims data provide new largely untapped sources for safety surveillance. Real-time access to sales data and social media may allow better determination of the population exposed to a drug and therefore better estimate the "expected" value for signal detection. Machine learning and other advanced computer science techniques will allow analyses that generate more, and faster, insights. Technology and analyses cannot replace scientific and medical judgment. However, judgement could be overwhelmed by increasing data and analytics. The future requires weighing the value of information, determining which sources have the most value, and providing the information that is most likely indicative of safety signals to experts for further examination.[15] A successful PV organization will combine analytics and the "brains" of signal management, the safety scientist, the safety physician, the statistician, the epidemiologist, and the bioinformatics expert, all collaborating to elucidate different parts of the safety puzzle.

The effort of experts applying knowledge to a particular analysis or a particular product within signal management is merely a portion of the overall activity within an organization responsible for PV. This activity may be repeated multiple times across multiple teams products. To maintain a cohesive reliable structure responsible for ensuring public health, proper governance across all signal management activities is necessary.

SAFETY GOVERNANCE IN PHARMACOVIGILANCE

Governance is the process by which decisions are evaluated, made, and implemented.[16] Good governance includes a system that is participatory, consensus oriented, accountable, transparent, responsive, effective and efficient, equitable and inclusive, as well as follows the rule of law.[16] Governance promotes individual and institutional integrity in the pharmaceutical sector,[17] particularly in the field of PV.

Safety governance ensures an integrated approach to drug safety by proactively monitoring drug safety from development through postmarketing product stages. Because drug safety is a shared responsibility across functions and has direct impact on patients, healthcare professionals, and regulators, it is essential that safety issues are managed efficiently and escalated appropriately. Safety governance should not be a box-checking activity; rather, it should strengthen safety roles, responsibilities, and processes across the enterprise.

There are many options for implementation of safety governance, and there is truly no one-size-fits-all solution. The following sections describe a structure that may address various governance functions within a pharmaceutical company. Although this example refers to a pharmaceutical company, there are analogous structures within other organizations that impact PV (e.g., regulatory authorities) (Box 2.7).

SAFETY GOVERNANCE FRAMEWORK

Safety governance varies across pharmaceutical companies, making it difficult to make comparisons or recommend a particular framework.[17] An example structure of the entities that might be included within a safety governance framework is shown in Fig. 2.9.

Collectively, these entities provide oversight of the safety of all drug products; however, the Safety Oversight Board represents the mechanism through which corporate due diligence and governance would occur with respect to safety. Each entity of the safety

governance framework will be discussed; however, it is important to note that to have a properly functioning safety governance framework, it must be adequately sustained by robust processes and support systems, which will also be discussed.

SAFETY OVERSIGHT BOARD (BOX 2.8)

The Safety Oversight Board is the highest executive management-level safety oversight body with regard to drug safety. The Safety Oversight Board is central to the safety governance framework and oversees cross-functional activities impacting the benefit-risk profile of any drug products in clinical development and those that are authorized and marketed. Therefore inclusion

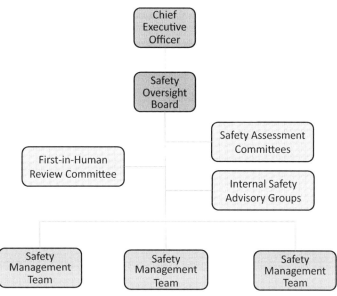

FIG. 2.9 Sample safety governance structure.

of senior-level management representatives from core functions relevant to benefit-risk assessments is critical. The Safety Oversight Board is responsible for the following:

- reviewing and responding to recommendations of Safety Management Teams by facilitating evidence-based decisions and consistent decision-making across teams with regard to safety;
- providing perspective on whether or not emerging safety issues carry a possible public health impact, thereby requiring accelerated evaluation and communication;
- overseeing and managing safety concerns arising from development/marketing partnerships, academic institutions, regulatory authorities, and legal procedures.

SAFETY MANAGEMENT TEAMS[18]

Safety Management Teams should be established for each drug product when preclinical studies are initiated and should remain in place throughout the product life cycle. Safety Management Teams are accountable to the Safety Oversight Board. Each team should be led by a physician who is ultimately responsible for understanding the product benefit-risk profile. Composition of teams should include representatives who are responsible for various aspects of product characterization. Teams monitor the product safety profile, which includes the continuous collection and evaluation of information relevant to the benefit-risk profile. If a team cannot reach consensus across functions, the topic may be escalated to the Safety Oversight Board for resolution (Box 2.9).

FIRST-IN-HUMAN REVIEW COMMITTEE[19,20]

After Good Laboratory Practice toxicology study data have become available, but before initiation of the first-in-human clinical trial, a committee of preclinical and clinical experts should review and approve proposed safety measures in the protocol to ensure adequate protection of clinical trial subjects. The Safety Management

---

BOX 2.9
Safety Management Teams

The Safety Management Team
- has the responsibility of understanding the benefit-risk profile throughout the product life cycle,
- ensures continuous collection and evaluation of information for product characterization,
- is accountable to the Safety Oversight Board.

BOX 2.10
Additional Safety Committees

- Additional safety governance entities may include a first-in-human review committee, internal safety advisory groups, and safety assessment committees.
- Safety governance framework is supported by a strategic partner responsible for material information flow, compliance, and project management.

Team should refer the proposed first-in-human study protocol to the committee for approval before initiation of the first-in-human trial. The committee functions under the governance of the Safety Oversight Board. When consensus cannot be achieved by the committee that the proposed safety margins adequately protect trial participants, there is provision to escalate to the Safety Oversight Board for resolution (Box 2.10).

INTERNAL SAFETY ADVISORY GROUPS

Owing to the variety of medical expertise across the enterprise, it is efficient to leverage that expertise and form internal safety advisory groups for areas of interest, e.g., hepatology experts for assessment of potential drug-induced liver injury. Safety Management Teams may leverage the medical expertise of an internal safety advisory group before discussing a potential safety issue with an external consultant panel, regulatory authority, or with the Safety Oversight Board.

SAFETY ASSESSMENT COMMITTEES[21]

During drug product development, regulatory authorities have issued guidance for the establishment of internal or external Safety Assessment Committees to review adverse events in an unblinded fashion. The objective of these committees is to identify a threshold for safety reporting based on aggregate analyses of adverse event rates not interpretable as single events for a drug product.

SAFETY GOVERNANCE SUPPORT

Because the Safety Oversight Board is central to the overall safety framework, it is essential to have a designated resource that may be a strategic partner and serve as a primary contact for the Safety Oversight Board and its governing entities. The responsibilities of this multifaceted role are to ensure an effective infrastructure for material information flow, oversee compliance with safety governance reporting requirements, provide project management support,[18] advise the Safety Management Teams on how best to communicate with the Safety Oversight Board, and escalate issues to the attention of the Safety Oversight Board Chair as appropriate.

SAFETY GOVERNANCE PROCESS (BOX 2.11)

Safety information required by the Safety Oversight Board must be well defined so that product teams understand when to communicate and escalate appropriately. Requirements for information may have some overlap in order to cover possible scenarios that may potentially impact patients, healthcare professionals, and regulatory authorities.

Safety topics of interest requiring communication or escalation fall into three main categories:
1. event-triggered activities
2. regulatory submission activities
3. studies/programs with safety oversight

Examples of safety topics of interest may include, but are not limited, to the following:

- product actions or regulatory notifications due to significant safety issues;
- safety issues for clinical development and marketed products, including any safety issues that may significantly impact the product benefit-risk assessment;
- significant compliance gaps or safety issues, e.g., label submissions, late reporting resulting in corrective action/preventative action, late aggregate reports, or critical findings/requests from regulatory authorities;
- additional risk minimization (global)/risk evaluation and mitigation strategies (in the United States);
- major PV regulatory inspections or Advisory Committee Meetings;
- product, device, or manufacturing quality issues that have the potential to impact safety.

Safety governance is appropriately informed by evidence and lessons learned, increasing the likelihood of continued success and improvement.[22] Evidence of a safety governance process is guaranteed to be highly scrutinized during audit or inspection, especially when key safety decisions have the potential to impact patients, healthcare providers, and regulatory authorities. Therefore it is imperative to capture key safety decisions and endorsement of such decisions at the appropriate levels. In addition, documentation of general oversight of the benefit-risk product assessment (See Chapter 13) and the associated safety topics of interest is an important component of a robust safety governance model. Lastly, but perhaps most importantly, the safety governance framework must have the necessary support systems and qualified personnel in place to ensure the process works as intended.

CONCLUSION

Signal detection, signal management, and governance are essential processes for a robust PV system. Proactively considering the broad context in which these activities take place and collaborating with numerous and varied subject-matter experts (epidemiologists, safety scientists, physicians, and statisticians) positions a PV organization for the future. A future where vastly increasing amounts of data and shortened drug development timelines demands a cross-functional agile team able to integrate data, technology, and human expertise to ensure public health.

LIST OF DEFINITIONS

Term	Definition	t0010
Case definition	Defining the medical concept of interest and determining which individual cases from a case series to include or exclude during the medical assessment.	
Case series	A group of individual case safety reports (ICSRs) selected by defined criteria (Standardized MedDRA Query (SMQ) or Preferred Term) used to assist in the validation and assessment of a safety signal.	
Confirmed signal	An adverse event of suspected causality that has been verified after the assessment of available data.	
Index case	An ICSR describing an adverse event(s) with some suspicion of a causal relationship to the use of a drug product in the absence of any confounding variables or other possible causes.	
Safety scientist	Safety science professionals responsible for pharmacovigilance activities related to the identification, validation, assessment, and prevention of adverse effects or any other medicine-related problem.	

BOX 2.11
Safety Governance Support

- Safety governance is supported by a well-defined process for communication and escalation.
- Requirements should cover all possible scenarios with potential safety impact.
- It is informed by evidence and lessons learned.

Term	Definition
Safety surveillance	Activities, both qualitative and quantitative, designed to identify previously unknown effects of a compound, or new aspects of known effects, in order to harness such effects (if beneficial) or prevent or mitigate them (if harmful).
Signal assessment	Evaluating the totality of available scientific evidence across all developmental phases of a drug product and from multiple sources.
Signal management	A set of activities performed to determine whether there are new risks causally associated with an active substance or medicinal product or whether known risks have changed. This includes signal detection, signal validation, signal assessment, and recommendation for action.
Signal sources	Signals may come from various sources that include, but are not limited to, • spontaneous reporting • solicited reporting • published literature • clinical trials • product quality/manufacturing • toxicology • legal • regulatory authorities • Internet and digital, including social media • independent organizations • academia
Signal validation	Process of evaluating the data supporting a detected signal in order to verify that the available documentation contains sufficient evidence demonstrating the existence of a new potentially causal association, or a new aspect of a known association, and therefore justifies further assessment of the signal.

REFERENCES

1. *ICH Harmonised Tripartite Guideline Pharmacovigilance Planning E2E*; 2004. Available from: http://www.ema.europa.eu/docs/en_GB/document_library/Scientific_guideline/2013/05/WC500143294.pdf.
2. *Safety of Medicines a Guide to Detecting and Reporting Adverse Drug Reactions: Why Health Professionals Need to Take Action*. Geneva: World Health Organization; 2002. Available from: http://apps.who.int/iris/bitstream/10665/67378/1/WHO_EDM_QSM_2002.2.pdf.
3. Harpaz R, DuMouchel W, LePendu P, Bauer-Mehren A, Ryan P, Shah NH. Performance of pharmacovigilance signal-detection algorithms for the FDA adverse event reporting system. *Clin Pharmacol Ther*. 2013;93(6):539−546.
4. Hauben M, Madigan D, Gerrits CM, Walsh L, Van Puijenbroek EP. The role of data mining in pharmacovigilance. *Expert Opin Drug Saf*. 2005;4(5):929−948.
5. Chan KA, Hauben M. Signal detection in pharmacovigilance: empirical evaluation of data mining tools. *Pharmacoepidemiol Drug Saf*. 2005;14(9):597−599.
6. Bate A, Evans SJ. Quantitative signal detection using spontaneous ADR reporting. *Pharmacoepidemiol Drug Saf*. 2009;18(6):427−436.
7. Quattrini G, Zambon A, Simoni L, Fiori G. Disproportionality measures used in signal detection: an assessment on pharmacovigilance adverse event reporting system data. *Value Health*. 2015;18(7):A720.
8. Hauben M, Zhou X. Quantitative methods in pharmacovigilance: focus on signal detection. *Drug Saf*. 2003;26(3):159−186.
9. Almenoff JS, LaCroix KK, Yuen NA, Fram D, DuMouchel W. Comparative performance of two quantitative safety signalling methods: implications for use in a pharmacovigilance department. *Drug Saf*. 2006;29(10):875−887.
10. Jokinen JD. *Determination of Change in Online Monitoring of Longitudinal Data: An Evaluation of Methodologies* [Dissertation]. Athens, OH: Ohio University; 2015.
11. Jokinen JD, Lievano F, Truffa M. *A Frequency-Based Method for Safety Signal Detection Data Mining*. 2017.
12. European Medicines Agency. *Guideline on Good Pharmacovigilance Practices (GVP) Module IX Addendum I — Methodological Aspects of Signal Detection from Spontaneous Reports of Suspected Adverse Reactions 2016*; 2016. Available from: http://www.ema.europa.eu/docs/en_GB/document_library/Regulatory_and_procedural_guideline/2016/08/WC500211715.pdf.
13. Pinheiro LC, Candore G, Zaccaria C, Slattery J, Arlett P. An algorithm to detect unexpected increases in frequency of reports of adverse events in EudraVigilance. *Pharmacoepidemiol Drug Saf*. 2017.
14. Banks PA, Bollen TL, Dervenis C. Acute Pancreatitis Classification Working Group. Classification of acute pancreatitis—2012: revision of the Atlanta classification and definitions by international consensus. *Gut*. 2013;62:102−111. https://doi.org/10.1136/gutjnl-2012-302779.
15. Heath A, Manolopoulou I, Baio G. A review of methods for analysis of the expected value of information. *Med Decis Mak*. 2017;37(7):747−758.
16. What is good governance? http://www.unescap.org/pdd/prs/ProjectActivities/Ongoing/gg/governance.asp.
17. *Good Governance for Medicines: Model Framework*. World Health Organization; 2014. http://apps.who.int/iris/bitstream/10665/129495/1/9789241507516_eng.pdf?ua=1&ua=1.
18. *Management of Safety Information from Clinical Trials, Report of CIOMS Working Group VI*; 2005. https://cioms.ch/wp-content/uploads/2017/01/Mgment_Safety_Info.pdf.
19. *US FDA Guidance for Industry, Estimating the Maximum Safe Starting Dose in Initial Clinical Trials for Therapeutics in Adult Healthy Volunteers*; 2005. https://www.fda.gov/downloads/drugs/guidances/ucm078932.pdf.

20. European Medicines Agency. *Committee for Medicinal Products for Human Use (CHMP) Guideline on Strategies to Identify and Mitigate Risks for First-in-human and Early Clinical Trials with Investigational Medicinal Products, Draft*; 2016. http://www.ema.europa.eu/docs/en_GB/document_library/Scientific_guideline/2016/11/WC500216158.pdf.

21. *Safety Assessment for IND Safety Reporting Guidance for Industry*; December 2015. https://www.fda.gov/downloads/Drugs/GuidanceComplianceRegulatoryInformation/Guidances/UCM477584.pdf.

22. Kohler, et al. *BMC Public Health*. 2014;63:14. http://www.biomedcentral.com/1471-2458/14/63.

FURTHER READING

1. *European Medicines Agency, Committee for Medicinal Products for Human Use (CHMP) Guideline on the Limits of Genotoxic Impurities*; 2006. http://www.ema.europa.eu/docs/en_GB/document_library/Scientific_guideline/2009/09/WC500002903.pdf.

2. *Practical Approaches to Risk Minimisation for Medicinal Products, Report of CIOMS Working Group IX.* 2014.

3. *Format and Content of a REMS Document, Guidance for Industry*; October 2017. https://www.fda.gov/downloads/Drugs/GuidanceComplianceRegulatoryInformation/Guidances/UCM184128.pdf.

4. *Practical Aspect of Signal Detection in Pharmacovigilance, Report of CIOMS Working Group VIII.* 2010.

CHAPTER 3

Product Safety Monitoring in Clinical Trials

THAO DOAN, MD • RADHIKA M. RAO, MD, MPH • KAROLYN KRACHT, MS •
JAMES M. PAUFF, MD, PHD • BARBARA A. HENDRICKSON, MD

INTRODUCTION

This chapter will discuss clinical trial safety planning, data collection and evaluation, and the reporting and communication of clinical trial safety information (Box 3.1). The planning for safety monitoring begins before the product enters the first-in-human clinical trials. Evolution of the safety monitoring plan occurs throughout clinical development as information accumulates from ongoing and completed clinical trials, in addition to other sources.

Defining the emerging safety profile of an investigational medicinal product (IMP) requires a systematic approach including the preparation of a development risk management plan (DRMP) or its equivalent. The DRMP documents the measures to characterize and minimize risks during clinical development. Creating a DRMP requires knowledge about the demographics of the study population, the disease condition and the rates of its associated comorbidities, the product's pharmacokinetic and toxicologic information, and the possible risks based on the class of the product.

The identification of safety signals during clinical development of a potential therapy requires organized data collection and evaluation using qualitative and quantitative analyses by an assembled team of cross-functional experts. Once a safety signal has been identified, the signal should be assessed using the totality of the available nonclinical and clinical data as well as relevant epidemiologic information. Safety events for which there is sufficient evidence to conclude a causal relationship with product administration are considered adverse reactions. Identified adverse reactions should be communicated to relevant regulatory authorities, site investigators, institutional review boards (IRBs), ethics committees (ECs), and trial subjects. The safety team evaluates ways to mitigate the risk at the individual subject or study population level and determines if changes to the reference product safety information (e.g., investigator's brochure, subject informed consent form) are required. From a regulatory perspective, safety reporting during clinical trials focuses on the expedited reporting of designated individual case safety reports (ICSRs) as well as periodic update reports that delineate significant safety information from the reporting period and the important risks determined for the product.

SAFETY PLANNING
Systemic Approach

The Council for International Organizations of Medical Sciences (CIOMS) has defined a signal (Box 3.2) as *"information that arises from one or multiple sources (including observations or experiments), which suggests a new, potentially causal association, or a new aspect of a known association between an intervention [e.g., administration of a medicine] and an event or set of related events, either adverse or beneficial, that is judged to be of sufficient likelihood to justify verificatory action".*[1]

An adverse event is any untoward medical occurrence in a patient or a clinical investigation subject, whether or not it is considered drug related. The term

---

BOX 3.1
Overview of Safety Monitoring

- Safety monitoring begins before the product enters clinical trials and continues throughout clinical development
- Identifying safety signals involves extensive collection, assessment, and reporting of data
- Safety reporting and risk management are done on an individual and study population level

---

> **BOX 3.2**
> **A Signal**
>
> - Defined as new information that implies a potential association between an intervention and an event (which can be either adverse or beneficial)
> - Should not be confused with an adverse reaction and/or risk
> - Surveillance for safety signals should be systematic and proactive throughout all stages of clinical development, involving a team of experts

> **BOX 3.3**
> **DRMPs and DCSI**
>
> - A DRMP requires knowledge of the disease or condition, the demographics of the study population, and the product's profile.
> - Along with a benefit-risk plan, a DRMP provides a crucial early record of identified or potential risks, plus plans for risk management.
> - A DCSI outlines the product's available safety information at each stage and records adverse drug reactions found during the clinical development program.

---

adverse reaction implies that a causal relationship has been established between the adverse event and administration of the medicinal product.

A risk is an undesirable clinical outcome for which there is scientific evidence either to suspect the possibility of a causal relationship with the medicinal product (potential risk) or to conclude that there is causal relationship with the medicinal product (identified or known risk).[2]

The identification of risks of an IMP starts with an assessment of the following:[3]

- the product's mechanism of action and the safety profile of products in the same class, if applicable;
- the product's potential to exacerbate events associated with the intended disease indication (i.e., an antidiabetic medication that raises blood pressure and therefore could worsen major adverse cardiac event rates);
- preclinical safety pharmacology assays that provide information about possible effects of the product on the cardiovascular, respiratory, and central nervous systems;
- in vitro assays that assess for possible binding to off-target receptors and the potential of small-molecule drugs to induce mutations or structural chromosomal aberrations;
- animal toxicology studies that identify organ systems targeted for adverse effects and the relationship of these effects to drug exposure;
- toxicology studies in animals that evaluate adverse effects on the fetus or reproductive function.

The implications of these findings to human administration of the IMP should be considered. These observations may inform the need for specific safety studies to precede or coincide with clinical trials for efficacy. A prospective plan (DRMP) should be developed to monitor for and minimize these potential risks in the clinical trials.[3]

Surveillance for safety signals should be systematic and proactive.[3] A team of experts (e.g., product safety team, safety management team) should be assembled to evaluate the emerging information about the safety of the product and make decisions regarding the management of any identified or potential risks. This safety team should function according to prespecified standard operating procedures and meet regularly to review any new safety concerns that may require further investigation. Clear roles and responsibilities should be delineated for data collection, analyses, and interpretation and implementation of safety actions.

Furthermore, the need for involvement of external experts who are independent of those conducting and managing the trials should be considered, such as expert adjudication of adverse events (the Adjudication or Endpoint Committee) or a data monitoring committee (DMC) that assesses the benefit versus risk of continuing the ongoing clinical trial(s) without modification.[3]

Development Risk Management Plan and Development Core Safety Information (Box 3.3)

During early development, typically after phase 1 or during phase 2, a benefit-risk plan can be constructed that includes an analysis of the disease/condition, current treatment options, and a preliminary understanding of the IMP's key benefits and risks.[4] The plan will serve as a starting point for the benefit-risk assessment to be prepared later in the development life cycle (see Chapter 13).

Additionally, a development risk management plan (DRMP) is prepared; the DRMP includes early documentation of identified or potential risks along with plans for minimizing these risks during development. This document eventually evolves into the risk management plan (RMP) that will accompany the product's registration application as well as support on-market usage.[3] (See Chapter 13)

The development risk management plan includes the following[3]:

- anticipated product profile
- epidemiology of the disease indication
- nonclinical safety experience
- clinical safety experience
- identification and assessment of known or anticipated risks
- identification and assessment of potential new risks
- actions and/or plans for mitigating risks

Finally, a program safety analysis plan is prepared to describe the collection and analysis of product-level safety data in more detail, including how the safety data across studies will be integrated as well as the characterization of safety events of interest (e.g., incidence rate, dose relationship, severity, time to onset, risk factors).[5] This program safety analysis plan will be used to inform the statistical analysis plan for the clinical safety summary that is included in the regulatory submission of the product for the intended indication.[5]

Adverse drug reactions identified during the clinical development program are included in the Development Core Safety Information (DCSI), which is recommended for investigational products in the current EU regulations as well as the proposed US regulations. The DCSI should provide the most updated safety information available for the product at each stage of development.[3]

Specific Safety Issues (Box 3.4)

When considering the safety of new products, the following issues should always be considered.

- Cardiac electrophysiology: QT prolongation is thought to increase the risk of torsade de pointes and/or sudden death and is mainly a concern for small-molecule drugs. Several drugs have been withdrawn from the market and development of some products was stopped due to drug-induced QT or QTc (i.e., QT corrected for heart rate) prolongation.

  Traditionally, evaluation for cardiac conduction effects has occurred in a specifically designed thorough QT/QTc (TQT) study.[6] However, more recently, exposure response analysis of QT effects in early clinical trials of healthy subjects has demonstrated promise for generating data that can negate the necessity of conducting a dedicated TQT study.[7]

- Hepatotoxicity: The potential for hepatotoxicity should be evaluated for all products in development[8] (see Chapter 4).

- Immunogenicity: In the development of biologics, a plan is needed to monitor potential immunogenicity (ability to induce a humoral and/or cell-mediated immune response), which can be associated with an increased risk of hypersensitivity reactions or immune complex disease.[9]

- Bone marrow toxicity: Hematologic adverse reactions are commonly encountered in drug development and should also be evaluated; the most severe effects being agranulocytosis and aplastic anemia.[3]

- Drug–drug and food–drug interactions: The potential for drug–drug interactions and food–drug interactions is important. Drug–drug interactions are based on what is known about the drug's metabolism, mechanism of action, and concomitant therapies for the indication. Food–drug interactions may be examined through clinical bioavailability and/or dedicated pharmacokinetic studies. Information on products in the same class also may be helpful.[3]

DATA COLLECTION AND EVALUATION

Data Collection (Box 3.5)

General principles and considerations

The clinical trial (principal) investigator (PI) is responsible for conducting the clinical trial at an investigative site. Clinical trial data, which includes subject medical history, adverse event reports, physical examinations, and laboratory and other evaluations as defined by the protocol, are collected using case report forms. The relevant information is entered into case report forms by the PI or their designee.

Data collection and evaluation during the clinical trials is critical to the process of safety monitoring. In addition to accuracy, timely acquisition of comprehensive

---

BOX 3.4
Specific Safety Issues

- Cardiac electrophysiology e.g. drug-induced QT prolongation
- Hepatotoxicity
- Immunogenicity (may be associated with hypersensitivity reactions or immune complex disease)
- Bone marrow toxicity (most seriously, agranulocytosis and aplastic anemia)
- Drug–drug and food–drug interactions

safety information is important to properly assess individual events and for aggregate safety data reviews.

Serious and nonserious adverse events from a trial are collected by the sponsor using a standardized approach.[3] Adverse events are considered serious if the event is fatal (death); is life-threatening; results in hospitalization, disability or permanent damage, or congenital anomaly; or is considered an important medical event. Serious adverse events are reported to the regulatory authorities on a form recommended by the CIOMS for the European Medicines Agency (EMA) or via a MedWatch format for the US FDA.

The study protocol should describe reasonable efforts to collect safety data for study subjects that discontinue treatment, regardless of whether discontinuation was due to a protocol-defined event or other reason (e.g., withdrawal of informed consent, or "lost to follow-up").[5]

Specialized data collection and adjudication
Baseline risk factor documentation. Adverse events reported in the clinical trial should be assessed in the context of the subject's baseline risk factors. Collecting relevant risk factors for safety events of interest is important for interpretation of the product safety data.[3]

Safety topics of interest. In addition to the general adverse event case report forms, the protocol could specify collection of additional information and events relevant to the disease population being studied for the IMP. This information helps facilitate the understanding of the role of the IMP in observed events in the clinical trial.[3]

For example, for patients experiencing hepatic adverse events the collected information should include history of alcohol use, concomitant medications, and herbal supplements; travel history; occupational toxin exposure; and family history of liver disease, as well as relevant diagnostic testing such as viral serologic tests.

Event adjudication. Individual PIs characterize the nature of adverse events experienced by the clinical trial

subjects through their verbatim reports, which are then coded by the company via a standardized Medical Dictionary for Regulatory Activities (MedDRA). A Maintenance and Support Service Organization has been created by the International Conference on Harmonisation (ICH) to govern the structure, content, and versioning of MedDRA. The extent to which information is available regarding the circumstances of the event, the accuracy of the conveyed information, and the expertise of the trial investigator all may influence the verbatim report and the subsequent MedDRA coding of the adverse event.

Adjudication of specified clinical endpoint events is believed to enhance the validity of clinical trial outcome measures.[10] For example, external cardiac adjudication committees are commonly employed to evaluate cardiovascular events in clinical trials involving patients at higher risk for events, such as patients with diabetes or rheumatoid arthritis. Adjudication of the events is conducted using prespecified procedures and medical concept definitions, typically outlined in a formal charter. The goal of independent adjudication may be solely to systematically classify reported events in a manner blinded to treatment assignment. Alternatively, independent expert panels may also provide judgments regarding the role of the IMP in the observed adverse events. Completion of supplemental case report forms and/or facilitation of attempts to obtain source records with key information is an important consideration when event adjudication committees are employed.

Data monitoring committee (Box 3.6)
As noted earlier, a DMC independent of the study team may be indicated for some clinical studies, such as large registrational trials.[3] The DMC consists of a group of experts with knowledge about the disease under study or particular safety events of interest (for example, experts with subspecialty training in cardiology, hepatology, or infectious diseases) and includes a statistician with

expertise in clinical trials. The roles, responsibilities, and procedures of the DMC are governed by a charter. The DMC meets at prespecified time points to evaluate the safety and/or efficacy data of the relevant clinical trial, typically in a manner unblinded to the treatment group. The DMC is charged with evaluating the benefit/risk of the ongoing clinical trial and making recommendations to sponsors regarding modifications needed to maintain a favorable benefit-risk profile for clinical trial participation or discontinuation of the trial for an unfavorable benefit-risk assessment. The DMC charter is critical to outline the procedures required to maintain data integrity, independence from the study team, and appropriate communication channels with the sponsor.[3]

Safety assessment committees

The FDA has issued a draft guidance that describes the concepts of a safety assessment (Box 3.7) committee and a safety surveillance plan.[11] The objective is for the clinical trial sponsor to identify events which meet the threshold for the investigational new drug (IND) safety reporting based on aggregate analyses of adverse event rates not interpretable as single events. However, the FDA has acknowledged circumstances where serious unexpected adverse reactions should be expedited based on a single report, including Stevens-Johnson syndrome, agranulocytosis, and acute liver failure.

Data Evaluation

Safety signals detected at each stage of clinical development are used to form the safety plan and influence the design of subsequent studies and trials. Adverse drug reactions that have a causal relationship with the IMP must be separated from adverse events that may have occurred in subjects irrespective of their participation in the clinical trial.[12,13] Evaluating safety signals that arise during the clinical trials requires both quantitative and qualitative analyses.

Quantitative analysis

Individual studies (Box 3.8). The data collected in clinical trials may be characterized into two types: categorical and continuous. Safety data such as adverse events, concomitant medications, prior medications, and medical history are considered categorical data. Laboratory assessments, ECG findings, and vital sign measurements are considered continuous safety data. When analyzing either type of data, many analysis options are available, depending on the questions under consideration.

The different analysis options for categorical safety data can be described by a contingency table presentation. Table 3.1 is a 2×2 contingency table layout for an adverse event.

The proportion of subjects who experience the event of interest on treatment is $(A/[A + B])$. This is referred to as the risk (or rate) of the adverse event. The magnitude of the differences between treatment risk and placebo risk is referred to as risk difference or the absolute difference in risk. The Fisher exact test and chi-square test may be used to test the difference in risk proportions (treatment vs. placebo). A significant P-value indicates that there is difference in the risk between the treatment and placebo groups. In addition to statistical tests, a 95% confidence interval (CI) may be calculated for the risk difference. A CI that includes 0 implies that there is no difference in risk between the treatment and placebo groups.

> **BOX 3.8**
> **Quantitative Analysis: Ways to Analyze Categorical Data**
>
> - Risk difference (measures treatment risk of adverse events vs. placebo risk)
> - Relative Risk and the odds ratio measure the magnitude of difference between the treatment and placebo
> - Exposure-adjusted event rate (event rate per patient per year)
> - The Kaplan-Meier survival plot

> **BOX 3.7**
> **Safety Reporting**
>
> - Expedited reports during clinical trials may be based on individual events or aggregate data analysis
> - Serious adverse reactions which are often associated with administration of drugs (e.g. agranulocytosis, drug induced liver failure) should be expedited based on single case reports
> - Safety signals are used to inform the safety plan and influence the design of later studies.

TABLE 3.1
Adverse Event Occurrence by Treatment Group

	Treatment	Placebo
Adverse event	A	C
No adverse event	B	D
Total	A + B	C + D

As an alternative to risk difference, relative risk and odds ratio may be calculated to measure the magnitude of the difference between the treatment and placebo groups. The odds of an adverse event occurring in the treatment group is (A/B). Furthermore, the odds of the event occurring in the placebo group is (C/D). The odds ratio, (A/B)/(C/D), may be calculated to measure the association between treatment exposure and adverse events. In addition, a 95% CI can be calculated for the odds ratio as well. If the CI contains 1, this implies that there is no difference in the odds ratio between the two groups.

Relative risk is simply the proportion of the risk ratios for an event of interest. The relative risk is defined as (A/[A + B])/(C/[C + D]). A 95% CI that contains 1 implies there is no difference in risk for the event of interest based on whether participants were exposed to the treatment or not.

Length of time on study is another factor that must be considered when assessing safety data. This is very important when combining multiple studies with different treatment durations. The exposure-adjusted rate provides a rate per person time. Table 3.2 illustrates how to calculate an exposure-adjusted event rate.

An exposure-adjusted event rate for treatment is calculated as (A/[a + b]). The results give the number of events per patient-year. To calculate the number of events per 100 patient-years, simply multiply $100 \times (A/[a + b])$.

Another way to assess the timing of an event is to calculate the survival probabilities using the Kaplan-Meier method (Fig. 3.1).[14] For example, one may calculate the median time to first occurrence of an adverse event such as anemia and its respective 95% CI. Additionally, a Kaplan-Meier survival plot may be created to graphically show the median time to onset of an event.

TABLE 3.2
Exposure-Adjusted Adverse Event Rate by Treatment Group

	Treatment	Treatment Duration (Patient Years)	Placebo	Placebo Duration (PT Years)
Adverse event	A	a	C	c
No adverse event	B	b	D	d
Total	A + B	a + b	C + D	c + d

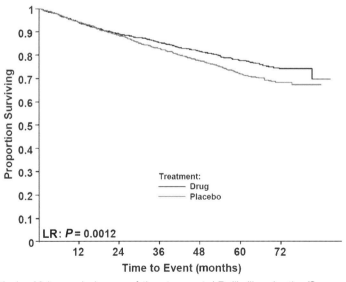

FIG. 3.1 The Kaplan-Meier survival curve of time to event. LR, likelihood ratio. (Source: FDA Guidance: Clinical Studies Section of Labeling for Human Prescription Drug and Biological Products. https://www.fda.gov/downloads/Drugs/GuidanceComplianceRegulatoryInformation/Guidances/UCM075059.pdf.)

Continuous data (Box 3.9), such as laboratory assessments, ECG findings, and vital sign measurements, are evaluated differently than categorical data. Simple summary statistics (mean, median, minimum, maximum, standard deviation, and 95% CI) can be calculated for each evaluation time point (for example, each study visit). The boxplot in Fig. 3.2 illustrates the change from baseline distribution by dose level. A similar series of boxplots (Fig. 3.2) may be constructed to show the change from baseline at each time point instead of dose.[14]

In addition to boxplots, line graphs may be used to illustrate a visual trend in the subject's laboratory, ECGs, and vital sign values. An example of a line graph is shown in Fig. 3.3.[14] This graph shows the percent change from baseline over time for three treatment groups. A graph like this may be used to show the change from baseline over time for a particular

laboratory or vital sign. Additionally, error bars or the number of subjects with data present at each time point can be displayed.

Another way to look for trends in continuous safety data is through shifts from baseline. A simple scatter plot of baseline versus minimum, maximum, or end of study results can be used. Deviations from the diagonal of the plot may indicate an important finding with regard to laboratory, ECG, or vital sign results. An example of a scatter plot is shown in Fig. 3.4.[14] This graph allows the reader to quickly understand the magnitude of difference between baseline and a time point of interest. Scatter plots like that in Fig. 3.4 are often used to help describe the magnitude of change between baseline and the maximum laboratory value observed in the trial.

Lastly, the "rule of three" (Box 3.10) can be applied to rare or infrequent events (i.e., events that would only be seen if tens of thousands of subjects were exposed to the drug).[3] The rule states that if no events are seen in x individuals, then the estimate for the risk is no more than $3/x$. For example, if no events were reported in 1000 subjects exposed to the drug, then the risk of occurrence of that event would be no more than $3/1000$ (0.3%) with 95% certainty. This principle is a good approximation and may be used to construct the upper bound of the 95% CI when zero events have been observed.

This section presented some examples of the many different ways to analyze and display data. There are

---

BOX 3.9
Quantitative Analysis: Ways to Analyze Continuous Data

- Boxplots
- Line graphs (to show a visual trend in a subject's measurements)
- Scatter plots (to show shifts from the baseline)
- Other graphics (forest plots, bar charts, spaghetti plots, etc.)

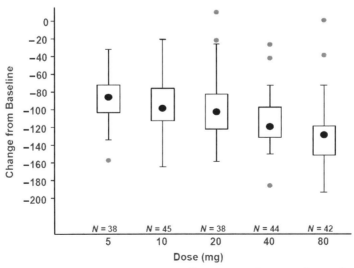

FIG. 3.2 Boxplots of response at endpoint by dose. (Source: FDA Guidance Clinical Studies Section of Labeling for Human Prescription Drug and Biological Products. https://www.fda.gov/downloads/Drugs/GuidanceComplianceRegulatoryInformation/Guidances/UCM075059.pdf.)

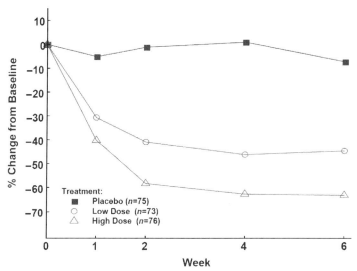

FIG. 3.3 Line graph: percent change from baseline by week. (Source: FDA Guidance: Clinical Studies Section of Labeling for Human Prescription Drug and Biological Products. https://www.fda.gov/downloads/Drugs/GuidanceComplianceRegulatoryInformation/Guidances/UCM075059.pdf.)

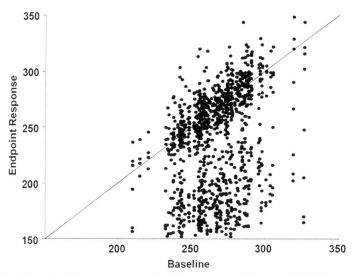

FIG. 3.4 Scatter plot: endpoint response versus baseline response. (Source: FDA Guidance: Clinical Studies Section of Labeling for Human Prescription Drug and Biological Products. https://www.fda.gov/downloads/Drugs/GuidanceComplianceRegulatoryInformation/Guidances/UCM075059.pdf.)

BOX 3.10
"Rule of Three"

- Rule of three in regard to rare events
- The rule states that if no events are seen in x individuals, then the estimate for the risk is no more than $3/x$

---

also many other graphic representations that can highlight changes in safety data. These include forest plots, bar charts, tree maps, dot plots, spaghetti plots, and many others. The CTSPEDIA website (https://www.ctspedia.org/do/view/CTSpedia) is a good reference for finding safety graphics.

Meta-Analysis (Box 3.11). Most clinical trials during the clinical development of a drug tend to be too small

BOX 3.11
Meta-Analysis

- Combines individual studies together in order to increase the ability to detect rare adverse events
- QUOROM lists factors (treatment duration, dose, patient population, etc.) that should be considered before combining data
- Statistical methods that account for study size should be used when combining data

BOX 3.12
Qualitative Analysis: Process Steps

- All available patient data should be aggregated and regularly reviewed.
- Previously identified safety concerns and pharmacokinetic and/or pharmacodynamic properties should be considered.
- Patient/population and disease characteristics should also be examined.

BOX 3.13
Responding to Potential or Identified Risks

- All investigators and participating sites must be notified.
- Any necessary changes to subject informed consent forms and the IB should be done.
- Risks should be included in the DSUR or IND reports submitted annually.
- Confirmed safety signals should be incorporated into the DRMP.

to detect rare or uncommon adverse events. Combining available studies together can increase statistical power and increase the ability to detect rare or uncommon adverse events. This is most often termed as a meta-analysis. The main purpose of performing a meta-analysis is to obtain a sufficient amount of data on rare and uncommon events that may not otherwise be obtained from a single trial.

Combining study-level data can be complicated; there is no absolute criterion as to which studies can and cannot be combined. The Quality of Reporting of Meta-analyses (QUOROM) guidelines referenced in CIOMS VI lists questions that should be considered when combining data. Dose, treatment duration, protocol design, patient population, and comparator arms are all elements that must be considered when combining studies for the sake of unified analysis.[3] Statistical methods that adjust for study size in a direct way should be used when combining two or more studies.[15] With the proper pooling techniques, inferences regarding the population of interest may be made. Carefully constructed meta-analytical approaches should be used routinely as part of drug development to examine data for potential safety signals.

Qualitative analysis (Box 3.12)

In addition to statistical quantitative methods, clinical judgment or qualitative analysis plays an important role in the detection and evaluation of safety signals.

Signal evaluation. In evaluating an event of interest the available patient-level data should be aggregated. The size of the studies contributing data and duration of drug exposure should be considered. In addition, the safety team should evaluate other relevant data, such as safety concerns identified in the preclinical studies or in related products, or the pharmacokinetic and/or pharmacodynamic properties known to be associated with the adverse reaction, including possible drug–drug interactions with concomitant medications.[3] Patient- and disease-specific factors

should then be considered, including the natural history of the disease being treated. For example, an older population with a life-limiting disease is likely to have a significant background rate of morbidity or mortality when compared with a younger study population. In general, such evaluation should ensure the following:[3]

1. All individual serious cases and any adverse event of special interest should be promptly evaluated by a member of the safety team.
2. Aggregate safety data from all available studies and trials (blinded where appropriate and including adverse events, laboratory data, and significant aberrancies in physical examination or imaging data), irrespective of causality assessment or seriousness, should be regularly reviewed.
3. Safety data from unblinded studies should undergo medical/clinical review on a regularly scheduled basis.

Safety actions in response to a confirmed signal—risk management (Box 3.13). If a safety signal is confirmed as a true risk to patients, the safety team needs to consider whether steps are needed to manage or mitigate the risk. Any ongoing risk to patients currently receiving the study drug is the most immediate concern. All investigators and participating sites must be notified about newly identified risks,

- ICSR consists of data from each adverse event.
- Causality assessment of the ICSR is required by the PI and the sponsor.
- The critical data points to consider in causality assessment of the ICSR are
  - temporal relationship
  - biological plausibility
  - medical history and concomitant medications
  - dechallenge
  - rechallenge
- Serious ICSR with reasonable possibility of association between IMP and adverse event and is not expected based on the known safety profile of the drug should be reported to the regulators expeditiously.

and for new important risks the impact on study conduct should be considered. The safety team should also make any necessary changes to subject informed consent forms and the investigator's brochure.[16]

A Development Safety Update Report (DSUR) is developed and updated for submission to regulators on an annual basis (see Section B Communication Safety Information where the DSUR is discussed in more detail). The DSUR has some analogy to the Periodic Safety Update Report for postmarketed products, although the exact content and timing of the DSUR varies widely.[3] According to the FDA regulations, the annual IND report includes line listings of the most serious and the most frequent adverse events as well as reasons for study drug discontinuation. However, the FDA accepts submission of the DSUR in place of an annual IND report.[17]

As drug development continues, confirmed safety signals should be incorporated into the DRMP.

REPORTING AND COMMUNICATION OF SAFETY INFORMATION
Expedited Reporting
Causality assessment of individual case safety report (Box 3.14)
The ICSR is the basic fundamental unit of safety analysis.[3] Medical review of an ICSR involves appropriately qualified professionals associated with the study, but it may also benefit at times from engaging external experts.

The PI has the responsibility to report the individual subject adverse events/abnormal laboratory values (as defined by the protocol) to the IRB and to the sponsor according to the timelines defined by the protocol (Fig. 3.5).

For any reported adverse event to be considered as a valid case report, the four criteria in Fig. 3.6 should be met.[18]

Adverse events are collected by the sponsor as a part of the clinical trial data. Adverse events are classified as serious or nonserious according to the ICH E2A guidelines.[19]

Clinical Scenario: A PI reports two events for one of his subjects in the clinical trial. The events are bullous rash and fever. The subject is admitted to the hospital for treatment of the bullous rash. Hence the event of bullous rash meets the seriousness criteria of hospitalization and should be reported as serious. The adverse event of fever that responded to oral medications did not meet any of the seriousness criteria and hence is noted as nonserious.

Causality: The next step in the review of adverse events is for the PI/sponsor to assess the causality toward the IMP. In order to assess whether the adverse event is associated with the use of the IMP, an in-depth review of all the critical data elements, along with the knowledge of the background disease and a clear understanding of the design of the study protocol, is essential.

Scientific approaches for causality assessment of an adverse event have been described by several regulatory agencies and healthcare entities. The most widely known of these approaches include the CIOMS Working Group, the Bradford Hill criteria, the Naranjo algorithm, and the World Health Organization criteria (see Chapter 4).

These scientific approaches to causality assessment have in common the following fundamental principles of review[18] (Fig. 3.7):

Temporal relationship: For an adverse event to be considered as caused by the IMP, the event should at least occur after the start of the IMP administration in a clinical trial. If the adverse event occurs before the start of the IMP administration, the event is considered temporally implausible.

Biological plausibility: A concept used to describe an adverse event that could possibly occur because of the known mechanism of action of the IMP.

concomitant medications: Review of all the current and recent concomitant medications used by the subject that could contribute to the occurrence of the adverse event.

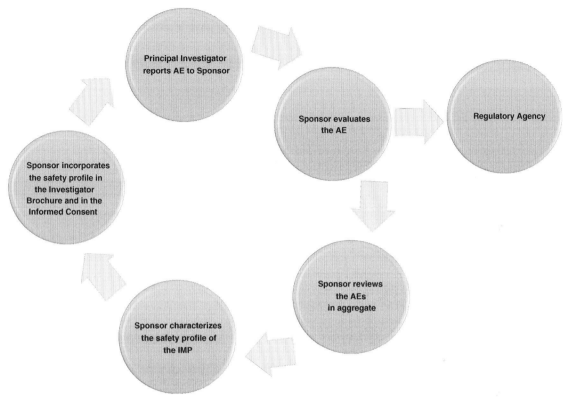

FIG. 3.5 Life cycle of an adverse event (AE). IMP, investigational medicinal product. (Created by Radhika M Rao for Elsevier to use.)

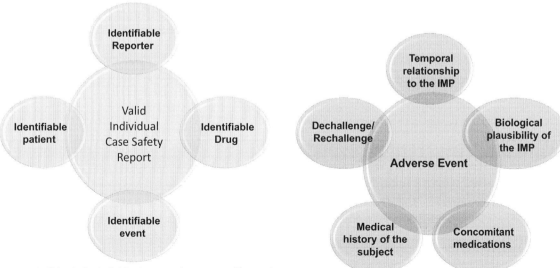

FIG. 3.6 Criteria for individual case safety report. (Created by Radhika M Rao for Elsevier to use. Ref: https://cioms.ch/wp-content/uploads/2017/01/Group5_Pharmacovigilance.pdf.)

FIG. 3.7 Data for causality assessment. IMP, investigational medicinal product. (Created by Radhika M Rao for Elsevier to use.)

past medical history: Review of the past medical history of the subject for any background disease risk factors that could contribute to the occurrence of the adverse event.

Dechallenge: Resolution of the adverse event with stopping the IMP administration supports the association of the adverse event with the IMP.

Rechallenge: Although this is sometimes not ethical or practical with clinically significant adverse events, the recurrence of the adverse event with the reintroduction of the IMP supports the association of the adverse event with the drug.

Clinical Scenario: The adverse event of bullous rash occurred 2 days after starting the study drug. There was no other medical history of allergies or dermatologic history. The subject has been taking all his concomitant medications for diabetes and hypertension for the past 5 years. No other new medications were started recently. The subject was admitted to the hospital; the study drug was discontinued and the bullous rash was treated with intravenous steroids. The rash resolved after X days. After discharge from the hospital and discussion with the PI, the subject resumed the study drug. Two days after resuming the study drug, the bullous rash recurred (positive rechallenge). The PI reports the event to the sponsor along with the assessment that this event has a reasonable possibility of being related to the study drug.

The sponsor evaluates all the data reported for the adverse event of bullous rash and comes to the same conclusion that this adverse event has a reasonable possibility of being related to the study drug.

Expectedness: After the ICSR is identified as serious or not serious, and assessed if the event is causally associated/not associated with the IMP, the next step is to assess if the event is expected or unexpected with the IMP. According to CIOMS V, expectedness refers to whether a similar serious adverse event was previously observed and considered associated (reasonable possibility) with that IMP[18] (Box 3.15).

Clinical Scenario: The event of "rash" is noted as "expected" per the investigator brochure (IB), but since the reported adverse event of "bullous rash" is more specific than a "rash" and also more severe because it required hospitalization, this adverse event of "bullous rash" is considered unexpected.

Thus based on the causality and expectedness assessment, a serious adverse event could be classified as shown in Fig. 3.8.

Expedited Reporting:

The reporting requirements for adverse events are based on current regulatory requirements. The FDA Guidance for safety reporting requirement for IND is the following.

- *"Under 21 Code of Federal Regulation (CFR) 312.32(c) the sponsor is required to notify the FDA and all participating investigators in an IND safety report (i.e., 7- or 15-day expedited report) about the potentially serious risks from clinical trials or any other source as*

BOX 3.15
Steps Involved in Evaluation of an ICSR

- Validity of the ICSR
- Seriousness criteria
- Causality
- Expectedness
- Reportability of the ICSR

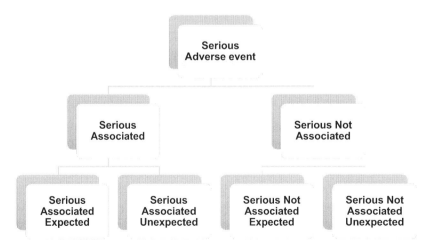

FIG. 3.8 Adverse event classification. (Created by Radhika M Rao for Elsevier to use.)

soon as possible, but no later than 15 calendar days after the sponsor receives the safety information and determines that the information qualifies for reporting.

- *Unexpected fatal or life-threatening suspected adverse reactions represent especially important safety information and, therefore, must be reported more rapidly to the FDA (21 CFR 312.32(c)(2)). The requirement for reporting any unexpected fatal or life-threatening suspected adverse reaction to the FDA is no later than seven calendar days after the sponsor's initial receipt of the information."*[20]

Communicating Safety Information (Box 3.16)

In addition to reporting the ICSRs within the regulatory timelines, there is a periodic aggregate review of the adverse events from clinical trials, particularly serious associated and unexpected adverse events. This aggregate review of the clinical trials' serious adverse events is summarized for the PI in the IB, for the regulatory agencies in the Development Safety Update Report (DSUR), and to the IRB or EC.

The IRB constitutes a group that has been formally designated to review and monitor biomedical research involving human subjects for designated clinical study sites. The IRB reviews the protocols, informed consents, and the adverse event reports of the research studies.[21] The EC is the European equivalent of the IRB. Members of the IRB/EC have the qualifications and experience to review and evaluate the science, medical aspects, and ethics of the proposed study.[22] Communication of safety information is shown in Fig. 3.9.

Informed consent. According to the US FDA 21 CFR, informed consent is the process of providing the prospective subject or their legal representative all the information about the study and study drug in a language that is understandable to most of the US population with a basic health literacy level.[21] This language should not contain any coercion or undue influence and any exculpatory language.

All the materials for informed consent, including the recruitment, should be approved by the IRB.

The informed consent should clearly describe the following:

- description of the clinical investigation
- risks and discomforts
- benefits
- alternative procedures or treatments
- confidentiality
- compensation and medical treatment in the event of medical injury
- voluntary participation

- Evaluations of aggregate safety data are communicated to the regulatory agency at periodic intervals in
  - IB
  - Development Safety Update Report
  - Informed consent
- Safety information is communicated to the PI/EC/IRB through
  - IB
  - Informed consent
  - Ad hoc communications

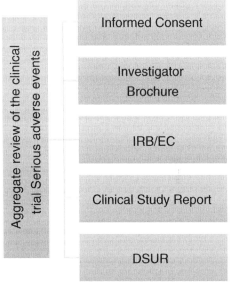

FIG. 3.9 Communication of safety information. EC, ethics committee; DSUR, Development Safety Update Report; IRB, institutional review board. (Created by Radhika M Rao for Elsevier to use.)

In the risks and discomforts section of the informed consent document, the sponsor should clearly explain the potential risks from the IMP and any comparator product being used in the study. These risks should be based on the information provided in the IB, protocol, and package labeling.

Investigator brochure. The IB is a document created by the sponsor summarizing all the known information about the IMP.[21] This document serves as a reference for the PIs, IRB, sponsor, and regulatory agencies. The IB includes information about the following:[22]

- physical, chemical, and pharmaceutical properties and formulations
- nonclinical studies
- nonclinical pharmacology
- pharmacokinetics and product metabolism in animals
- Toxicology
- effects in humans
  - pharmacokinetics and product metabolism in humans
  - safety and efficacy
  - marketing experience
  - guidance for the investigator

As the clinical trial data increases owing to greater enrollment in the clinical studies, the sponsor periodically reviews the data in aggregate and communicates the safety information in the IB. The sponsor is required to update the IB yearly (or sooner if there is new safety information) and to provide an updated IB to the PI.

Development Safety Update Report. A DSUR is an annual aggregate review of adverse events from all the clinical trials conducted by the sponsor with a particular IMP.[23]

Every IMP has a date of first authorization to conduct a clinical trial in any country that is called the "Development International Birth Date" (DIBD). One year from the DIBD is taken as the first data lock point (the cutoff period for all the clinical trial adverse events). The DSUR should be reported no later than 60 calendar days from a DSUR data lock point (which occur annually).

The DSUR includes a systematic review of both cumulative and interval safety data from the clinical trials in that 1-year period, such as
- deaths
- discontinuations
- serious unexpected associated adverse events
- preclinical toxicology study findings
- literature review
- safety information from the same class of drugs
- noninterventional study data
- completed and ongoing clinical trials
- overall safety assessment
- interim analysis
- conclusion
- summary of important risks

A DSUR is required every year that clinical trials are being conducted.

CONCLUSION

Safety planning requires an assessment of the available information relevant to the safety of the product, including nonclinical and clinical data and related product information. Ongoing benefit-risk assessments of the IMP are achieved through safety surveillance and evaluation of data from all available sources. Quantitative and qualitative analyses are performed on individual clinical trial data and aggregate product-level data using statistical methodologies and clinical medical judgment. These analyses aim to distinguish adverse drug reactions from adverse events and to determine the important risks associated with the product. Regulatory reporting and communication of safety information to the health authorities, IRB/EC, clinical trial investigators, and subjects are required. A systematic approach to product safety monitoring throughout clinical development is critical to characterize the evolving safety profile of the IMP.

REFERENCES

1. *Practical Aspects of Signal Detection in Pharmacovigilance Report of CIOMS Working Group VIII. Geneva.* 2010.
2. *EMA/838713/2011 Rev 2* Guideline on Good Pharmacovigilance Practices (GVP) Module V — Risk Management Systems (Rev 2).* March 28, 2017.
3. *Council for International Organizations of Medical Sciences (CIOMS) Working Group VI, Management of Safety Information from Clinical Trials. Geneva.* 2005.
4. *Structured Approach to Benefit-Risk Assessment in Drug Regulatory Decision-Making Draft PDUFA V Implementation Plan.* February 2013.
5. Crowe BJ, Xiab HA, Berlin JA, et al. Recommendations for safety planning, data collection, evaluation and reporting during drug, biologic and vaccine development: a report of the safety planning, evaluation, and reporting team. *Clin Trials.* 2009;6:430−440.
6. U.S. FDA Guidance for Industry. E14 clinical evaluation of QT/QTc interval prolongation and proarrhythmic potential for non-antiarrhythmic drugs. In: *Proceedings of the International Conference on Harmonisation; ICH Topic;* 2005. https://www.fda.gov/downloads/Drugs/GuidanceComplianceRegulatoryInformation/Guidances/UCM073153.pdf.
7. Darpo B, et al. CSRC White paper: can the thorough QT/QTc study be replaced by 'early QT assessment' in routine clinical pharmacology studies? Scientific update and a research proposal for a path forward. *Am Heart J.* 2014; 168:262−272 [PubMed].
8. U.S. FDA Guidance for Industry. *Drug-Induced Liver Injury: Premarketing Clinical Evaluation; Drug Safety;* July 2009. https://www.fda.gov/downloads/Drugs/.../Guidances/UCM-174090.pdf.

9. Tovey MG, Lallemand C. Immunogenicity and other problems associated with the use of biopharmaceuticals. *Ther Adv Drug Saf*. 2011;2(3):113−128.

10. Seltzer JH, et al. Centralized adjudication of cardiovascular end points in cardiovascular and non cardiovascular pharmacologic trials: a report from the Cardiac Safety Research Consortium. *Am Heart J*. 2015;169(2):197−204.

11. *U.S. FDA Safety Assessment for IND Safety Reporting Guidance for Industry*. December 2015.

12. Hsu PH, Stoll RW. Causality assessment of adverse events in clinical trials: I. How good is the investigator drug causality assessment? *Drug Inf J*. 1993;27:377−385.

13. Hsu PH, Stoll RW. Causality assessment of adverse events in clinical trials: II. An algorithm for drug causality assessment. *Drug Inf J*. 1993;27:387−394.

14. *Clinical Studies Section of Labeling for Human Prescription Drug and Biological Products*; January 2006. https://www.fda.gov/downloads/Drugs/GuidanceComplianceRegulatoryInformation/Guidances/UCM075059.pdf.

15. Crowe BJ, Wang W, Nilsson ME. *Advances in Collating and Using Trial Data*. Future Science Ltd.; 2014.

16. Yao B, Zhu L, Jiang Q, Xia HA. Safety monitoring in clinical trials. *Pharmaceutics*. 2013;5:94−106. https://doi.org/10.3390/pharmaceutics5010094.

17. *U.S. Code of Federal Regulations 21CFR312.33: Investigational New Drug Application Annual Reports*; Revised as of April 1, 2004. http://www.accessdata.fda.gov/.

18. Current Challenges in Pharmacovigilance: Pragmatic Approaches. Report of CIOMS Working Group V. https://cioms.ch/wp-content/uploads/2017/01/Group5_Pharmacovigilance.pdf.

19. ICH E2A CLINICAL SAFETY DATA MANAGEMENT: DEFINITIONS AND STANDARDS FOR EXPEDITED REPORTING E2A. https://www.ich.org/fileadmin/Public_Web_Site/ICH_Products/Guidelines/Efficacy/E2A/Step4/E2A_Guideline.pdf.

20. U.S. FDA Guidance for Industry and Investigators. *Safety Reporting Requirements for INDs and BA/BE Studies; Drug Safety*; December 2012. https://www.fda.gov/downloads/Drugs/Guidances/UCM227351.pdf.

21. U.S. FDA Informed Consent Information Sheet Guidance for IRBs. *Clinical Investigators, and Sponsors; Draft Guidance*; July 2014. https://www.fda.gov/downloads/Regulatory Information/Guidances/UCM405006.pdf.

22. *U.S. FDA E6(R2) Good Clinical Practice; ICH Harmonised Guideline*; June 2015. https://www.fda.gov/downloads/Drugs/Guidances/UCM464506.pdf.

23. *EMA ICH Topic E2F Development Safety Update Report; Note for Guidance on Development Safety Update Report*; 2008. http://www.ema.europa.eu/docs/en_GB/document_library/Scientific_guideline/2009/09/WC500002827.pdf.

CHAPTER 4

Causality Assessment and Examples of Adverse Drug Reactions (Drug-Induced Liver Injury, Renal, Skin, and Major Adverse Cardiac Events)

CHARLES SCHUBERT, MD, MPH • MONALI DESAI, MD, MPH •
MEENAL PATWARDHAN, MD, MHSA • FABIO LIEVANO, MD •
SYED S. ISLAM, MBBS, MPH, MSPH, DR.PH • DEEPA H. CHAND, MD, MHSA •
HANS PETER BACHER, MD, PHD • SUZANNE PAULINE GREEN, MD, MBCHB, FFPM •
ARSALAN SHABBIR, MD, PHD • JAWED FAREED, PHD, DSC, FAHA •
VERGHESE MATHEW, MD, FACC, FSCAI

INTRODUCTION

In medicine, the benefits of a drug/vaccine are often clear. Examples include decreased occurrence of transmissible diseases due to vaccination, increased life expectancy after anticancer therapy, and prompt recovery without infectious complications following surgical procedures with the judicious use of antibiotics. However, understanding the side effects of a drug/vaccine poses many challenges. Side effects and their severity vary from individual to individual, and some may only occur after the medicine is taken for a long period or even well after stopping the medicine (delayed onset). It may be difficult to discern if a side effect is truly caused by a drug or is confounded by the patients' medical condition(s) and/or concomitant medications. Healthcare professionals (HCPs) often rely on published literature and drug prescribing information to help them (1) chose the right medicine for the right patient, (2) counsel their patients on the side effects of the drug, (3) prevent and monitor side effects, and (4) understand how to treat side effects when they occur. Although clinical trials are one of the most important sources for collecting safety information and characterizing the risks of a medicine, safety information can come from a variety of other sources. These sources include, but are not limited to, side effects observed in other drugs in the same or similar class of medicines, direct reporting of side effects by patients or HCPs (spontaneous reports), and published literature. Pharmaceutical companies and regulatory agencies gather information from these sources, analyze the data, and communicate the relevant information to healthcare providers and patients, with the intent of creating awareness of adverse effects and providing information aimed at reducing or helping to manage side effects when they occur.

An (Box 4.1) adverse drug reaction (ADR) is an adverse event (side effect) whose cause can be directly attributed to a drug and its physiologic properties. By definition, an ADR is a response to a drug that is noxious and unintended and occurs at doses normally used in humans for prophylaxis, diagnosis, or therapy for disease or for the modification of physiologic function.[1]

As a general rule, ADR determination is an art using the totality of evidence from various sources, with an assessment that is based on the strength of the evidence and incorporates appropriate medical judgment and common sense. There are a variety of systematic approaches to identify ADRs, including the following:

1. The Council for International Organizations of Medical Sciences (CIOMS) Working Group Criteria[2]
2. The Bradford-Hill Criteria[3]
3. The Naranjo algorithm[4]: This scale is often used when reporting suspected ADRs as case reports in the published literature. The algorithm contains 10

> **BOX 4.1**
> **Determination of Adverse Drug Reactions**
>
> - An adverse drug reaction (ADR) is a response to a drug that is noxious and unintended, and it occurs at doses normally used in humans for prophylaxis, diagnosis, or therapy for disease
> - ADR determination is an art using the totality of evidence coming from various sources and incorporating appropriate medical judgment
> - Several systematic approaches/frameworks (e.g., CIOMS Working Group Criteria) may be used to guide the assessment of an adverse reaction and its potential relationship to a pharmaceutical agent

items with 3 possible responses ("yes," "no," or "do not know or not done") and points are assigned for each response. The items are based on certain criteria such as temporal relationship, objective evidence (e.g., drug levels), other potential causes, and dechallenge/rechallenge observations. One can then conclude whether an adverse event is "definite," "possible," "probable," or "doubtful" based on the cumulative score. The simplicity of the score makes it a useful tool for everyday clinical practice when a known or unknown drug-related adverse event is suspected.

4. WHO-Uppsala Monitoring Centre causality assessment adverse event scoring system[5]: This scale ranks adverse events as "certain," "probable/likely," "possible," or "unlikely" based on criteria such as laboratory parameters and biological plausibility. It requires that all criteria for a certain causality term be met, which may lead to more ambiguity when assigning a probability.

The first two approaches are presented in more detail here.

THE CIOMS WORKING GROUP CRITERIA

The CIOMS Working Group Criteria can be very useful for helping to assess whether an event meets the definition of an ADR. There are several factors that need to be considered when determining an ADR. Although most reliable data come from well-designed placebo-controlled trials, a single well-documented case report can be sufficient to determine an ADR. Irrespective of the source, a well-documented positive dechallenge (i.e., the event resolves after stopping therapy) and positive rechallenge (i.e., the event reoccurs after restarting therapy) provides strong evidence of a drug-effect correlation. A positive dose-response (i.e., more frequent or severe side effects with increasing dose) observed in clinical trials is also strongly suggestive of an ADR. Furthermore, a side effect occurring in relatively close proximity to administration of a medicinal product, especially within minutes, hours, or days (temporal association), may provide evidence of a possible drug-effect relationship. Other factors may contribute to the overall understanding of a possible side effect and its relationship to a drug. Consistencies in patterns of presenting symptoms, frequencies, and time to onset within a population receiving the drug provide supportive evidence. Previous knowledge of the side effects observed in the same class of drugs (class effects), biological plausibility, and similar effects observed in animal models can contribute to the weight of evidence pointing to a drug-effect correlation.

THE BRADFORD-HILL CRITERIA

For more than 50 years, nine "aspects of association" provided by Sir Austin Bradford Hill have been used to evaluate hypothesized relationships between occupational/environmental exposures and disease outcomes.[6,7] Although safety science is dynamic and many statistical tools are available, the nine "aspects" (strength of association, consistency, specificity, temporality, biological gradient, plausibility, coherence, experiment, and analogy) continue to provide a solid foundation to consider a possible drug-event relationship.[7] These criteria are best used as a framework to think through, as opposed to a rigid checklist. The following diagram illustrates this framework,[3] which is described later in more detail.

1. Strength (effect size): A small association does not mean that there is not a causal effect; however, the larger the association, the more likely that it is caused by the medicine.

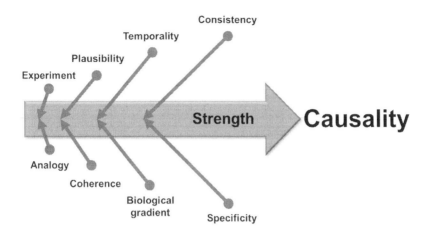

2. Consistency (reproducibility): Consistent findings observed by different persons in different places with different samples (e.g., clinical trials with the same medicine or class of medicine) strengthens the likelihood of an effect.
3. Specificity: Causation is likely if there is a very specific population at a specific site and disease with no other likely explanation. The more specific an association between a medicine and a side effect is, the bigger the probability of a causal relationship.
4. Temporality: The side effect has to occur after the medicine has been administered.
5. Biological gradient: Greater exposure of the medicine (higher dose) should generally lead to greater frequency or severity of side effects. However, in some cases, such as an anaphylactic reaction, the mere presence of the medicine (even in lower doses) can trigger the side effect.
6. Plausibility: The side effect can be explained based on current knowledge of the mechanism of action of the medicine.
7. Coherence: There is coherence between epidemiologic information about the medicine and/or laboratory findings following administration of the medicine and the side effect.
8. Experiment: Safety studies can be designed to experiment with administering the medicine and observing for side effects.

9. Analogy: The effect of similar factors may be considered.

When used in totality, these key aspects of association can assist in understanding and identifying an ADR.

The remainder of this chapter is dedicated to the examination of selected organ systems and the key issues involved in identifying ADRs in those areas.

LIVER: CAUSALITY ASSESSMENT IN DRUG-INDUCED LIVER INJURY IN ADULTS

This section provides a structured approach to perform a causality assessment in cases of suspected drug-induced liver injury (DILI). The background, etiology, and treatment of DILI are beyond the scope of this section and are well described in the literature and regulatory guidance documents.[8]

DILI is a rare ADR and can result in jaundice, liver failure, and, in extreme cases, death. DILI may be asymptomatic (Box 4.2) but often presents as an acute viral hepatitislike syndrome (fatigue, malaise, nausea, vomiting, and right upper quadrant pain), without symptoms that specifically point to a drug-induced cause, unless rash or other cutaneous manifestations reinforce the suspicion of drug toxicity.[9] The clinical spectrum of DILI can mimic almost every other liver disorder.[10] DILI is a diagnosis of exclusion, and thus careful history taking and a thorough workup for alternative causes are essential for its timely diagnosis. The varied clinical presentations, latency, laboratory profiles, histologic findings, and lack of sensitive and specific clinical tests to diagnose, predict, and monitor drug-induced injury to the liver are the major hurdles in the diagnosis of DILI.[11] Polypharmacy and the use of herbal and dietary supplements is common, which increases the complexity of determining the causal relationship for any one particular agent in a case of suspected DILI.

DILI is characterized as either intrinsic or idiosyncratic. Intrinsic DILI is caused by drugs that predictably cause liver injury when given in sufficiently high doses (e.g., acetaminophen). Idiosyncratic DILI (iDILI) is less common, affects only susceptible individuals, has a less consistent relationship to dose, and is more varied in its presentation.[11]

According to the US Drug-Induced Liver Injury Network (DILIN) registry, antibiotics account for 45.4% of all cases of iDILI, followed by herbal and dietary substances (16.1%), drugs acting on the central nervous system (9.8%), hypolipidemic agents (3.7%), and others (25.7%).[12] Of (Box 4.3) note, cancer patients are more likely to have multiple comorbidities and concomitant medications relative to other populations and are therefore at greater risk for hepatotoxicity.[13] This patient group is increasingly being treated with newer molecular targeted agents, many of which have been identified to be associated with liver injury. Hepatotoxicity occurs in one-third of patients treated with a protein kinase inhibitor, with fatal outcomes being reported for pazopanib, sunitinib, and regorafenib.[12] About 10% of patients treated with immune checkpoint inhibitors, notably ipilimumab, develop liver injury with high rates of recurrent liver injury upon rechallenge; 18.5% of patients treated with the epidermal growth factor receptor (EGFR) tyrosine kinase inhibitor (TKI) gefitinib experience hepatotoxicity, and cases have occurred for all EGFR TKIs.[14]

Characterizing the liver injury by latency, pattern of injury (e.g., R-value), mortality risk (Hy's law), and outcome (resolution vs. chronic) is critical in evaluating DILI.[12] The consensus criteria for DILI as published by Aithal et al.[10] are

1. alanine aminotransferase (ALT) $\geq 5\times$ upper limit of normal (ULN) or
2. alkaline phosphatase (ALP) $\geq 2\times$ULN or
3. ALT $\geq 3\times$ULN with simultaneous elevation in total bilirubin (TBL) $> 2\times$ULN

Considerations must be made for concomitant elevations in γ-glutamyltransferase levels and/or presence of bone issues resulting in increased ALP levels. Hy's law states that if hepatocellular injury causes jaundice in a patient during a phase 3 trial, then for every 10 patients with jaundice, 1 will develop acute liver failure (ALF).[12] Generally a pure hepatocellular injury sufficient to cause hyperbilirubinemia is an ominous indicator of the potential for a drug to cause serious liver injury. Hy's law is fulfilled when the following three criteria are all met:

1. Serum ALT or aspartate aminotransferase (AST) $> 3\times$ULN
2. Serum TBL $> 2\times$ULN, without initial findings of cholestasis (elevated serum ALP levels)
3. No other reason can be found to explain the combination of increased levels of aminotransferases and bilirubin, such as viral hepatitis A, B, C, or other preexisting or acute liver disease

In clinical trials, Temple's corollary refers to an imbalance in the frequency of ALT values greater than three times the ULN between the active treatment and control arm(s). Cases that fall within Temple's corollary are usually assessed carefully to determine whether the drug has a potential to cause liver injury.[12]

When there are elevations in the pretreatment serum ALT levels, change from baseline ALT values may provide a more quantitative and individualized measure of ALT elevation relative to using the ULN of ALT for the detection of liver injury and definition of stopping rules (Box 4.4). The ULN has been shown to vary across laboratories according to the methodology and the choice of reference population used to define the limits.[14]

There are three patterns of liver injury in DILI: hepatocellular, cholestatic, and mixed injury. The type of injury is determined by the R-value, which is calculated by (ALT/ULN) ÷ (ALP/ULN). The hepatocellular injury has an R-value >5; cholestatic injury, <2; and mixed injury pattern, between 2 and 5.[13] The pattern of injury helps define the possible differential diagnoses to be

excluded during the diagnostic workup of a suspected DILI case.[12]

DILI remains a diagnosis of exclusion based primarily on a detailed history and judicious use of blood tests, hepatobiliary imaging, and liver biopsy. The following steps outline the approach to evaluate a potential case of DILI.

Step 1: Take History and Perform a Physical Examination

The importance of a thorough history in suspected DILI cannot be overemphasized. An accurate history of medication exposure and the onset and course of liver biochemistry abnormalities is crucial. Herbal and dietary supplements, particularly those used for body building and weight loss, are an increasing cause of DILI. Usually, DILI events tend to occur within the first 6 months after starting a new medication, but some compounds have a propensity to cause DILI after a longer latency (e.g., nitrofurantoin, minocycline, and statins). The minimum data elements to collect in a diagnostic workup of suspected DILI are summarized in the following table.[15]

BOX 4.4
Diagnosis of DILI

Drug-induced liver injury is a diagnosis of exclusion based primarily on a detailed history and judicious use of blood tests, hepatobiliary imaging, and liver biopsy.

In patients with liver disease, the change in alanine aminotransferase (ALT) levels from baseline is a more reliable indicator of liver injury than using the upper limit of normal of ALT.

Minimum Elements of a Diagnostic Evaluation in the Workup of Suspected Drug-Induced Liver Injury

Gender	Important for competing disorders (e.g., primary biliary cirrhosis)
Age	Important for competing disorders (e.g., hepatitis E virus)
Race	Important for competing disorders (e.g., sarcoidosis, sickle cell–related biliary stone disease, oriental sclerosing cholangitis)
Indication for use of drugs	
Concomitant disease	Important disorders are sepsis, heart failure, hypotension episodes, recent general anesthesia, parenteral nutrition, and cancer
Rechallenge	Timing of rechallenge, if performed
History of other drug reactions	Certain cross-reactivities may exist (e.g., antiepileptic drugs)
History of other liver disorders	Chronic viral hepatitis, nonalcoholic fatty liver disease, hemochromatosis, alcoholic liver disease, primary sclerosing cholangitis, primary biliary cirrhosis, liver cancer
History of alcohol abuse	Past versus present, estimated grams per day; sporadic versus binge drinking versus regular (daily or weekly)
Exposure time "latency"	Start and stop dates or total number of days, weeks, or months taken
Symptoms and signs	Presence or absence, time of onset, type (fatigue, weakness, abdominal pain, nausea, dark urine, icterus, jaundice, pruritus, fever, rash)
Physical findings	Fever, rash, hepatomegaly, hepatic tenderness, signs of chronic liver disease
Medications and HDS	Complete list of medications or HDS with particular attention to those started in the *previous 6 months*
Laboratory results	Day of first abnormal liver biochemistry; liver biochemistry findings, eosinophil counts at presentation

Continued

Minimum Elements of a Diagnostic Evaluation in the Workup of Suspected Drug-Induced Liver Injury—cont'd	
Gender	Important for competing disorders (e.g., primary biliary cirrhosis)
Viral hepatitis	Anti-HAV IgM, HBsAg, anti-HBc IgM, anti-HCV serologic tests, HCV RNA (quantitative measurement)
Autoimmune	Antinuclear antibody and anti–smooth muscle antibody serologic tests, IgG level
Imaging	US ± Doppler, CT, or MRI ± MRCP
Histology, if available	Timing of biopsy in relation to enzyme level elevation and onset
Dechallenge data	Follow-up liver biochemistry tests
Clinical outcome	Resolution, transplant, death, and timing of each

CT, computed tomography; *HAV*, hepatitis A virus; *HCV*, hepatitis C virus; *HDS*, herbal and dietary supplements; *Ig*, immunoglobulin; *MRCP*, magnetic resonance cholangiopancreatography; *MRI*, magnetic resonance imaging; *US*, ultrasonography.
Modified from Agarwal VK, et al.

Step 2: Calculate the R-Value

The diagnostic approach to DILI can be tailored according to the pattern of liver injury at presentation. There are three patterns of liver injury in DILI: hepatocellular, cholestatic, and mixed injury. The type of injury is determined by the R-value, which is calculated by $(ALT/ULN) \div (ALP/ULN)$. The hepatocellular injury has an R-value >5; cholestatic injury, <2; and mixed injury pattern, between 2 and 5. The pattern of injury helps determine differential diagnoses and further evaluation; however, the R-value may change as DILI evolves.

Step 3: Exclude Differential Diagnoses

The differential diagnoses for acute hepatocellular injury includes acute viral hepatitis, autoimmune hepatitis, ischemic liver injury, acute Budd-Chiari syndrome, and Wilson disease. Acute cytomegalovirus, Epstein-Barr virus, and herpes simplex virus infection may present with elevations in liver biochemistry findings and systemic manifestations such as lymphadenopathy, rash, and atypical lymphocytosis. Autoimmune hepatitis should be considered in the differential diagnosis of all cases of DILI. Serum autoantibodies and immunoglobulin G levels should be routinely obtained. Low levels (e.g., titers less than 1:80 dilutions) of autoantibodies are not helpful in differential diagnosis because ~30% of adults, especially women, may have positive autoantibodies. Although rare, one should screen for Wilson disease with a serum ceruloplasmin level, particularly in patients younger than 40 years. The Budd-Chiari syndrome may sometimes mimic DILI and should be considered, especially if tender hepatomegaly and/or ascites are present.

Alternative findings in individuals with suspected cholestatic DILI are pancreaticobiliary in nature and can be either extrahepatic or intrahepatic. Extrahepatic findings, such as choledocholithiasis or malignancies (e.g., pancreatobiliary or lymphoma), can be readily identified with abdominal imaging tests, including ultrasonography, computed tomography, or magnetic resonance imaging. Intrahepatic findings mimicking DILI must be excluded based on careful history and physical examination (e.g., sepsis, total parenteral nutrition, or heart failure), serologic testing (antimitochondrial antibody for primary biliary cirrhosis), or imaging (infiltrating disorders or sclerosing cholangitis). The role of endoscopic retrograde cholangiography in individuals with suspected DILI is largely limited to instances where routine imaging is unable to exclude impacted bile duct stones or primary sclerosing cholangitis with certainty.

The role of liver biopsy in the evaluation of DILI is limited. Liver biopsy may be useful to differentiate autoimmune hepatitis from DILI, in cases of worsening liver functions despite withdrawal of the suspect agent, and in cases where the clinical need for the suspect medication is high and a rechallenge is considered. Biopsy may also be considered if peak ALT levels have not decreased by $>50\%$ at 60 or 180 days for cases of unresolved acute hepatocellular or cholestatic injury.

The diagnosis of DILI in patients with chronic liver disease (CLD) requires a high index of suspicion and exclusion of other, more common, causes of acute liver injury, including a flare-up of the underlying liver disease. The most common causes of CLD in the general US population are nonalcoholic fatty liver disease

(NAFLD), alcoholic liver disease, chronic hepatitis C virus (HCV) infection, and chronic hepatitis B virus (HBV) infection.[10] Some forms of CLD can present with an icteric flare (e.g., alcoholic hepatitis, autoimmune hepatitis, chronic HBV) that may be mistaken as DILI. Most patients with NAFLD and HCV do not experience icteric flares in disease activity, although liver biochemical indices may wax and wane from two- to fivefold ULN.[10]

Rechallenge is best avoided in DILI, especially if the initial liver injury was associated with significant aminotransferase level elevation (>5×ULN, Hy's law, jaundice). The only exception to this is in life-threatening situations where there is no suitable alternative.[10]

Step 4: Literature Review

A literature search should be performed for published reports of hepatotoxicity with the suspected product.

There are also various online resources that contain information on potentially hepatotoxic products, such as LiverTox (http://www.livertox.nih.gov).

Step 5: Clinical Judgement for Final Drug-Induced Liver Injury Diagnosis

Diagnostic algorithms based on clinical scoring systems (e.g., Roussel Uclaf Causality Assessment Method [RUCAM] and Maria and Victorino) are available and perform reasonably well in comparison to the "gold standard" of expert consensus opinion.[12] RUCAM is used by regulators, the industry, and clinicians; however, there are some ambiguities on how to score certain sections of RUCAM, as well as suboptimal retest reliability (reliability coefficient of 0.51, upper 95% confidence limit 0.76). A study showed that the concordance between RUCAM and the DILIN causality scoring system, which is based on expert consensus opinion, is modest ($r = 0.42$, $P < .05$).[12] Despite these limitations, RUCAM provides a framework for the diagnostic evaluation of suspected DILI. The RUCAM and Maria and Victorino causality worksheets can be found at https://livertox.nih.gov/rucam.html and https://livertox.nih.gov/MVcausality.html.

Step 6: Expert Consultation if Doubt Persists

If uncertainty persists following a thorough history and evaluation for alternative causes, clinicians should consider seeking expert consultation to ascertain the diagnosis of DILI and to attribute causality to a suspected agent.

Clinical Case Examples

Cholestatic hepatitis from amoxicillin-clavulanate (Modified from a case in the database of the DILIN).[16]

A 75-year-old man with a history of prostate cancer and regular alcohol use (two to three drinks daily) was given amoxicillin-clavulanate (500 mg/125 mg) for chronic maxillary sinusitis. Because of persistent symptoms, the antibiotic was continued for 31 days. When seen in follow-up 2 weeks later, he complained of jaundice and was admitted to the hospital for evaluation. He had symptoms of dark urine, weakness, and poor appetite. Blood test results showed a TBL level of 42.7 mg/dL, ALT level of 194 U/L, AST level of 107 U/L, and ALP level of 257 U/L. Tests for acute hepatitis A, B, C, and E were negative. Ultrasound of the abdomen showed no evidence of biliary obstruction or gallstones. During hospitalization, he developed profound anemia and thrombocytopenia, requiring blood and platelet transfusions, and was further treated with corticosteroids and cyclophosphamide. His serum bilirubin levels peaked at 48.8 mg/dL and remained elevated for several months while aminotransferase and ALP levels were only modestly elevated. The prothrombin time was elevated (international normalized ratio, 1.4−1.6) transiently and he developed mild confusion that was believed to be due to hepatic encephalopathy; he was treated with lactulose. During hospitalization, he developed renal failure and required dialysis. A liver biopsy was performed and findings were consistent with amoxicillin/clavulanate hepatotoxicity. He was hospitalized for 2 months and required another 2 months to recover fully. When seen 4 months after onset of jaundice, he was back to his usual state of health and had normal laboratory test results, including normal aminotransferase and ALP levels, normal serum bilirubin and creatinine levels, and normal hemoglobin and platelet counts.

Acetaminophen hepatotoxicity

Harmless at low doses, acetaminophen has direct hepatotoxic potential when taken as an overdose and can cause acute hepatocellular injury and death from ALF. Currently, acetaminophen is the major cause of ALF in the United States, Europe, and Australia. Even in therapeutic doses, acetaminophen can cause transient serum aminotransferase level elevations. Acetaminophen is largely converted to nontoxic glucuronate or sulfate conjugates and secreted in the urine. A minor amount of acetaminophen is metabolized via the cytochrome P450 system to intermediates that can be toxic, particularly *N*-acetyl-*p*-benzoquinone imine. Ordinarily, this intermediate is rapidly conjugated to reduced glutathione, detoxified, and secreted. If levels of glutathione are low or the pathway is overwhelmed by high doses of acetaminophen, the reactive intermediate accumulates and binds to intracellular macromolecules that can lead to cell injury, usually through apoptotic pathways.

Severe acute acetaminophen hepatotoxicity after an intentional overdose (Acute Liver Failure Study Group Patient #2281).[17]

A 27-year-old woman took an overdose of acetaminophen (30 tablets of 325 mg each) in a suicide attempt. The following day she was nauseated and vomited several times, but she waited another day before presenting to an emergency room, approximately 48 hours after the ingestion. She had no other significant medical problems and denied a history of liver disease, alcohol abuse, or risk factors for viral hepatitis. On presentation, she was oriented but drowsy. Her vital signs included pulse of 125 beats/min, blood pressure (BP) of 100/65 mmHg, respirations 25/min, and a temperature of 37°C. She had mild jaundice but had no rash or signs of CLD. The total serum bilirubin level was 4.4 mg/dL; ALT level, 3570 U/L; AST level, 7377 U/L; and ALP level, 109 U/L. A urine toxicology screen was positive for benzodiazepines and cocaine. Serum acetaminophen levels were 31 mcg/mL, and serum acetaminophen adducts were positive (23.8 nmol/mL). She was admitted to the intensive care unit and given intravenous *N*-acetylcysteine. Tests for hepatitis A, B, and C were negative, as were autoantibodies. Abdominal ultrasound showed no evidence of biliary obstruction. Over the next few days, she had mild hepatic encephalopathy. She was placed on a liver transplantation waiting list, but began to improve spontaneously, and was transferred to a psychiatric service after a week in the hospital. When finally discharged several weeks later, all liver test results had returned to normal.

RENAL

The hallmark manifestations of ADRs within the kidneys are commonly termed acute kidney injury (AKI). The risk of drug-induced AKI has been estimated at 3.2% based on published data.[18] While the risk increases with age, especially in those over 60 years old, other comorbidities and concomitant medications can increase this risk.[19,20] AKI typically presents clinically with elevation in serum creatinine levels; however, evaluating the precise mechanisms of kidney injury can be helpful in managing these events. By definition, AKI

> **BOX 4.5**
> **Acute Kidney Injury (AKI)**
>
> - Predisposing risk factors for acute kidney injury (AKI) should be evaluated in anticipation of potential injury.
> - AKI can result from prerenal, renal, or postrenal insults.
> - The most common causes of AKI are antimicrobials, nonsteroidal antiinflammatory drugs, angiotensin-converting enzyme inhibitors, angiotensin-receptor blockers, and diuretics.

implies reversibility; however, it can be classified anatomically as prerenal, renal, or postrenal to allow for a greater understanding of the pathophysiology.

Before discussing the mechanisms of injury, it is imperative to recognize certain underlying medical conditions that can predispose one to AKI. These (Box 4.5) include chronic kidney disease, diabetes mellitus, cardiovascular (CV) disease, CLD, and autoimmune disorders. Alternatively, pathologic states in which perfusion is decreased, such as heart failure or hepatic failure, may predispose a patient to AKI, as the patient is in a "low-flow" state. These conditions must be recognized early so as to potentially avoid compounding the injury with additional pharmacologic agents. Furthermore, polypharmacy with concomitant medications, such as CV medications (antihypertensive agents, lipid-lowering medications, antiarrhythmics, and diuretics), antineoplastic agents, antimicrobials, and radiographic contrast dyes, can contribute to the risk of AKI. Of note, the most frequently implicated medications include antimicrobials, nonsteroidal antiinflammatory drugs (NSAIDs), angiotensin-converting enzyme inhibitors, angiotensin receptor blockers, and diuretics.[18]

Prerenal injury implies a lack of perfusion to the kidneys. This can be related to pharmacologic agents whose mechanisms of actions include systemic vasodilation, such as calcium channel blockers, or hydralazine. Many agents can be adjusted by either dose reduction or a decrease in the frequency of dosing to prevent renal injury. Reinstatement of adequate perfusion pressure often results in reversal of renal impairment. However, with prolonged use, the damage may result in irreversible fibrosis. Prerenal injury most often manifests as proteinuria, elevation of creatinine levels, and/or oliguria.

Some pharmaceutical agents can cause direct renal injury to kidney components including the glomeruli, tubules, or interstitium. Examples of renal toxicity include tubulointerstitial nephritis (often induced by antimicrobial agents or NSAIDs), vascular injury from thrombotic microangiopathy (from agents such as tacrolimus, muromonab-CD3, or clopidogrel), and tubulopathies from antineoplastic agents (such as cyclophosphamide, ifosfamide, and cisplatin). Drug-induced systemic lupus erythematosus results from nephrotoxicity associated with an immune-mediated mechanism and can be associated with agents such as hydralazine, isoniazid, and procainamide. The clinical presentation can vary from an increase in serum creatinine levels to proteinuria, azotemia, etc.

Postrenal injury occurs in the setting of tubular obstruction. The most common pharmacologic form involves crystal-induced injury caused by drug precipitation, such as with acyclovir, methotrexate, or sulfonamides. Alternatively, medications such as topiramate can induce renal calculi formation, resulting in urinary

obstruction. Affected patients often present with microscopic and/or gross hematuria, dysuria, or severe flank pain.

An (Box 4.6) algorithm for the assessment of drug-induced renal injury is illustrated in Fig. 4.1. Clinical evaluation begins with obtaining a comprehensive history and performing a thorough physical examination. The practitioner should make note of aberrations in relevant vital signs, such as BP. Hypertension and hypotension may be associated with renal impairment. Similarly, obtaining information regarding concomitant medications and potential drug–drug interactions is imperative. With potential nephrotoxicity, physical examination findings may be lacking and the patient's symptoms are often constitutional and may include fatigue, malaise, nausea, etc.

Laboratory evaluation should include a comprehensive metabolic profile, including assessment of electrolytes, acid–base status, and renal function. Metabolic acidosis should alert the practitioner to possible pathologic conditions, including volume depletion, diabetic ketoacidosis, lactic acidosis, etc. A urinalysis can further help evaluate fluid status (specific gravity), diabetic control (glucosuria), and proximal tubular function (amino aciduria, glucosuria). Furthermore, the presence

> **BOX 4.6**
> **Evaluation of AKI**
>
> When evaluating acute kidney injury, the process should involve obtaining a thorough history and physical examination, laboratory evaluation, and critical evaluation of all available information.

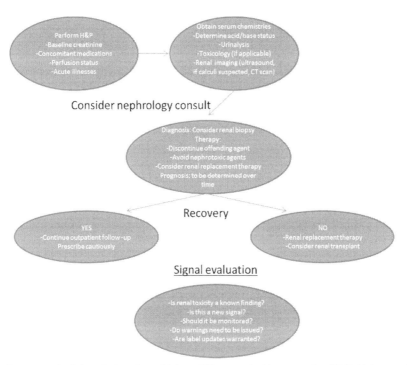

FIG. 4.1 Assessment of drug-induced renal injury. *CT*, computed tomography; *H&P*, history and physical examination.

of certain casts (white blood cell casts, red blood cell casts, muddy brown casts) can be indicative of specific pathologic conditions.

As is true of any pharmacologic agent, key associations that should be considered include time interval between exposure and onset of event, known safety profile of the product, the severity and frequency of the event, etc. However, unique to nephrotoxicity is the fact that renal physiology is ever-changing, and abnormalities can impair drug absorption, distribution, metabolism, and elimination based on circulating blood volume, intrinsic physiologic changes related to age, and uremic changes within other organs in situations of abnormal renal function. For example, uremia can result in gastrointestinal malabsorption, which can decrease the absorption of a medication, leading to a suboptimal effect. If significant systemic edema is present, the patient's volume of distribution may be compromised, as the altered increase in volume may result in lowered plasma drug concentrations. Drug metabolism may be compromised as well, especially because of the slowing of hydrolysis and various metabolic reactions. Similarly, if the renal function is reduced, there may be significantly less clearance of a medication, potentially resulting in toxicity.[21] With this in mind, many pharmacologic agents require dose adjustment based on renal impairment and the drug's biochemical properties.

When approaching the potential implication of a medicinal agent with nephrotoxicity, it is important to recognize that renal failure often is a very comprehensive term. For example, the Medical Dictionary for Regulatory Activities (MedDRA) coding for "acute renal failure" can include 44 different terms. When evaluating a case, it is imperative to evaluate specific preferred terms whenever available. This can provide great insight into the mechanism of action of a potential adverse event. Adverse events may be reported through clinical trials, postmarketing spontaneous reporting, literature, or solicited reports. During a clinical trial, it may be easier to obtain relevant clinical information regarding circumstances surrounding the event due to continued interactions between the physician and patients. Obtaining as much information as possible, such as comorbid conditions, concomitant medications, precipitating events, and temporal relationship to drug administration, can be tremendously helpful. In the postmarketing setting, obtaining additional information can prove to be a challenge, especially because of limited practitioner–patient interaction or if the findings were as a result of review of a literature source.

Nevertheless, obtaining as much information as possible is critical.

Often, correlation with known toxicologic properties of the agent can also provide useful information regarding biochemical properties inherit to absorption, distribution, metabolism, and elimination. While this information is provided in the product information guide in various forms, it should be reevaluated based on the frequency and severity of safety issues identified. Updates to information provided to practitioners should be made as necessary. Similarly, healthcare providers should reference these materials when prescribing agents to determine if modifications to the prescription regimen are warranted.

Clinical Case Examples

Acute kidney injury in chronic kidney disease

A 73-year-old woman was admitted to the hospital from the nursing home with acute bacterial pneumonia. She had been treated with oral ciprofloxacin for a urinary tract infection approximately 2 weeks prior. Owing to suspicion of infection due to methicillin-resistant *Staphylococcus aureus*, vancomycin therapy was initiated. Her other medical problems include diabetes mellitus and hypertension. Her initial vital signs included a temperature of 39°C, pulse of 130 beats/min, respirations 25/min, and BP of 90/56 mmHg. Her urine output over the subsequent 3 days decreased progressively to 50 mL/day. Her serum creatinine level was 1.6 mg/dL on admission, increased to 2.4 mg/dL 1 day after admission, and peaked at 4.5 mg/dL 3 days after admission. She was administered diuretics without an increase in urine output. After three doses of vancomycin administered every 12 hours, a serum trough level was noted to be 40 mg/L (desired level is 15–20 mg/L). Despite continued efforts to restore adequate perfusion, she was initiated on renal replacement therapy and ultimately renal function did not recover. She died of overwhelming sepsis approximately 1 week after admission.

Case assessment

This case highlights the need to adjust medication dosing for baseline renal deficits if the medication is excreted through the kidneys. In this scenario, the patient has a decrease in baseline renal function based on serum creatinine levels. A calculated estimated glomerular filtration rate can provide a creatinine clearance upon which the dosing should be adjusted based on prescribing guidelines.

Interstitial nephritis from nonsteroidal antiinflammatory drugs

A 27-year-old woman with a history of mild infrequent migraine headaches presents for treatment of a headache that has been present for the past 3 days. She states she has not been eating or drinking well owing to vomiting associated with the headaches. She has been taking oral 800 mg of ibuprofen every 8 hours for the past 2 days, without relief from her headaches. Her vital signs were stable and physical examination was significant for photophobia; otherwise, she was neurologically intact. Routine renal function panel was obtained, which revealed the following:

$Na^+ = 135$ mmol/L, $K^+ = 4.6$ mmol/L, $Cl = 99$ mmol/L, $HCO_3 = 25$ mmol/L, blood urea nitrogen $= 30$ mg/dL, and creatinine $= 2.6$ mg/dL.

She was provided intravenous hydration with 1 L of normal saline. A repeat serum creatinine 6 hours later was 2.5 mg/dL. Ibuprofen was discontinued. Four days later, her serum creatinine levels decreased to 1.4 mg/dL and was 0.7 mg/dL 1 week later with full recovery.

Case assessment

This case highlights interstitial nephritis, which is often associated with the use of NSAIDs. In someone with normal baseline renal function, full recovery from interstitial nephritis should occur with discontinuation of the offending agent. Antimicrobial agents are also known to cause interstitial nephritis, which also typically reverses upon discontinuation of the offending agent. If signs and symptoms of intravascular volume depletion are present, hydration can help with excretion of the medication and its metabolites, if applicable.

SKIN

Skin (Box 4.7) is one of the most common targets of ADRs. Adverse cutaneous drug eruptions are observed in 0.1%–1% of subjects in premarketing trials of drugs, including placebo groups.[22] Owing to underreporting in the postmarketing setting, the rate of events may be higher. In one series, on a general internal medicine service, adverse skin reactions occurred in 2.7% of 48,000 patients hospitalized over a 20-year period.[23] Maculopapular exanthemas (91.2%), urticaria (5.9%), and vasculitis (1.4%) were the reactions most commonly observed. Moreover, approximately 2% of dermatologic adverse cutaneous drug eruptions are considered serious according to the World Health Organization.[24] Stevens-Johnson syndrome/toxic epidermal necrolysis (SJS/TEN) and drug reaction with eosinophilia and systemic symptoms are examples of serious adverse

> **BOX 4.7**
> **Cutaneous ADRs**
>
> - Skin is one of the most common targets of adverse drug reaction
> - Case assessment utilizes an approach based on clinical characteristics, chronologic factors, and a literature search

cutaneous drug eruptions. Although not always possible, cutaneous drug eruptions should be categorized based on a drug having a high, medium, or low probability of being responsible for the observed reaction. Case assessment begins with a logical approach based on clinical characteristics, chronologic factors, and a literature search (see Table 4.1).

An (Box 4.8) initial approach to case assessment starts with an accurate description of skin lesions, their distribution and number, mucous membrane involvement, and associated signs and symptoms. A skin biopsy is frequently helpful (and for severe reactions mandatory) to validate the diagnosis and exclude nondrug causes of a cutaneous eruption. If a specific diagnosis is proposed, it is important to know if it has been made (or confirmed) by a dermatologist. Data gathered from the patient should include all medications taken (including prescription, over-the-counter [OTC] and alternative/complementary treatments), past medical history (PMH) (including previous cutaneous reactions observed), and a complete review of systems. Importantly, the dates of administration of any drugs taken by the patient should be noted. The time between drug initiation and onset of the eruption is a very important element in identifying the offending drug, as most immunologically mediated drug eruptions occur within 8–21 days after starting the offending drug. The major characteristics of the most commonly encountered cutaneous drug eruptions are listed in Table 4.2.

The following examples illustrate some typical drug-induced cutaneous reactions that are observed both in clinical practice and described in clinical study/spontaneous reports received by pharmaceutical professionals.

Clinical Case Examples
Case 1: Exanthematous drug eruption

A spontaneous report is received concerning a 42-year-old woman receiving a company's newly marketed asthma drug (Drug X) who presented to her primary care provider with an itchy rash that started 1 day ago. It started on her trunk and spread to her extremities. She was seen 1 week ago at an urgent care where she

TABLE 4.1
Case Assessment Strategy

Clinical characteristics	• Type of primary lesion (macule, papule, maculopapular, pustules, bullae, urticaria) • Number and distribution of lesions (extremities vs. thorax/abdomen; photodistributed vs. covered areas) • Mucous membrane involvement • Associated signs and symptoms (fever, pruritus, lymph node involvement, visceral involvement)
Chronologic factors	• Document all drug exposures (include over-the-counter, alternative and excipients) • Note time interval between date of drug administration and date of eruption • Response to dechallenge and rechallenge
Literature and database search	• FDA MedWatch, drug alert registry, EudraVigilance • Extrapolation based on drug class • Safety information collected by pharmaceutical companies • Medline for case reports, case series, etc.

BOX 4.8
Assessment of Cutaneous ADRs

- The initial assessment starts with a description of the skin lesions, their distribution, mucous membrane involvement, and associated signs and symptoms
- Data gathered should include concomitant medications (including prescription, over-the-counter drugs, and other supplements), medical history, and a complete review of systems
- Temporal relationship between the onset of the reaction and drug initiation is important and should be correlated with the typical time to onset of the suspected reaction

was diagnosed with acute pharyngitis and started on an antibiotic for empiric treatment. She has also been taking OTC medications to treat the acute pharyngitis.
- PMH: asthma
- Medications: see timeline below
- Allergies: no known drug allergies
- Family history: mother with history of basal cell carcinoma
- Social history: married, works as a realtor
- Health-related behaviors: no tobacco, alcohol, or drug use
- Review of systems: no fevers, sweats, chills

- Physical examination: diffuse maculopapular eruption involving trunk and extremities (see Image 1). No mucous membrane involvement. No fever and no lymphadenopathy. Laboratory results are all within normal limits.

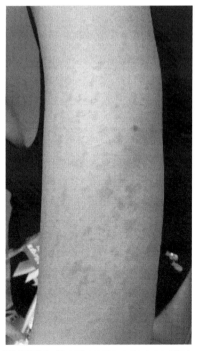

IMAGE 1 Exanthematous drug eruption.

TABLE 4.2
Major Characteristics of Common Cutaneous Drug Eruptions

Drug Eruption Types	Clinical Signs and Symptoms (s/s)	Time to Onset After Drug Ingestion	Common Culprit Drugs
Exanthematous	Dermatologic s/s: Polymorphic erythematous macules and minimally raised papules (morbilliform) symmetrically distributed on the trunk and proximal extremities. Systemic s/s: Low-grade fever, pruritus.	4–14 days	Amoxicillin, ampicillin, cephalosporins, sulfonamides, anticonvulsants, allopurinol
Urticaria (drug induced <10% of cases)	Transient erythematous and edematous papules/plaques that last less than 24 h.	Minutes to hours	Penicillins, cephalosporins, sulfonamides, tetracyclines, aspirin, NSAIDs, monoclonal antibodies, contrast media
Drug rash with eosinophilia and systemic symptoms	Dermatologic s/s: Commonly presents with a morbilliform eruption that may become more edematous; ± vesicles, tense bullae, erythroderma; commonly involves face, upper trunk, and extremities; facial edema is the hallmark finding. Systemic s/s: Fever, enlarged lymph nodes, and internal organ involvement (elevated eosinophils, elevated liver function tests (LFTs), interstitial nephritis, etc.).	2–6 weeks	Aromatic anticonvulsants, sulfonamides, lamotrigine, minocycline, abacavir
Acute generalized exanthematous pustulosis	Dermatologic s/s: Nonfollicular sterile pustules in a background of edematous erythema. Superficial desquamation in 1–2 weeks. Typically occurs on the face and intertriginous area and subsequently spreads to trunk and upper extremities. Systemic s/s: Fever, leukocytosis, neutrophilia, eosinophilia.	Hours to days	β-lactam antibiotics, Macrolides, calcium channel blockers, antimalarials
Fixed drug eruption	Sharply demarcated erythematous/violaceous, edematous plaques with dusky hue, ± blisters; occur at same site with each exposure. Lesions can be found anywhere on the body but favor the lips, face, hands, feet and genitalia; six or fewer lesions present, frequently one.	First exposure: 1–2 weeks, reexposure: <48 h, usually within 24 h	TMP/SMX, NSAIDs, tetracyclines, pseudoephedrine
Photosensitivity (phototoxic/photoallergic)	Phototoxic: appearance of an exaggerated sunburn ± blisters, followed by hyperpigmentation. Photoallergic: lesions are pruritic and resemble dermatitis or lichen planus.	Phototoxic: minutes to hours Photoallergy: 24–72 h	Phototoxic: tetracyclines, NSAIDs, fluoroquinolones, amiodarone, psoralen, Phenothiazines Photoallergic: thiazide diuretics, sulfonamides, sulfonylureas, phenothiazines

Continued

TABLE 4.2
Major Characteristics of Common Cutaneous Drug Eruptions—cont'd

Drug Eruption Types	Clinical Signs and Symptoms (s/s)	Time to Onset After Drug Ingestion	Common Culprit Drugs
Cutaneous small-vessel vasculitis (drug-induced ~10% of cases)	Nonblanchable purpuric papules primarily on the lower extremities.	7–21 days	PCN, NSAIDs, sulfonamides, cephalosporins, thiazides, furosemide, allopurinol, phenytoin, fluoroquinolones
EM minor and major (drug induced, less than 10% of cases)	Dermatologic s/s: EM (major when mucous membranes are involved) is characterized by typical concentric "target" lesions acrally distributed, with limited blisters (detachment rarely involves more than 2%–3% of the body surface area). Systemic s/s (present in EM major only): fever, asthenia, arthralgias.	3–14 days	Anticonvulsants, barbiturates, ciprofloxacin, NSAIDs, penicillins, phenothiazines, sulfonamides, and tetracyclines
Stevens-Johnson syndrome/toxic epidermal necrolysis	Begins with poorly demarcated dusky erythematous or purpuric macules, papules, patches, or plaques that subsequently result in frank epidermal detachment; often starts on trunk and spreads to face, proximal extremities, and neck; always presents with painful mucosal erosions/ulcerations; ± respiratory and gastrointestinal involvement.	7–21 days	Anticonvulsants (aromatic), sulfonamides, allopurinol, NSAIDs, lamotrigine

EM, erythema multiforme; *NSAIDs*, nonsteroidal antinflammatory drugs; *TMP/SMX*, trimethoprim/sulfamethoxazole.

Case 1: Medication timeline

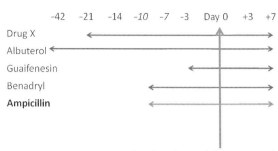

Day 0 = when rash first appeared

Case assessment

From the history and physical examination, the skin eruption is maculopapular, starting on the trunk and spreading to the extremities. There is no systemic involvement. This is consistent with an exanthematous drug eruption, which develops between 4 and 14 days after medication initiation. Examination of the drug timeline reveals that ampicillin has the highest likelihood of being the culprit medication. Indeed, ampicillin is one the most common causes of exanthematous drug eruptions.

Case 2: Fixed drug eruption

A case report is received from a phase I clinical trial of a company's targeted cancer therapy (Drug Y) in patients with advanced solid tumors. The report describes a 32-year-old woman with stage IV ovarian cancer. She received her first dose of Drug Y and the following day developed a "spot" on her arm. She has also recently taken several OTC herbs and complementary medications; however, these were discontinued before starting the trial.

- PMH: no major illnesses or hospitalizations
- Medications: see timeline below
- Allergies: no known drug allergies
- Family history: father with history of hypertension
- Social history: recently married, works as a sales representative
- Health-related behaviors: no tobacco, alcohol, or drug use
- Review of systems: no fevers, sweats, chills
- Physical examination: single erythematous plaque with blisters (see Image 2). No mucous membrane involvement. No fever and no lymphadenopathy. Laboratory results are all within normal limits.

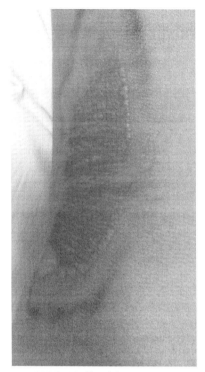

IMAGE 2   Fixed drug eruption.

Case 2: Medication timeline

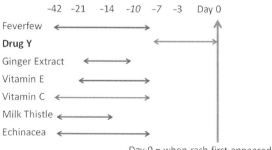

Day 0 = when rash first appeared

Case assessment

From the history and physical examination, the skin eruption is a solitary erythematous plaque with blisters. There is no systemic involvement. This is consistent with a fixed drug eruption, which typically develops in 7–14 days on first exposure and less than 24 hours on reexposure. History and examination of the drug timeline reveals that Drug Y has the highest likelihood of being the culprit medication.

Case 3: Stevens-Johnson syndrome/toxic epidermal necrolysis

- This case report is received from a phase II clinical trial for a company's drug (Drug Z) for psoriasis. The report describes a 54-year-old male who presented to the local emergency room with a painful, expanding, and "sloughing" rash. He began treatment in the clinical trial 6 weeks ago. During the interview, he experiences respiratory distress and is immediately intubated. His wife is called and told to bring his medications to the hospital.
- PMH: hypertension, recent urinary tract infection, knee arthritis
- Medications: see timeline below
- Allergies: none
- Family history: adopted, unknown
- Social history: social drinker, no drugs or smoking
- Review of systems: unknown
- Physical examination: erythematous erosions, mainly localized on the face, upper trunk, and hands, involving ~25% body surface area (see Image 3). Erosions on the mouth and nose. Pathologic examination reveals full-thickness necrosis throughout the specimen.

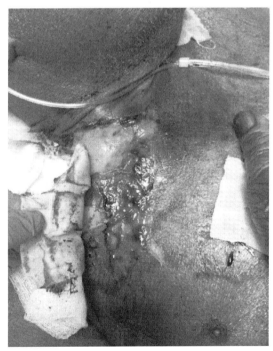

IMAGE 3 Stevens-Johnson syndrome/toxic epidermal necrolysis.

Case 3: Medication timeline

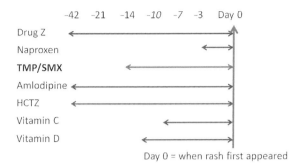

Day 0 = when rash first appeared

Case assessment

From the history and physical examination, the patient has erosions involving approximately 25% of his body surface area. He has mucous membrane involvement and likely respiratory epithelium involvement, given his respiratory distress. The pathologic examination shows full-thickness necrosis throughout. This is consistent with SJS/TEN, which develops between 7 and 21 days after drug initiation. Examination of the drug timeline reveals that trimethoprim/sulfamethoxazole (TMP/SMX) has the highest likelihood of being the culprit medication. Literature review further confirms that TMP/SMX is the frequent cause of SJS/TEN. Although much less likely, a causal association with the study drug cannot be completely excluded.

CARDIOVASCULAR

This section provides an overview of CV adverse events that may be associated with drug treatment.

Specific types of events to be discussed include major adverse CV events (MACE) and QT prolongation associated with serious arrhythmias. As with many other body systems, it can be challenging to determine whether a CV side effect of a specific drug is due to the drug or by individual risk factors (i.e., hypertension, diabetes, dyslipidemia, smoking, etc.) in the person experiencing the event. However, given the public health impact if it were attributable to drug treatment, a skilled evaluation of the data to ascertain causality is required.

Major Adverse Cardiovascular Events (Box 4.9)

MACE is an acronym that captures CV endpoints that can be measured in clinical trials and includes myocardial infarction (MI), stroke, and all-cause death or CV death. This composite endpoint was originally used to measure important clinical outcomes in CV research, whether they were associated with lifestyle, procedural, and/or drug treatment (i.e., for hypertension, dyslipidemia, diabetes, etc.) interventions. It can also be used to assess whether a drug can adversely cause the same outcomes. It is often the end result of the five etiopathologic mechanisms: atherosclerosis, thromboembolism, hemorrhagic events, events related to changes in electrophysiology of heart, and events related to cardiomyopathy or myocarditis. Given the insidious nature of some of these events, it is critical to assess the impact of the drug on intermediate endpoints, such as lipid changes, changes in BP, effect on renal function, impact on platelet function, and levels of atherosclerosis, to determine if there is a causal association between use of the drug and observation of MACE.

Following are few practical points/indicators that help determine a drug–CV event relationship.

Distribution and pathophysiology of MACE were well studied both in drug-treated and drug-untreated population. It is general knowledge that cardiac events associated with atherosclerosis occur mainly in older adults. A cardiac event occurring in a young healthy volunteer following administration of a drug without known risk factors would immediately point to a causal association between drug and CV event, whereas a cardiac event occurring in an older patient with several CV comorbidities would be much more difficult to point to a causal association.

Drugs Associated with MACE or Components of MACE (Box 4.10). One mechanism by which drugs may cause MACE is by increasing BP, especially in patients with other risk factors for MACE, such as diabetic patients or those with dyslipidemia. There is considerable evidence that certain non-CV drugs (such as vascular endothelial growth factor inhibitors, calcineurin inhibitors, erythropoiesis-stimulating agents, NSAIDs), as well as commonly used OTC drugs, herbal preparations, supplements, foods, and substances such as alcohol, can increase BP,[25] either directly or through their effect on renal function. Similarly, a new category of NSAIDs such as the cyclooxygenase inhibitors has been removed from the market or had its use restricted because of the increased risk of MACE via platelet aggregation or prostaglandin effects. Potential mechanism for MACE secondary to drug treatment varies by drugs, and examples are provided in the following table and further described in the following paragraphs.

BOX 4.9
Key Aspects of Major Adverse Cardiovascular Events (MACE)

- Captures measurable cardiovascular (CV) endpoints, including myocardial infarction, stroke, and all causes of CV death
- Used to assess whether a drug is causally associated with adverse outcomes or whether those outcomes are associated with lifestyle, age, or other factors

---

BOX 4.10
MACE Mechanism Example: Increased Blood Pressure

- Drugs may cause MACE by increasing blood pressure, especially in already-susceptible patients (e.g., diabetics)
- Common agents include calcineurin inhibitors, erythropoiesis-stimulating agents, and nonsteroidal antiinflammatory drugs
- Certain over-the-counter drugs, herbal preparations, supplements, foods, and alcohol can also increase blood pressure

Class of Drug or Drug Name	Mechanism of Action Predisposing to Major Adverse Cardiovascular Events	References
CNS stimulants, such as catecholamines and amphetamines, including dextroamphetamine and methylphenidate	Increase systolic and diastolic blood pressure and heart rate via sympathomimetic properties including stimulation of the β-receptors of the heart and α-receptors in vascular smooth muscle	Gottfridsson C et al.[25]
Nonsteroidal antiinflammatory drugs such as rofecoxib (Vioxx), which is a COX-2 inhibitor	Inhibition of prostaglandins, thromboxanes, prostacyclins, and platelet aggregation	O'Connor AD et al,[26] Angell PJ et al,[27] Agrawal PR et al,[28] Gunter BR et al.[29]
Chemotherapeutic agents	Damages to cardiomyocytes	Maria A et al.[30]
Opioids, anabolic steroids, particularly when used in high doses, and clenbuterol	Abnormal myocardial contractility, conduction, and possibly reperfusion	Yulia Khodneva et al.[31]
Thiazolidinediones, particularly rosiglitazone	Increased LDL-C, fluid retention	Erdmann et al.[32] Nissen et al.[33]

LDL-C, low-density lipoprotein cholesterol.

BOX 4.11
MACE Mechanism Example: QT Prolongation

- Drugs may cause MACE by prolonging the QT interval (normal corrected QT [QTc] interval is <430 ms for males and <450 ms for females)
- An increased QT interval can lead to cardiac arrhythmias, such as torsades de pointes, which can progress to ventricular fibrillation and sudden death
- Various antipsychotics, antiarrhythmics, antidepressants, and miscellaneous drugs (e.g., diphenhydramine, quinine, terfenadine) are known to alter or prolong the QTc interval
- However, other risk factors (drug–drug interactions, preexisting conditions, advancing age, etc.) must also be considered

QT Prolongation as an Indicator of Drug-Related Adverse Events Associated with MACE (Box 4.11)

Another mechanism by which a drug can cause MACE is through prolongation of the QT interval, which represents the duration of ventricular depolarization and subsequent repolarization, and is measured from the beginning of the QRS complex to the end of the T wave. The normal corrected QT (QTc) value for males and females are <430 and <450 ms, respectively. The QT interval represents electrical depolarization and

repolarization of the ventricles, and its prolongation is a measure of delayed ventricular repolarization. Excessive delay in cardiac repolarization, often described as a QTc of >500 ms,[34] can predispose the myocardium to cardiac arrhythmias such as torsades de pointes (TdP), other ventricular tachycardias that can progress to ventricular fibrillation, leading to sudden death. It is standard practice during drug development to study the impact of a drug on the QT interval through conducting a thorough QTc study.[35]

The following table provides data from a study that connected QTc prolongations to sudden cardiac death (SCD).[36] The classification of QT interval in men and women was derived separately.

QTc Times in Association with Clinical Outcome Risk

QTc Category (ms)	Men	Women
Normal	≤430	≤450
Borderline	431–450	451–470
Abnormal	>450	>470

As the QTc interval is dependent on heart rate, two commonly used formulas are used to provide a mathematical correction to achieve individual standards for each patient.[37,38]

Bazett formula: $QTcB = QT/\sqrt{RR}$
Friedericia formula: $QTcF = QT/\sqrt[3]{RR}$

Any abnormal increase in QT interval must be considered in the context of preexisting cardiac conduction disorders and concomitant medications. Therefore critical assessment of ADR, such as TDP events leading to SCD, must be assessed using not only the QT interval criteria but also the underlying causes of QT interval abnormality.

The results of the thorough QTc study are included in the package insert allowing clinicians to be aware of any inherent arrhythmogenic potential at therapeutic doses. However, in some situations, owing to drug–drug interactions, the patient is exposed to the toxic level of a drug (which at normal doses may not cause QTc prolongation), increasing the likelihood of ventricular arrhythmias (i.e., Seldane along with a popular antibiotic, erythromycin, or with a common antifungal drug, ketoconazole). Alternatively, if the drug is used in the setting of significant electrolyte imbalances such as hypokalemia or hypomagnesemia, or in patients with reduced ability to metabolize the drug (i.e., advanced liver disease), arrhythmogenic activity may also be potentiated.

The following table provides a list of important drugs known for altering/prolonging the QTc interval.

If the drug is used in the setting of significant risk factors, arrhythmogenic activity may also be potentiated. The following table summarizes the risk factors that may aggravate QTc prolongation.[34,39–42]

Unmodifiable Risk Factors	Potentially Modifiable Risk Factors
Female gender (present in 70% of cases)	Hypokalemia or severe hypomagnesemia
Increasing age	Absolute or relative bradycardia (including recent conversion from atrial fibrillation)
Genetic predisposition	Drug interactions
Congenital long QT syndrome	Use of >1 QT prolonging medicine
Family history of sudden death	Medicines that inhibit the metabolism of another QT prolonging medicine
History of previous drug-induced QT prolongation	Medicines that cause electrolyte abnormalities or may cause renal or hepatic dysfunction
	Starvation or obesity
Structural heart disease/left ventricular dysfunction	
Impaired elimination due to renal or hepatic disease	High drug concentrations due to overdose or rapid intravenous administration

Antipsychotics	Antiarrhythmics	Antidepressants	Others
• Chlorpromazine	• Quinidine	• Amitriptyline	• Diphenhydramine
• Haloperidol	• Procainamide	• Doxepin	• Astemizole
• Droperidol	• Disopyramide	• Imipramine	• Loratadine
• Quetiapine	• Flecainide	• Nortriptyline	• Terfenadine
• Olanzapine	•Encainide	• Desipramine	• Chloroquine
• Amisulpride	• Sotalol	• Mianserin	• Hydroxychloroquine
• Thioridazine	• Amiodarone	• Citalopram	• Quinine
		• Escitalopram	• Macrolides
		• Venlafaxine	• Erythromycin
		• Bupropion	
		• Moclobemide	

Clinical Case Example

Drug-induced MACE or components of MACE

A 50-year-old man working as a truck driver complained at his HCP visit about increasing joint pain in the right knee over the past 6 months, which hardly improved taking OTC ibuprofen up to 3×200 mg/day. Besides his body mass index of 28, he had no other significant medical conditions. Further diagnostic tests revealed a moderate case of arthritis in the right knee, not requiring joint replacement surgery. The patient was told to discontinue ibuprofen and start 25 mg rofecoxib tablets (Vioxx). A follow-up visit was scheduled 2 months later.

At the follow-up visit, the pain had somewhat improved, but the patient's arthritic symptoms persisted. Rofecoxib, 25 mg/day, was well tolerated. The HCP increased the dosage to 50 mg/day and arranged for a follow-up call. At the follow-up call, the patient reported no or little pain. The patient returned to the normal annual follow-up and received 1 year of rofecoxib, 50 mg/day.

About a year later the patient presented to the emergency room with severe, acute chest pain, problems breathing, and cold sweat on the forehead. He was diagnosed with an MI, underwent stent placement, and survived.

Background: During the development of rofecoxib, certain beneficial effects, mainly on the gastrointestinal tract, were noted and further study, the VIGOR (Vioxx Gastrointestinal Outcomes Research) Study, was conducted, which compared the efficacy and safety profiles of rofecoxib and naproxen in patients who required chronic pain therapy. The trial revealed a fourfold increased risk for MI (0.4% vs. 0.1%, RR 0.25) over the 12-month study time. The elevated risk began at the second month, and the risk of MI seems to be more pronounced when the drug was used with higher doses and for a longer time. Subsequently Vioxx was voluntarily removed from the market.

In conclusion, it is important to understand that rare events may be difficult to detect during routine clinical development programs, as the programs are too small to observe a rare event (see "Rule of Three" in Chapter 3). However, if major events, such as death or MIs, are observed in smaller studies, they need to be taken seriously, and all data during the clinical development (pharmacokinetics, pharmacodynamics) must be evaluated carefully to fully understand potentially early safety signals.

CONCLUSION

Determining the causal relationship of a drug to an observed adverse effect requires a careful examination of the totality of evidence from various sources. Although there are several frameworks/approaches designed to be used as guides to aid in this assessment, one must always utilize appropriate medical judgment. Regardless of the adverse event being observed, certain factors are critical in making this assessment, including (1) a thorough understanding of the patient's underlying disease state, medical history, concomitant medications and (2) the details regarding the drug(s) and its administration to the patient, such as known adverse effects, mechanism of action, time to onset relative to drug administration, and whether or not the reaction abates after stopping the drug (dechallenge) or recurs upon readministration (rechallenge). In addition, it is important to understand the key issues involved in identifying ADRs specific to particular organ systems, as demonstrated by the descriptions of such reactions in this chapter and elsewhere in the published literature. When the totality of this information is applied in a systematic fashion, the HCP can effectively assess such reactions and, ultimately, gain an understanding of the important risks posed by a pharmaceutical agent. Only by understanding these risks is it possible to take steps to address or mitigate these issues and ensure the safety and well-being of the patient.

REFERENCES

1. *Guideline on Good Pharmacovigilance Practices (GVP) — Annex I (Rev 4)*. October 2017.
2. *Guidelines for Preparing Core Clinical-Safety Information on Drugs Second Edition — Report of CIOMS Working Groups III and V*. 2nd ed. 1999.
3. Hill AB. The environment and disease: association or causation? *Proc R Soc Med*. 1965;58(5):295–300. PMC 1898525 PMID 14283879.
4. Naranjo CA, Busto U, Sellers EM, et al. A method for estimating the probability of adverse drug reactions. *Clin Pharmacol Ther*. 1981;30:239–245.
5. The Uppsala Monitoring Centre. The Use of the WHO-UMC System for Standardised Case Causality Assessment; 2018. Available: https://www.who-umc.org/media/164200/who-umc-causality-assessment_new-logo.pdf (accessed Jan 24, 2018).
6. Fedak KM, et al. Applying the Bradford Hill criteria in the 21st century: how data integration has changed causal inference in molecular epidemiology. *Emerg Themes Epidemiol*; 2015. https://www.ncbi.nlm.nih.gov/pmc/articles/PMC4589117/.

7. Kundi M, et al. Causality and the interpretation of epidemiologic evidence. *Environ Health Perspect*; July 2006. https://www.ncbi.nlm.nih.gov/pmc/articles/PMC1513293/.

8. *FDA Guidance for Industry Drug-Induced Liver Injury: Premarketing Clinical Evaluation*. July 2009.

9. Kullak-Ublick GA, Andrade RJ, Merz M, et al. Drug induced liver injury: recent advances in diagnosis and risk assessment. *Gut*. 2017;66:1154–1164.

10. Aithal GP, Watkins PB, Andrade RJ, et al. Case definition and phenotype standardization in drug-induced liver injury. *Clin Pharmacol Ther*. 2011;89:806–815.

11. Rasi G. *Letter of Support for Drug-Induced Liver Injury (DILI) Biomarker*. September 30, 2016. http://www.ema.europa.eu/docs/en_GB/document_library/Other/2016/09/WC500213479.pdf.

12. Chalasani, et al. ACG clinical guideline: the diagnosis and management of idiosyncratic drug-induced liver injury. *Am J Gastroenterol*. 2014;109:950–966. https://doi.org/10.1038/ajg.2014.131.

13. Alempijevic T, et al. Drug-induced liver injury: do we know everything? *World J Hepatol*. 2017;9:491–502. https://doi.org/10.4254/wjh.v9.i10.491.

14. Kullak-Ublick G, et al. Liver safety assessment in special populations (hepatitis B, C, and oncology trials). *Drug Saf*. 2014;37(suppl 1):S57–S62. https://doi.org/10.1007/s40264-014-0186-3.

15. Agarwal VK, McHutchison JG, Hoofnagle JH. Important elements for the diagnosis of drug-induced liver injury. *Clin Gastroenterol Hepatol*. 2010;8:463–470.

16. https://livertox.nlm.nih.gov//AmoxicillinClavulanate.htm.

17. https://livertox.nlm.nih.gov//Acetaminophen.htm.

18. Pierson-Marchandise M, Gras V, Moragny J, et al. French National Network of Pharmacovigilance Centres. The drugs that mostly frequently induce acute kidney injury: a case – noncase study of a pharmacovigilance database. *Br J Clin Pharmacol*. 2017;83(6):1341–1349. https://doi.org/10.1111/bcp.13216. Epub 2017 Mar 14.

19. Feest TG, Round A, Hamad S. Incidence of severe acute renal failure in adults: results of a community based study. *BMJ*. 1993;306:481–483.

20. Groeneveld AB, Tran DD, van der Meulen J, Nauta JJ, Thijs LG. Acute renal failure in the medical intensive care unit: predisposing, complicating factors and outcome. *Nephron*. 1991;59(4):602–610.

21. Aronoff G, Berns J, Brier M, et al. *Drug Prescribing in Renal Failure*. 4th ed. 1999:1–12.

22. Arndt KA, Jick H. Rates of cutaneous reactions to drugs. A report from the Boston Collaborative Drug Surveillance Program. *JAMA*. 1976;235(9):918–923.

23. Hunziker T, et al. Comprehensive hospital drug monitoring (CHDM): adverse skin reactions, a 20-year survey. *Allergy*. 1997;52(4):388–393.

24. McKenna JK, Leiferman KM. Dermatologic drug reactions. *Immunol Allergy Clin North Am*. 2004;24(3):399–423, vi.

25. Gottfridsson C, et al. Drug-induced blood pressure increase–recommendations for assessment in clinical and non-clinical studies. *Expert Opin Drug Saf*. 2017;16(2):215–225. https://doi.org/10.1080/14740338.2017.

26. O'Connor AD, et al. Cerebrovascular and cardiovascular complications of alcohol and sympathomimetic drug abuse. *Med Clin North Am*. 2005;89(6):1343–1358.

27. Angell PJ, et al. Performance enhancing drug abuse and cardiovascular risk in athletes: implications for the clinician. *Br J Sports Med*. 2012;46(Suppl 1):i78–84.

28. Agrawal PR, et al. Current strategies in the evaluation and management of cocaine-induced chest pain. *Cardiol Rev*. 2015.

29. Gunter BR, et al. Non-steroidal anti-inflammatory drug-induced cardiovascular adverse events: a meta-analysis. *J Clin Pharm Ther*. 2017;42:27–38.

30. Mitry Maria A, Edwards John G. Doxorubicin induced heart failure: phenotype and molecular mechanisms. *IJC Heart & Vasculature*. 2016;10:17–24.

31. Khodneva Yulia, et al. Prescription opioid use and risk of coronary heart disease, stroke, and cardiovascular death among adults from a prospective cohort (REGARDS study). *Pain Medicine*. 2016;17:444–455.

32. Erdmann E, Charbonnel B, Wilcox R. Thiazolidinediones and cardiovascular risk — a question of balance current cardiology reviews. 2009;5:155–165.

33. Nissen E, Wolski K. Effect of rosiglitazone on the risk of myocardial infarction and death from cardiovascular causes. *N Engl J Med*. 2007;356:2457–2471.

34. Heist EK, Ruskin JN. Drug-induced proarrythmia and use of QTc prolonging agents: clues for clinicians. *Heart Rhythm*. 2005;2(11):S1–S8.

35. FDA Guidance for Industry. *E14 Clinical Evaluation of QT/QTc Interval Prolongation and Proarrhythmic Potential for Non-antiarrhythmic Drugs*. 2005.

36. Medscape. *QTc Prolongation and Risk of Sudden Cardiac Death: Is the Debate Over?* 2006. https://www.medscape.com/viewarticle/522879.

37. Bazett HC. An analysis of the time-relations of electrocardiograms. *Heart*. 1920;7:353–370.

38. Fridericia LS. The duration of systole in the electrocardiogram of normal subjects and of patients with heart disease. *Acta Medica Scand*. 1920;53:469–486.

39. Viskin S. Long QT syndromes and torsades de pointes. *Lancet*. 1999;354:1625–1633.

40. Al Khatib SM, et al. What clinicians should know about the QT interval. *JAMA*. 2003;289(16):2120–2127.

41. Morissette P, et al. Drug induced long QT syndrome and torsade de pointes. *Can J Cardiol*. 2005;21(10):857–864.

42. Fraley MA, et al. Obesity and the electrocardiogram. *Obes Rev*. 2005;6:275–281.

CHAPTER 5

Role of Epidemiology in the Biopharmaceutical Industry

DENISE M. OLESKE, PHD • SYED S. ISLAM, MBBS, MPH, MSPH, DR.PH

INTRODUCTION

Epidemiology is defined as the study of the distribution and determinants of diseases, disabilities, and injuries in the human population. Epidemiology aims to characterize the natural history of disease, the burden of disease upon human population, and the public health impact of diseases as well as determine the potential causes of a disease and factors that influence its progression. Using the results of epidemiologic studies, effective population-based public health measures are planned for the distribution of resources for healthcare and prevention of diseases and their complications. Utilizing the epidemiologic methodology a subspecialty called "pharmacoepidemiology" was developed. It is defined as the science of studying the use and effects (harmful or beneficial) of drugs and devices in the human population (Box 5.1).

Harmful effects of drugs have been known for a long time. In 1937, more than 100 people died from renal failure as a result of taking a drug called Elixir of sulfanilamide to treat a variety of conditions from gonorrhea to sore throat. In response, the 1938 Food, Drug, and Cosmetic act was passed, requiring preclinical toxicity testing for all drugs.[1] In the winter of 1961, the infamous "thalidomide disaster" was publicized. Epidemiologic studies confirmed the cause of this birth defect to be in utero exposure to thalidomide. In the United Kingdom, this resulted in the creation of the Committee on Safety of Medicines in 1968. In other circumstances, we might wait for a long period to detect an adverse effect. For example, subacute myelo-optic neuropathy was

found to be caused by clioquinol, a drug marketed in the early 1930s, but its severe neurologic effect was not detected until the 1970s.[2] Similarly, clear cell adenocarcinoma of the vagina after in utero exposure to diethylstilbestrol was not detected until two decades passed after the drug was approved for market distribution.[3]

The role of pharmacoepidemiology is rapidly evolving. This is driven by the need to increase the focus of what is best not only for the individual patient but also for optimizing the safety and efficacy of treatments for populations at need and the overall public health impact. New data sources, methodologies, technologies, and regulations requiring real-world data are drivers in this evolution.

Pharmaceutical product development follows systematic steps for the identification of compounds that affect the pathophysiology of a disease and lead to curing the disease or altering the disease symptomatology and prognosis. These steps include molecular studies of the compound's ability to target the biological site or pathway of the disease of interest, investigation of potential adverse reproductive effects and toxicology in animal studies, first-in-human testing to determine pharmacokinetics in healthy volunteers, randomized clinical trials to determine efficacy, and finally, continued assessment of effectiveness in larger populations through observational studies. Most pharmaceutical products are approved after studying a limited number of subjects; therefore, safety and efficacy may not be possible to be fully examined. Specific safety and effectiveness issues may emerge after market authorization, which require characterization and evaluation in a population-based context (Box 5.2).

The specific activities conducted by epidemiologists throughout the drug/biopharmaceutical life cycle are summarized in Table 5.1. These activities and the resultant data compiled fill gaps in the evidence characterizing the indication, its use, and benefit to patients relative to

> **BOX 5.1**
> **Definition**
>
> • Pharmacoepidemiology is the science of studying the use and effects (harmful or beneficial) of drugs and devices in the human population.

the risk of use of the new drug/biopharmaceutical product. These data not only aid in decision-making but also contribute to updating the epidemiology and drug utilization for regulatory documents, risk management plan (RMP) updates, updated benefit-risk assessment when needed, periodic benefit-risk evaluation Reports (PBRER) required by the EMA, and Periodic Adverse Drug Event Reports (PADER) submitted to the FDA.

EPIDEMIOLOGY ACROSS THE DRUG LIFE CYCLE
Disease/Target Indication Selection

It is essential to understand disease epidemiology before any drug development is undertaken. This early assessment includes the components discussed in the following sections.

Disease definition and validation

Diseases targeted for treatment with a drug are often not homogeneous with regard to etiology, pathology, response to treatment, and/or prognosis. Therefore when defining a disease, one must consider potential etiopathologic and diagnostic heterogeneity and develop clear-cut parameters to capture a homogeneous group of patients with the disease. No matter how a disease is defined, an agreed-upon validation method is needed to compare the criteria for determining a case against a gold standard (which is not always available and is derived from clinical experience or coding algorithms).

Incidence, prevalence, and mortality

Describing the target population requires understanding the distribution of the disease and its severity in populations and subpopulations. The epidemiologic measures used to describe the frequency of a disease or health problem in a population are the incidence, prevalence, and mortality rates. Knowledge of the incidence, prevalence, and mortality rates by person (age, gender, and other characteristics), place (country, urban area), and time (month, year, decade) is critical. Epidemiologic measures are used for identifying potential geographic areas for study sites, assessing the burden of disease in a population, determining sample sizes for clinical trials and observational studies, and putting any potential safety signals into a population-based context. Incidence and prevalence measures are also classified as "morbidity measures," meaning the frequency of occurrence of disease, injury, and disability in a specific population.

Incidence is defined as the number of *new cases* of a disease that occur during a specified *period* in previously disease-free ("at-risk") individuals. The determination of an incidence rate requires data on (Box 5.3) history to determine if the target population was free of the disease of interest during some previous period (i.e., meaning the disease event is a new occurrence).

An incidence rate may be numerically expressed in three ways: (1) incidence proportion, the number of new cases of disease during a specified time interval divided by the total number of disease-free population at the start of the time interval; (2) cumulative incidence, the number of new cases divided by the total number of disease-free population multiplied by the average duration of follow-up; and (3) incidence density, the number of new cases of disease among disease-free population multiplied by each person's actual follow-up time (each person's time of observation before the occurrence of the disease event or death or end of study without disease event is calculated and summed up to derive the denominator). The generalized formulae for incidence rates are

$$\text{Incidence proportion (or percent)} = \frac{\text{Number of new events during a specified time period}}{\text{Number of persons at the start of that period}} \times 100$$

$$\text{Cumulative incidence} = \frac{\text{Number of new cases during a specified time period}}{\text{Number of persons at risk of developing the disease at the beginning of follow} - \text{up} \times \text{Average duration of follow} - \text{up period}} \times 100$$

$$\text{Incidence density} = \frac{\text{Number of new cases during a specified time period}}{\text{Person} - \text{time at risk (disease} - \text{free time of entire cohort) during specified time period}} \times 100$$

TABLE 5.1
Role of Epidemiology Throughout the Drug/Biopharmaceutical Life Cycle

Pre-Clinical phase: Information needed at the time of compound selection target disease	Clinical testing phase: Phase 1, Phase 2. Phase 3 trials	Market authorization and post marketing phase
1. Disease definition 2. Incidence, prevalence, mortality 3. Trends and projection of disease incidence, prevalence and mortality 4. Natural history of disease 5. Disease risk factors 6. Genotype phenotype distribution 7. Recurrence and progression pattern 8. Co-morbidities 9. Current available treatment 10. Unmet medical need (population sub-population level)	1. Define target population for effective treatment. 2. Determine if the clinical trial population is representative of target population. 3. Assess location and the size of the trial population based on distribution in the real world data. 4. Background rates of specific safety events, comorbidities, and treatment patterns in populations similar to the clinical trial population to understand the safety context.	During NDA: 1. Submission dossier 2. Risk Evaluation and Mitigation Strategy (REMS) 3. Risk Management Plan (RMP) Post-Marketing monitoring: 1. Drug use in population subgroups 2. Post marketing observational studies to establish background rates, monitoring laboratory values, drug-drug interactions. 3. Formal Hypothesis testing studies to address specific safety and effectiveness questions.
• real world data • special cohort analysis • other epidemiologic studies	• predictive analytics and modeling • cohort building using real world data • estimate background rates • Cohort analysis and other epidemiologic studies	
		• Using claims/EMR/registry data, estimate background rates • develop algorithm for safety, effectiveness and test hypothesis using epidemiologic study design

EMR, electronic medical record; *NDA*, new drug application.

These fractions can be multiplied by some factor of 100 to 100,000 to express incidence as a rate depending on convention (multiplied by 100,000 used in vital statistics or multiplied by 100 or 1000 in most pharmacoepidemiology studies). When the incidence rate is not stratified by age, gender, or other characteristics, it is called a *crude incidence rate*. When we compare the incidence rate of one population with the other, the crude incidence rate may give us a flawed comparison if the rate varies by age and gender. In such situations, we sometimes calculate standardized incidence rates.

The cumulative incidence or incidence proportion is also considered as the measure of "risk" or probability of an event. Both incidence rate and risk are key epidemiologic measures used in safety assessment regardless of the stage in the drug life cycle (Box 5.4), as they help us in the estimation of disease burden as well as risk.

Prevalence represents a "snapshot" or the number of both new and existing cases. Prevalence is a function of both the incidence of disease and its expected duration. So when a disease has a high incidence and long duration in a population (e.g., asthma), the prevalence can be expected to be high. When expressed relative to a population at risk for the event, the result is termed the prevalence rate or prevalence percent. This is calculated as follows:

The prevalence rate may be expressed as either a *point prevalence*, the number of disease cases in a population at a single point in time, or a *period prevalence* (over a period of e.g., 5 years). Prevalence rate is a common epidemiologic measure to determine the "burden of disease" for orphan drug designations, accelerated assessments, and new drug filings. Prevalence measurement is very useful for chronic diseases that are not rapidly fatal and is often used in the planning of health resources.

Mortality rate refers to the number of deaths in a population. The death certificate is the source of information for cause of death from any diseases or circumstances (e.g., trauma). Demographic information such as age, sex, and residence of decedent are also on the death certificate. In the computation of mortality rate, deaths comprise the events in the numerator. The denominator is the population at risk and those data are obtained from the census of the population in the same geographic area and same time period as when the death events of interest occurred. The fraction resulting from the number of deaths divided by the population at risk is then multiplied by 100,000 to form the mortality rate and expressed as follows:

$$\text{Mortality Rate} = \frac{\text{Number of deaths in a time period}}{\text{Number at risk for the death event in the same time period}} \times 100,000$$

The mortality rate is another measure of risk and the most common measure of disease frequency and severity used in epidemiology. This is due to the registration of all deaths on death certificates as a global public health practice.

All these descriptive epidemiologic rates are called crude rates. They are overall rates averaged over many subgroups. The assessment of incidence, prevalence, or mortality rates in population subgroups (e.g., for

$$\text{Prevalence Rate} = \frac{\text{Number of new and existing cases at a point (or period) in time}}{\text{Population at risk at the same point (or period) in time}} \times 100$$

ages 18−49, 50−64, and 65+ years; males; females) is termed specific rates. However, it is important to determine if there are sufficient data to examine variations in the rates by subpopulations, at the very minimum by age group, and sex. When comparing rates over time or across geographic areas where the demographic composition of the populations may differ, the specific rates should be weighted by the numbers or

---

BOX 5.5
Standardized Rates and Why it Is Important

- Crude or averaged over subgroup rates should not be compared between groups if there are differences in the distribution of certain characteristics that influence the rate. In such situations a standardized rate should be calculated accounting for those characteristics.

BOX 5.6
Confidence Interval

- A 95% CI is the boundaries on a point estimate of an epidemiologic measure, such as a mortality rate. It means if the study is repeated many times, the true point estimate of the measure will be within the specified upper and lower values 95% of the time. Only 5% of the time the true point estimate measure may be outside that range. The wider the confidence interval, the less certainty there is about the true value of the point estimate.

---

proportions of persons in the corresponding groups in some reference population in a similar time period (e.g., population of the world) by age, sex, or other variables. This weighting is referred to as an adjusted rate or standardized rate (Box 5.5).

A ratio is another epidemiologic measure critical to understand risk. A ratio of incidence or mortality rates (incidence density ratio) or relative risk (risk ratio) can be used to assess if the likelihood of occurrence of an event is higher for one drug than another drug. A ratio greater than 1 may suggest association of a drug and an event. Further assessment of the significance of the ratio would require the examination of the confidence interval (CI) of (Box 5.6) the point estimate of that ratio and the statistical significance of the ratio. A ratio of twofold or greater in a well-designed epidemiologic study with adequate confounding control typically signals potential association that requires detailed assessment for causality. Examples of safety signals

generated through the use of epidemiologic ratio measures are found in Table 5.2.

In each of the studies cited, the rate ratio exceeded 2 and would warrant a closer look to assess the possibility of causality of an exposure–outcome relationship. The initial step in assessing evidence for causality in an epidemiologic study is to determine if the study design supports the computation of a *measure of risk* (Box 5.7) of the event of interest (see Table 5.2). The Bradford Hill criteria are then used to determine if there is evidence that the measure of association is supported by other criteria and results.[4] The Bradford Hill criteria also aid in assessing causality of an exposure–outcome relationship in pharmacovigilance (PV) practice of assessing spontaneous and solicited reports of adverse events.

TABLE 5.2
Examples of Safety Signals Generated and Assessed With Databases Using Pharmacoepidemiologic Methods

Author, Year	Database	Drug and Comparator	Event Assessed	RR: Users of Specific Drug vs. Comparator (95% CI)
Garcia Rodriguez et al., 1996	GPRD	Amoxicillin plus clavulanic acid vs. amoxicillin alone	Hepatic injury	RR 6.3 (3.2–12.7)
Jick et al., 1998	GPRD	Appetite suppressant users vs. nonusers	Cardiac valve regurgitation	~ infinity 35/10000 users vs. 0/10000 non-users
Straus et al., 2004	Integrated primary care information project	Antipsychotic users vs. nonusers	Sudden cardiac death	RR 3.3(1.8–6.2)
Ray et al., 2004	Tennessee Medicaid data	Tricyclic antidepressant user vs. nonusers	Sudden cardiac death	RR 2.5 (1.04–6.1)

GPRD, General Practice Research Database; RR, relative risk; CI, Confidence Interval.
Adapted from Stricker B, Psaty B. Detection, verification, and quantification of adverse drug reactions. *BMJ*. July 3, 2004;323:46.

> **BOX 5.7**
> **Various Rates and Ratios Used in Epidemiology**
>
> • Epidemiologic measures of risk of an event include incidence rate, relative risk, risk ratio, and mortality rate.

> **BOX 5.8**
> **Confounding–What it Is**
>
> • Confounding is a key concept in understanding the true association between a risk factor and a disease/event outcome. A factor is a confounder if it is causally independently related to a disease/event and correlated with the exposure of interest and is not in the causal pathway between exposure of interest and disease/event outcome.

These criteria and their application in PV are discussed in detail in Chapter 4.

Natural history of a disease

Natural history of a disease involves an understanding of the probabilities of the disease progressing as well as the factors (prognostic factors) that influence the transition probabilities. Epidemiologic measures used in assessing the natural history include survival rate and recurrence rate. Knowledge of the natural history aids assess gaps in unmet need for treatment and frames the understanding if a potential safety event is due to expected disease progression (clinically or nonclinically detectable) or that may be prevented or controlled by drug therapy or other prevention measures. The rate of disease progression may vary by age of onset of the disease, the stage at which the disease is diagnosed, behavioral factors (e.g., smoking, alcohol consumption), comorbidities, or other factors. The natural history of the disease may also identify population subgroups progressing and responding to treatment in different ways (e.g., by genotype).

Risk factors

Most diseases/events are results of multifactorial etiology, with more than one true risk factor associated with it. When assessing the risk of disease due to a specific factor, it is desirable to assess its independent association with the risk, while accounting for contribution of other causal factors. For example, smoking is an independent risk factor for myocardial infarction (MI), meaning the risk of MI is higher in smokers than nonsmokers even in the population not using drug A. When assessing the relationship of drug A with the subsequent development of MI and when it is known that the population of drug A users have a higher proportion of smokers than its comparator, then smoking must be considered while assessing the association between drug A and MI. Smoking needs to be controlled for as

it is a confounder in the association between drug A and outcome of MI (Box 5.8). Therefore if a risk factor is causally related to a disease/event (based on biological knowledge and statistical association) as well as correlated with exposure (risk factor of main interest) and is not in the causal pathway between exposure to disease/event, it is called a confounder that distorts the true association between exposure of interest and disease/event outcome. These confounders may be environmental factors (occupational exposure, air pollution, etc.), behavioral factors (smoking, alcohol use, diet), or disease-related factors (hypertension giving rise to chronic kidney disease) and are important in determining the risk independent of exposure to the drug. Disease-related risk factors may also be comorbidities, which are typically referred to as chronic conditions when appearing at the same time as the disease of interest. The presence or absence of risk factors influences the magnitude of event rates that may be seen in a target population.

Current state of disease management (treatment patterns)

In order to develop new drugs that will be superior to current standards of care or to treat diseases for which there are currently no known treatments to alter the disease course, it is essential to know the diagnostic and treatment pattern in the real-world clinical practice. Treatment patterns may also reveal how the patient is managed in the healthcare system. This is especially important for conditions for which there are no known treatments to impact the disease course, such as many neurodegenerative disorders. Guidelines advocated by governmental agencies, payer consortiums, professional organizations, and national and international societies representing clinical specialties are potential sources of information. These entities not only would provide statements on drugs and dosing but also may have recommendations on screening, diagnosing, and monitoring patients who have certain diseases or are receiving treatments for them. In order to evaluate real-world compliance and use of drugs in populations, pharmacoepidemiologic studies are needed. The drug utilization (use of drugs in the populations) data may be generated from market research (e.g., sales data), surveys of target populations, or now more commonly through querying large electronic health databases.

The abovementioned epidemiologic measures, concepts, and methods are summarized in Table 5.3.

Epidemiology in Clinical Drug Development

The assessment of unmet need guides drug research and development. The role of epidemiology in drug development focuses on the identification of the number of persons in the overall target population, estimated from epidemiologic measures. Potential inclusion and exclusion criteria based upon knowledge of risk factors, comorbidities, and prognostic factors are applied to aid

TABLE 5.3
Epidemiologic Measures, Concepts, and Methods for Assessing Burden of Disease and Causality

BURDEN OF DISEASE

Epidemiologic concept or measure	Definition	Major potential bias in assessing or interpreting
Incidence rates	New cases of a disease/disorder/indication in a time period divided by the population at risk in the same time period	New cases may not come to diagnostic attention; diagnostic criteria, methods, and classification systems may change over time
Prevalence rates	All cases in a point of time or in a time period divided by a population at risk for the disease/disorder/indication in the same time period	May only be based on cases coming to diagnostic attention; not suitable for rapidly fatal diseases
Mortality rates	Deaths in a population at risk over a time period divided by the population at risk in the same time period	Geographic variation in coding and coder knowledge of patient affect reason for death
Risk factors	Potentially modifiable (e.g., alcohol intake) and nonmodifiable factors (e.g., demographics) that contribute to the disease origins	Exposure to risk factors is highly variable among subpopulations and nations
Natural history including prognostic factors	Identification of how disease severity changes over time and those factors, potentially modifiable and nonmodifiable, that influence the rate of disease continuation are prognostic factors (e.g., the emergence of hepatic steatosis, old age)	Knowledge often based on clinical cohorts and requires long term follow-up
Comorbidities	A coexisting or co-occurring, usually a chronic one, condition in the same person at the same time as the indication	May be not be identified until presenting for the indication and may have a complex or broad definition (e.g., renal failure, an autoimmune disorder)
Treatment patterns	Current standard of care as defined by professional societies and/or governmental agencies based on knowledge of efficacy of treatments	Geographic variation in healthcare standards (driven by availability of diagnostic tools, treatment modalities, local formulary, insurance plans, and regulations) may affect use/nonuse of a treatment modality

Continued

TABLE 5.3 Epidemiologic Measures, Concepts, and Methods for Assessing Burden of Disease and Causality—cont'd		
Unmet need	Providing therapy for a condition for which treatment or diagnosis is not addressed adequately by available therapy, usually for a condition that is serious or life-threatening. May be expressed as prevalence or percentage not treated or responding to treatment	Social and political environment and complexity of condition may bias the prevalence of unmet need downward (e.g., liver-targeted antiviral agents in persons with coexisting metabolic, renal, or cardiac disease)
Drug utilization	Exposure to a biopharmaceutical product measured by sales data, shipments, prescriptions filled, self-report, or prescriptions written	May not have patient-level data for specific indication if using sales or shipment data, or if available, limited to a few variables such as age and sex of patient if using prescription data
METHODS: STUDY DESIGNS TO ASSESS CAUSALITY		
Observational study	Investigation presenting and statistically testing a hypothesis of the relationship of exposure and outcome(s) without the investigator applying either an intervention or a treatment directly to a patient	Potential confounder information may be unavailable or inadequate leading to bias in the estimation of relative risk
Cross-sectional study	Investigation of exposures to drugs and outcome event at one point or a period, without distinguishing if the outcome was preexisting	Risk of an outcome from exposure may not be determined in this approach.
Cohort (longitudinal, prospective)	Patients without the outcome of interest are followed over a defined period consistent with the expected latency period for the emergence of the outcome. The rate of the outcome is then compared between those exposed and those not exposed.	Large sample size and need to consider latency period. Potential lost to follow can be a problem, exposure can change. Multiple exposures make causality difficult to assess. If data are not deidentified, there may be privacy issues. Time to obtain information about the disease and exposure, cost, and time to complete the study are potential disadvantages.
Retrospective cohort	A cohort is created retrospectively, typically from an existing database of persons who received healthcare services.	Exposure is created from an algorithm that may lack sensitivity and specificity to dose ranges, formulations, and duration of use. Members of the cohort may not be representative of the population at risk, only those who had access to or treatment for health conditions.
Case-control	Cases with the disease or other health outcome of interest are compared with a comparator group without the disease or other health outcome of interest during a time window, with the objective of retrospectively assessing and comparing the frequency of an exposure in both groups.	The incidence rate and relative risk cannot be computed from this design. It is suitable for assessing significance of rare disease and exposures. Temporal relationship of exposure and disease is sometimes difficult to establish. The potential for biases is much higher than that in a longitudinal cohort study because of the available cases and controls for assessment may depend on survival differences, recall bias when collecting data, and loss of precision due to sampling.

in refining the estimated size and location of populations potentially eligible for study. This allows the clinical development team to focus on more specific populations and plan for effective recruitment.

The establishment of the disease profile also provides essential background for assessing the safety of medicines during drug development programs. Patients on medications may experience health events while taking medication or after completing the course of their medications. These events may be due to a patient's comorbidity or comedication, genetic susceptibility, or environmental exposures. It is important to take into account major confounders (Box 5.9) that may distort the association between a specific medication and health events and produce unconfounded true association. As the first step, assessment of background rates of specific events in various subgroups of patients may provide an important piece of information leading to identification of confounding that may have to be accounted for in the monitoring and interpretation of clinical safety data.

Epidemiology also evaluates published research on background rates (if available) or conducts postmarketing studies to provide the context of risk among the drug-exposed population. In addition, epidemiology may also conduct hypothesis-driven observational studies to address specific safety issues using real-world clinical practice data (e.g., health insurance claims, electronic medical records) or special data collection via disease, drug, device, or pregnancy registries (see Chapter 3).

Role of Epidemiology in Obtaining and Maintaining Market Approval

Epidemiologic data are essential for various regulatory dossiers including accelerated approval, orphan drug applications, pediatric investigational plan waivers, RMPs, and ad hoc regulatory requests. These data may be derived from the literature, rapid incidence surveillance data, or well-designed observational studies. These epidemiologic assessments aid in identifying if a similar potential event occurs in an untreated population with the indication, its magnitude, if it is restricted

to a certain subset of the population (e.g., persons with a certain genotype) and if the event is associated with or explained by the presence of comorbidities (e.g., the risk of MI is only found in those with diabetes). The widespread availability of electronic health data and recognition of the need for real-world impact on public health regarding the safety and effectiveness of the drug beyond utilization will prompt more original epidemiologic descriptive and observational studies to be included in regulatory documents. This has led to an increasing number of postmarketing studies required by regulatory authorities. Having epidemiology data available before making any regulatory decisions can increase the efficiency of a response to any communications from regulatory authorities.

Similar principles apply in the postmarketing setting. Epidemiology plays a critical role by continuously monitoring the uptake (exposure) of approved drugs and biopharmaceutical products. The assessment of utilization of the product is done through the use of sales data. But with the increasing availability of real-world electronic health data, the use of a product by age and gender and other important clinical conditions can be determined. When the uptake is sufficient, data on background rates of potential safety events of interest in the indicated population may be determined, as well as in specific subpopulations at risk for such events. This vigilance role of epidemiology is essential because clinical trials often do not have the sample size to detect rare events, such as torsade de pointes, that may have an impact on the safety profile of a drug. Moreover, clinical trial populations are primarily selected and sized in terms of inclusion and exclusion criteria to maximize an understanding of the efficacy of a drug. This limitation in knowledge of the extent or real-world exposure at time of approval will remain an important issue in the era of personalized medicine, as drugs are increasingly being approved based on sub-populations of a disease (i.e., specific genotypic variations of cancers), yet are often used more broadly after approval.

In summary, the knowledge and shared understanding of the fundamental epidemiology of the indication, regardless of the life cycle stage, position the epidemiologist as a strategic partner in the regulatory environment, impacting decisions both internal and external to the company. Providing consultation and contributions to various regulatory documents requires knowledge of important guidances, regulations, and initiatives currently underway, which may impact the success of drug development and subsequent sustenance in the marketplace. For example, consultations and contributions of epidemiology are almost routine

---

BOX 5.9
Impact of Confounding

- A confounder is something that is associated with both the exposure and the outcome. If not identified and controlled in the analysis, magnitude and direction of the association may be false.

during the signaling process, filing of a new drug application, accelerated approvals, RMPs, waiver requests, postapproval safety studies, postapproval efficacy studies, and postmarketing research studies (voluntary and imposed) by regulatory bodies.

Examples of current initiatives by regulatory authorities impacting epidemiology practice in the pharmaceutical industry are displayed in Table 5.4. For example, the FDA, as part of its Sentinel Initiative, is generating assessments on a distributed database formatted according to a Common Data Model. Assessments are publically posted and include drug utilization patterns, reports of medical error, and incidence rates of selected health outcomes from exposures, as well as reports of new methodologies for assessing safety in postmarket settings utilizing electronic health databases (Box 5.10).

Epidemiologic data and studies can have a significant impact on drug labels. Examples of how epidemiologic insights have impacted regulatory decisions in the drug life cycle are illustrated in Table 5.5 (Box 5.11).

BOX 5.10
Sentinel Initiative of the FDA

- The Sentinel Initiative is a public–private partnership to develop a system to obtain information from electronic healthcare data from multiple sources to assess the safety and extent of use of approved medical products. This active surveillance approach to detection of safety signals complements the longstanding, passive approach of review of spontaneously reported adverse events.

CRITIQUING THE EPIDEMIOLOGIC EVIDENCE

A critical assessment of the peer-reviewed literature presenting epidemiologic data and interpretation is needed for decision-making or fulfilling a regulatory request. In each of the aforementioned stages of the life cycle of the pharmaceutical product, scientific

TABLE 5.4
Examples of Regulatory Initiatives Impacting the Role of Epidemiology in the Industry

Initiative	Description/Website	Impact on Epidemiology
FDA Sentinel	Active surveillance on linked CDM formatted databases for active surveillance of health outcomes from treatment, https://www.sentinelinitiative.org/	Understand functionality of CDM-formatted databases and Sentinel Modular Programs Querying Tools for active surveillance including signal refinement
Guidelines	FDA: "Best Practices for Conducting and Reporting Pharmacoepidemiologic Safety Studies Using Electronic Healthcare Data Sets," https://www.fda.gov/downloads/drugs/guidances/ucm243537.pdf	Best practices for conducting and reporting on pharmacoepidemiologic safety studies that use electronic healthcare data sets, which include administrative claims data and electronic medical record data
Guidelines	EMA: ENCePP Guide on Methodological Standards in Pharmacoepidemiology, http://www.encepp.eu/	Elements for conducting pharmacoepidemiologic studies Posting of observational protocols and their status in public registers
Accelerated pathways for drug/biopharmaceutical approval	EMA PRIME: http://www.ema.europa.eu/docs/en_GB/document_library/Leaflet/2016/03/WC500202670.pdf	Epidemiologic and observational data supplement clinical trial data
Accelerated pathways for drug/biopharmaceutical approval	21st Century Cures Act (Public Law 114-255) https://www.gpo.gov/fdsys/pkg/PLAW-114publ255/pdf/PLAW-114publ255.pdf	New observational study designs can facilitate drug approval; establishment of surveillance systems for antibiotic use

CDM, Common Data Model; *ENCePP*, European Network of Centres for Pharmacoepidemiology and Pharmacovigilance.

TABLE 5.5
Examples of Signals Assessed From Epidemiology Methods Affecting the Life Cycle of a Drug

Safety Signal	Description of Epidemiologic Action to Assess Problem	Epidemiologic Data Source	Result
Possible increased risk of fractures of the hip, wrist, and spine with the use of PPIs	Six cohort studies, two of which showed dose-response with longer use of PPIs	FDA[5]	Communication to HCPs regarding potential risk of fractures if PPIs are used at higher doses for long periods of time.
Teratogenic effect of antiepileptic drugs	Patient registries developed to obtain information on specific drugs (product, dose, timing of use during pregnancy), and prevalence of major congenital pregnancy outcomes assessed	North American Antiepileptic Drug Pregnancy Registry Hernandez-Díaz et al.[6]	Black box for certain indications

PPIs, proton pump inhibitors; *HCP*, health care professionals.

BOX 5.11
Real-World Health Data

- The use of large electronic health data sets of real-world clinical practice provides an opportunity for epidemiologists to assess potential safety signals, thereby addressing limitations in sample sizes and generalizability of clinical trials.

publications (including epidemiologic research) must be compiled and reviewed. The purposes of such review may be varied, including identifying changes in diagnostic criteria and publication of new results from large studies impacting the course of a disease of interest. Regardless of the purpose, the level of evidence must be considered and interdisciplinary evaluations, including those of an expert epidemiologist, may be needed.

The Literature Review

The literature review is a comprehensive survey of publications and information (online sources, online queries, etc.) based on selected terms, time periods, and languages. The initial step in the literature review process is selection of terms relevant to the purpose of the search and the specific question asked. Take for example the question, "What is the background rate of hepatic decompensation among persons treated with directly acting antiviral (DAA) agents for hepatitis C viral infection?" Terms for a search would need to represent the medical concept (e.g., "ascites," "portal hypertension"), population of interest (treated with DAA agents), and study designs that would yield rate information

(cohort study, incidence rate, epidemiology). The MeSH (Medical Subject Headings) browser is an online vocabulary lookup aid available for use in selecting key terms and descriptors of possible interest and their hierarchic relationship. The end result of a literature search is a list of references. The references may include individual publications, a systematic review, a meta-analysis, conference reports and abstracts, and downloaded data tables from online. The priority for selection is review articles, systematic reviews, meta-analyses, major reports, and primary research publications in peer-reviewed journals in time periods during which the diagnostic methods follow accepted practice. The review should consider both negative and positive associations. Summarized in Table 5.6 are the steps in compiling the literature to be reviewed and/or included.

What is a systematic review?

A systematic review is a structured methodology to assemble, critically appraise, and synthesize original studies whose reports have individuals meeting predefined criteria similar to that of the target population for indication. The databases are targeted and commonly include MEDLINE, Embase, CINAHL, and Scopus along with a predefined time period, language designation, and list of keywords. Reference lists from relevant review articles are also searched. Selection criteria are applied to minimize bias in the assembly of relevant studies, such as a scoring system for article quality and to ascertain the level of evidence that article could provide.[7] Detail is provided in a table of the studies summarized, which include author, year, population size and characteristics, methods for obtaining the sample, description of the intervention (or exposure), and how the outcomes were quantified (Box 5.12).

TABLE 5.6
Steps in the Literature Review Process

- Define the key question(s)
- Identify contextual objective of search (e.g., natural history, incidence of adverse event among comparators, risk factors)
- Specify the target population
- Define the medical concept related to the question
- Determine how the medical concept should be measured (e.g., surveys of self-report, ICD-10 diagnoses or procedure codes, combinations of methods)
- Define the exposure
- Determine the acceptable means for how exposure should be measured (e.g., filled prescriptions, written prescriptions, doses from a clinical trial)
- Choose search words, terms, and their synonyms for your listing of keywords
- Develop the searching algorithm (Boolean logic example: hepatitis C AND (epidemiology OR incidence OR prevalence); Wildcard example: congenital anomaly ⇒ anomal*, malform*)
- Identify the data source/databases/websites to be sourced for epidemiologic literature information (MEDLINE, Embase, CINAHL, Scopus, Cochrane; CDC, WHO, FDA, EMA, NIH)
- Consult a subject-matter expert for additional authors, studies, publications
- Critically appraise the study's relevance for safety practice (e.g., is the information provided truly a measure of risk in a relevant comparator population?)
- Evaluate how the relationship between exposure is analyzed
- Recognize the strengths and limitations of the reference for product safety, particularly for the validity of exposure and measurement of safety endpoints

*(for searching alternative spellings of the same words).

BOX 5.12
Systematic Review of Scientific Studies

- A systematic review is a formal research study that follows a predefined structure to locate, retrieve, evaluate, and summarize publications of studies that have all tried to answer a similar question. Studies selected meet certain predefined criteria of quality and data granularity.

What is a meta-analysis?

A meta-analysis is a statistical summary and analysis of results of pooled primary data of sufficient detail from published comparator studies (i.e., studies that have the same exposure or class of exposure). The process of obtaining the studies for the analysis follows the abovementioned process for a systematic review. However, there are additional steps: (1) determine which publications contain study designs that provide the highest level of evidence and granularity of data for analysis and (2) determine what data are abstracted for pooled quantitative analysis, blinding as to the study title and author should be maintained for both the abstraction and analysis. The quantitative output should include a summary of measures for each study included, overall summary of the measure of the effect (e.g., risk difference) or association (odds ratio or relative risk) and their respective CIs, and the evaluation of heterogeneity (expressed as I^2) of the individual studies. The less the heterogeneity among the study measures of effect or association, the higher the likelihood that the outcome occurring from the exposure or intervention is true, within a certain level of confidence. The pooling or combining of raw data from individual studies may be done, but it may require the institutional review board approval if the Health Insurance Portability and Accountability Act of 1996 requirements are not met.

Both the systematic review and meta-analysis require a written protocol and a minimum set of items for reporting/including an article in the analysis of evidence. Illustrating this point is the PRISMA (Preferred Reporting Items for Systematic Reviews and Meta-Analyses) flowchart used to summarize the results of the articles to be included from a literature review. Depending on the study objective and type of study design, the articles may be included in only the systematic review; some may only meet the criteria for inclusion in a meta-analysis (Fig. 5.1). Individual articles meeting the desired quality may then be included in safety assessments and various regulatory documents and responses.

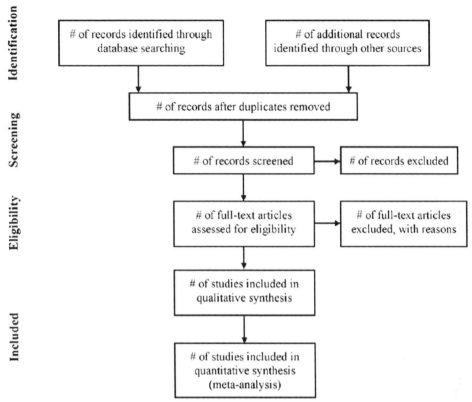

FIG. 5.1 Schematic of flow of information through the different phases of a systematic review or meta-analysis. (Reproduced from: Moher D, Liberati A, Tetzlaff J, Altman DG, The PRISMA Group. Preferred reporting items for systematic reviews and meta-analyses: the PRISMA statement. *PLoS Med*. 2009;6(7): e1000097. https://doi.org/10.1371/journal.pmed.1000097.)

How Is a Study From a Publication Critiqued?

Not all articles obtained from a literature search may have all the elements necessary for assessing safety. The questions to be asked for selecting an epidemiologic article or study for safety assessment are displayed in Table 5.7. A checklist is a useful aid for critiquing an article or a study. Those selected for a PV assessment, systematic review, or meta-analysis depend on the purpose of the article (e.g., evaluating a new diagnostic method, determining the risk of an event in a treated population) and study design. Box 5.13 lists some checklists.

The study sample: is it relevant to the population exposed to the drug of interest?

Seldom is an entire population studied; usually, only a sample is examined. For this reason, caution must be taken in determining if the sample is representative of the population and if the disease entity in the sample is relevant to the safety assessment. Evaluation of the

adequacy of a sample should include a well-characterized definition of the disease of interest, a description of the location for sample selection (by geographic boundaries, restricted to clinic referral, convenience, etc.), how the sample was selected (a random process or by convenience), and what proportion of the population was represented in the sample (or how many were in the sample). For example, one of the studies on the prevalence of dementia in Alzheimer disease in Canada was the Canadian Study of Health and Aging (CSHA).[9] This was a survey that covered five regions across Canada through a random sample of 10,263 persons in community and institutional settings. The CSHA used random sampling, stratified for age, sex, region, and place of residence (community or institution) to ensure representativeness of the sample. However, if the purpose of the study was to assess the prevalence of mild cognitive impairment due to early Alzheimer disease, data from this sample may not be relevant.

TABLE 5.7
Critiquing an Epidemiologic Article or Study: Points to Consider

SOURCE/ABSTRACT/INTRODUCTION

- What is the journal quality?
- What are author credentials, affiliations, and sources of funding?
- Can this article be used in signal detection or signal strengthening?
- Are the public health impacts addressed (magnitude of problem, severity, morbidity, mortality, utilization, trend)?
- Are the critical articles referenced for context?
- Was there a hypothesis?

METHODS

- Is the population similar to your target population of interest?
- Is the sample size adequate? Can the size of the sample allow for conclusions to population subgroups?
- Generalizability to the target population of interest
- Are the reliability and validity in classifying exposure and health outcome(s) assessed? Were objective or self-reported measures used? Are these methods assessed to pick up changes over time?
- What level of evidence can the study design provide?
- Are the statistical methods appropriate to the questions asked and the study design, level of measurement of exposure and outcome, and sample size, and are they adequately controlled for confounding?

ANALYSIS

- How similar or different are the nonresponders from the responders? How similar or different are those in the study compared to those who dropped out or lost to follow-up?
- Is the statistical analysis appropriate for the level of measurement of the exposure and health outcome, the sample size, and hypothesis?

RESULTS

- Are the sample characteristics presented in sufficient detail?
- Are the bivariate results presented for all the main terms?
- What terms are included in multivariate models? What terms in these models address confounding?
- Which are statistically significant? What are the magnitudes of the point estimates and associations?
- What are the widths of the confidence intervals?

DISCUSSION

- What is the main conclusion? Is this supported by the data and their analyses? Is it consistent with the abstract?
- What is the evidence for causality between exposure and outcome?
- How are bias and confounding addressed?

BOX 5.13
Some Checklists to Aid in Critique of Peer-Reviewed Articles

- Diagnostic/prognostic studies: STARD
- Case reports/case series: CARE
- Observational studies: STROBE
- Comparative effectiveness studies: GRACE
- Randomized trials: CONSORT
- Systematic reviews: PRISMA
- Meta-analysis: MOOSE

BOX 5.14
Example of a Null Hypothesis:

- There is no association between exposure to drug A and the occurrence of event B in the population receiving treatment with drug A.

Is there a study hypothesis? (Box 5.14)
Presentation of a clearly defined hypothesis allows for the reader to assess if the outcome of interest and its measurement, study population, exposure sources, and statistical methods are appropriate for a safety assessment. The statement of a hypothesis includes the type of relationship examined (association, correlation, difference) with the independent (or exposure) variable followed by the dependent or outcome variable of interest. It is recommended to state the hypothesis in a neutral or null manner to avoid subjective bias when interpreting study results.

Are the appropriate epidemiologic measures provided?

If the study question pertains to the burden of disease, the prevalence rate of that disease may be the most relevant overall measure. However, if the goal is to assess the risk of an outcome related to an exposure, a longitudinal (or prospective) study is required. In both cases, another consideration is whether or not the epidemiologic measure appropriately captures the frequency of disease occurrence in population subgroups or one that is specific to the indication of interest.

Are the study design, sampling method, and sample size clearly described and appropriate to the question asked?

The study design must be appropriate to generate the epidemiologic measurement. The study should target obtaining information from the entire population or a sample determined to be representative of the population of interest (indicated for specific drug treatment). The result should be that the study sample represents the condition in the population of interest that would be targeted for the drug treatment. Certain diseases are known to vary in prevalence or incidence across different geographic regions and population sectors. For example, persons older than 85 years and those residing in institutions are expected to have higher prevalence rates of dementia. For some health problems, rates for women may differ from those for men. Sociodemographic variables, such as educational status, may vary between countries. Therefore the study sample needs to be described in enough detail so that other researchers can determine if it is comparable to their population of interest. Data on a comparison of study participants with those who refused or were ineligible can help others determine for whom the study group is representative and if the descriptive or relative measure is biased in some manner.

How are the health outcomes classified and measured?

Health outcomes are defined as those events occurring as a result of an intervention. These may be measured clinically (physical examination, laboratory testing, imaging), self-reported, or observed (such as gait or movement fluctuations seen by a healthcare provider or caregiver). Some health outcomes require complex assessments to determine if they are present or absent. For example, some conditions, such as dementia, can be classified differently in studies depending on the country of the study population. The United States uses the *Diagnostic and Statistical Manual of Mental Disorders* (DSM), the continental Europe uses the International Classification of Diseases, and the United

Kingdom refers to CAMDEX (Cambridge Mental Disorders of the Elderly Examination). Other measurement scales of dementia and professional practice guidelines, with changes over time, can affect the classification of dementia as well as many other diseases. Attention must be given to the version for disease classification cited in a study in order to assess its relevance to safety assessment. In the American Framingham study, presence of dementia was determined through the Mini-Mental State Examination and a panel that included a neurologist and a neuropsychologist.[10] Many health problems are not easily diagnosed or defined, and some include stages where mild cases are not always easily distinguished until post mortem, such as many of the neurodegenerative disorders.

Is the health outcome measured in an unbiased fashion?

Considerable judgment by assessors or interviewers is required to determine the presence of some health outcomes under scrutiny; thus, it is best that trained assessors are independent and not aware (i.e., blinded) of the subjects' clinical status or, sometimes, even the purpose of the study. It is important that the subjects under assessment include those thought to be negatives as well as positives. If more than one rater is used, interobserver and/or intraobserver reliability of clinical assessments must be high and should be noted in the articles published. The interviewers or assessors must all use the same criteria, including specifics related to each health problem, such as its duration. This is especially pertinent when diagnosing an illness such as Alzheimer disease that requires multiple cognitive measurements or assessments that need to be conducted to rule out other health conditions.

Is the response rate adequate?

Missing data is an important issue. If data are missing on a large number of the study selected subjects (Box 5.15), it may affect the epidemiologic measurement profoundly leading to lack of validity of the assessment exposure and outcome relationship. A

> **BOX 5.15**
> **Missing Data Impact**
>
> • Missing data affects the magnitude and the direction of the exposure–disease association. The pattern of missing data is important to understand, as it may pose a threat to validity. Is the missing data random or is there a pattern (e.g., healthier people may have more missing lab data than those with an illness).

response rate in population surveys of two-thirds to three-quarters has been suggested to be generalizable to the population samples. Therefore a response rate of 70% is accepted for many surveys. In the case of dementia a significant proportion of those persons not responding to a survey might be suffering from dementia, which could lead to an underestimate of its prevalence. Because a large number of dropouts, refusals, or "not-founds" among the subjects selected may jeopardize a study's validity, the authors should describe the reasons for nonresponse and compare persons in the study with those not in the study as to their sociodemographic characteristics. If the reasons for nonresponse seem unrelated to the health outcome measured and the characteristics of those individuals not in the sample are comparable with those in the study, researchers may be able to justify a more modest response rate.

What is the duration of follow-up?

To determine incidence, all study subjects should be followed and measured to prevent bias in a time period consistent with the estimated latency of the effect of the treatment or its side effects, such as a period consistent with the doubling of the half-life of exposure (or in the case of a potential malignancy, cases exposed to a drug intervention may be followed up for up to 10 years). If persons die during the period of the study, the cause of death must be ascertained. It is necessary to follow subjects over a clinically sensible period, depending on the illness under study and the age of the population.

How are the results interpreted (Box 5.16)?

Conflicting results identified from studies in a literature review may arise from several factors. These include differences in the populations studied (underlying differences in comorbidities and exposures not related to the drug), period of study, study designs, variations in technique for obtaining health outcome, methods for

classifying exposure or health outcomes, and measurement reliability and validity. These factors will influence whether a statistically significant association is found. Confounding may also influence how results are interpreted. Confounding is a variable that distorts the estimate of the risk to upward, downward, or the null. For example, in an observational cohort study of cardiovascular risk, there was no risk (when adjusting for confounding factors) associated with sibutramine use in the study populations of two nations, whereas in a randomized open-label trial, an increased risk was observed.[11,12] For these reasons, it is important to note the point estimates, CIs of point estimates, and the degree of precision of the point estimates. CIs represent the minimum and maximum range of point estimates one can expect after repeated measures are obtained, usually expressed as a 95% CI. This means that 95% of the time, the true measure (e.g., incidence, relative risk) can fall within that range. Small samples and rare events can generate very wide CIs. A rule of thumb is that when a statistically significant association between exposure and outcome is found, there will be no overlap of either the higher or lower value of the 95% CI between the exposed and unexposed groups and the CI will include the null association value of 1 (Box 5.17). When an epidemiologic study, even with a large sample size, conflicts with the results of previous open-label, randomized, or other postmarket studies, attention should be given to the frequency of events of interest or sample size of each individual study. The analysis of composite events (e.g., assessing "cardiac outcomes" vs. "QTc prolongation") may not adequately drill down to the medical concept to determine the statistical significance of a potential safety event for action.[13] This would then limit the ability of risk management in addressing mitigation efforts. A framework for evaluating and interpreting the results of hypothesis testing is displayed in Fig. 5.2. After an article has been critiqued, a level of evidence should be assigned. One such assignment approach proposed by the authors is displayed in Tables 5.7 and 5.8. This will aid in triaging the articles reviewed for their value to a safety assessment.

BOX 5.16
Conflicting Study Conclusions Are Due to Differences in

- population characteristics
- period of study
- study designs
- disease classification changes
- access of population for diagnosis
- methods and criteria for diagnosis
- exposure measurements
- inter-rater data collection

BOX 5.17
Interpretation of Confidence Interval

- When confidence interval for risk ratio or relative risk include 1, or confidence interval for risk difference include zero, it is supportive of null hypothesis of no association.

Summary of interpretation of Epidemiologic hypothesis testing

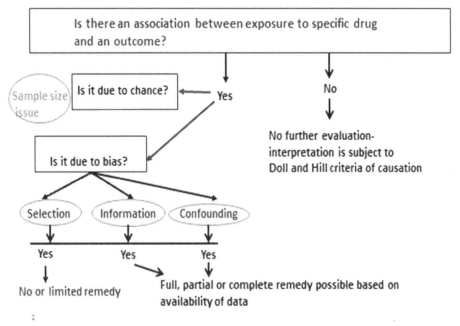

FIG. 5.2 Flow diagram for interpreting the results of hypothesis testing.

DATA SOURCES FOR EPIDEMIOLOGY PRACTICE IN THE INDUSTRY

The safety assessment's quantitative evaluations are enhanced through the use of data, particularly electronic health data that provide context. The data source selected for this purpose depends on how the signal is defined (e.g., laboratory value, medical concept) and the population from which it arose (e.g., elderly, those with renal impairment). Common data sources used by epidemiologists in PV include the following:

- vital statistics,
- population demographic data,
- public health surveillance systems,
- population surveys,
- patient registries,
- medical claims databases of patient encounters,
- electronic health records,
- prescription databases.

Accessing the data may be Web-based, available for purchase, or generated via a third-party contractual arrangement. In some situations, data sources may be linked. For example, the linkage of medical claims data to an electronic file of deaths for the purpose of determining the mortality rate among those who used

TABLE 5.8
Levels of Evidence

Level	Type of Evidence
I	Randomized clinical trial
II	Well-designed controlled intervention study without individual patient randomization (a quasi-experiment)
III	Well-designed observational prospective longitudinal study (a cohort study)
IV	Historical (retrospective cohort) study or case-control study
V	Case series
VI	Expert opinions

Adapted from Burns PB, Rohrich RJ, Chung KC. The levels of evidence and their role in evidence-based medicine. *Plast Reconstr Surg.* 2011;128(1):305–310.

a specific prescription. For confidentiality, linkage of data sets may be required to be performed through a third party. Caution is advised when drawing conclusions from electronic health databases, as differences in populations covered (size, geography, financial

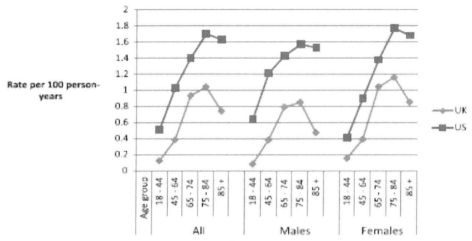

FIG. 5.3   An example of different databases yielding different primary hip replacement rates per 100 person-years among persons with knee osteoarthritis by gender, age, and country. (Reproduced from: Oleske, et al. 2014.[15])

payments for treatments, person-time in database) and local standards of care may affect conclusions. This is illustrated in the study by Oleske et al.[15] in which differences in joint replacement rates by age and sex are strikingly different between the United States and the United Kingdom for the same indication (Fig. 5.3). This may be due to differences in access to healthcare, exposure to risk factors, treatment practices, and other factors. Chapter 3 provides further discussion of the uses of electronic health databases in conducting observational studies for assessing a potential safety signal.

COMPETENCIES AND CRITERIA OF A SUCCESSFUL EPIDEMIOLOGIST IN THE INDUSTRY

The formal reporting structure of an epidemiologist may be different in each pharmaceutical company depending on its size and pipeline. Commonly, the epidemiology group resides in PV or health economics and outcomes research, but it can also be found in market access or other planning and commercial departments or in multiple units within a company.

Regardless of the position within the company structure, there are core competencies required for success. This requires at the minimum technical skills and knowledge related to epidemiology, including credentialed knowledge of advanced epidemiologic methods and statistics, experience with proposal development and complex project management, competency with statistical software, and hands-on use of large electronic databases. This technical and educational background is essential for many reasons. Given the fast-paced

environment of the biopharmaceutical industry, the epidemiologist must quickly understand the scientific issue within the broader picture, frame the targeted questions, operationalize the targeted questions by detailing the problem and approach to address the problem, and guide the decision-making for a proactive approach. Other requirements include excellence in both oral and written communication skills, particularly to audiences with diverse professional backgrounds. Collaboration and contributions are expected to reach across company divisions including PV, commercial, regulatory, statistics, clinical development, medical affairs, legal, and public affairs. For this reason, in addition to technical competence in epidemiology, the pharmacoepidemiologist must be able to demonstrate the ability to work in matrix environments, participate in teams as both a leader and a participant, and embrace the value that patients and their safety are the focus of their role. People management abilities are highly desirable. Participation and membership in professional and relevant therapeutic area focus are also key to gain depth of knowledge about new methods and advances in the biology of the indication supported. The International Society for Pharmacoepidemiology, the International Society For Pharmacoeconomics and Outcomes Research, a clinical specialty professional organization (e.g., American Society for Clinical Oncology), and keeping current with practice standards, guidances, and regulations which affect epidemiology practice. Knowledge of global health trends, even if the host company targets market authorization in only one country, may be gained from these memberships through structured offerings and networking.

FUTURE OF PHARMACOEPIDEMIOLOGY

There will be an evolving change in the model of epidemiology in the industry, from an exclusive support function to a leadership role at all phases of the biopharmaceutical life cycle. This will be due to the increasing complexity of scientific knowledge about a disease, its risk factors, and new methodologies for investigating these; increasing availability and number of electronic health databases (including molecular and genetic databases) and tools for querying these; and the recognition of the multifactorial nature of the risks that could emerge from treatment. Use of new analytic techniques and methods (e.g., natural language processing) to explore unstructured data such as social media, as well as the ability to integrate both new and different data sources, will greatly facilitate the application of epidemiology to PV practice. Lastly, the emergence of and acceptance for new study designs, such as the pragmatic design used in the Salford Lung Study[16] and other study designs endorsed in the 21st Century Cures Act aimed at simultaneously assessing drug safety and effectiveness in population-based settings, will require epidemiologic concepts and methods in the design, implementation, and interpretation studies.

REFERENCES

1. Wax PM. Elixirs, diluents, and the passage of the 1938 federal food, drug and cosmetic act. *Ann Intern Med.* 1995; 122:456−461.
2. Meade TW. Subacute myelo-optic neuropathy and clioquinol an epidemiological case-history for diagnosis. *Br J Prev Soc Med.* 1975;29:157−169.
3. Herbst AL, Ulfelder H, Poskanzer DC. Adenocarcinoma of the vagina: association of maternal stilbesterol therapy with tumor appearance in young women. *N Engl J Med.* 1971;284:878−881.
4. Fedak KM, Bernal A, Capshaw ZA, Gross S. Applying the Bradford Hill criteria in the 21st century: how data integration has changed causal inference in molecular epidemiology. *Emerg Themes Epidemiol.* 2015;12:14. https://doi.org/10.1186/s12982-015-0037-4.
5. US Food and Drug Administration. *FDA Drug Safety Communication: Possible Increased Risk of Fractures of the Hip, Wrist, and Spine with the Use of Proton Pump Inhibitors.* March 23, 2011.
6. Hernandez-Díaz S, Smith CR, Shen A, et al. Comparative safety of antiepileptic drugs during pregnancy. *Neurology.* 2012;78:1692−1699.
7. Dreyer NA, Velentgas P, Westrich K, Dubois R. The GRACE checklist for rating the quality of observational studies of comparative effectiveness: a tale of hope and caution. *J Manag Care Pharm.* 2014;20(3):301−308.
8. Moher D, Liberati A, Tetzlaff J, Altman DG, The PRISMA Group. Preferred reporting items for systematic reviews and meta-analyses: the PRISMA statement. *PLoS Med.* 2009;6(7):e1000097. https://doi.org/10.1371/journal.pmed.1000097.
9. The Canadian Study of Health and Aging Working Group. The incidence of dementia in Canada. *Neurology.* 2000;55: 66−73.
10. Satizabal CL, Beiser AS, Chouraki V, et al. Incidence of dementia over three decades in the Framingham Heart Study. *NEJM.* 2016;374:523−532.
11. James WPT, Caterson ID, Coutinho W, et al. Effect of sibutramine on cardiovascular outcomes in overweight and obese subjects. *N Engl J Med.* 2010;363:905−917.
12. Tyczynski JE, Oleske DM, Klingman D, Ferrufino CP, Lee W-C. Safety assessment of an anti-obesity drug (sibutramine) a Retrospective Cohort Study. *Drug Saf.* 2012; 35(8):629−644.
13. Strom BL, Eng SM, Faich G, et al. Comparative mortality associated with ziprasidone and olanzapine in real-World use among 18,154 patients with schizophrenia: the Ziprasidone Observational Study of Cardiac Outcomes (ZODIAC). *Am J Psychiatry.* 2011;168:193−201.
14. Burns PB, Rohrich RJ, Chung KC. The levels of evidence and their role in evidence-based medicine. *Plast Reconstr Surg.* 2011;128(1):305−310.
15. Oleske DM, Bonafede MM, Jick S, Ji M, Hall JA. Electronic health databases for epidemiological research on joint replacements: considerations when making cross-national comparisons. *Ann Epidemiol.* 2014;24:660−665.
16. Woodcock A, Bakerly NA, New JP, et al. The Salford Lung Study protocol: a pragmatic, randomized phase III real-world effectiveness trial in asthma. *BMC Pulm Med.* 2015;15:160. https://doi.org/10.1186/s12890-015-0150-8.

CHAPTER 6

Real-World Epidemiologic Studies and Patient Registries

JERZY EDWARD TYCZYNSKI, PHD • RYAN KILPATRICK, PHD

DATA SOURCES FOR OBSERVATIONAL STUDIES

Real-World Data Sources

Although there is a common agreement that randomized clinical trials (RCTs) are the "gold standard" for assessing efficacy and safety of new drug candidates in the drug development process, RCTs have known limitations in providing a comprehensive effectiveness and safety profile. These limitations include the following: Restricted study population (defined by inclusion and exclusion criteria), short follow-up after treatment termination, and limited sample size. Hence, marketing authorization of investigational medicines is supported by data that provide efficacy and safety information with high internal validity but whose generalizability to a general population of patients may be limited.[1,2] Often, registrational clinical trials are single-arm studies with no comparator data available to assess efficacy and safety of the product against other treatments or placebo. This creates a need for assessing safety of medicinal products in real-life use based on observational studies (Box 6.1).

Observational (epidemiologic) studies may use either data collected prospectively for the purpose of the particular study (de novo data collection), i.e., primary data collection, or data that were already collected for another purpose (e.g., as part of administrative records or patient healthcare), which is called secondary data.[2]

There are several types of real-world data (RWD) (secondary data sources) that can be used for conducting observational studies. In general, there are two broad categories of such data sources, i.e., medical records and administrative claims.[2] Different data sources have different characteristics in terms of coverage, follow-up, or ability for linkage with other sources. Table 6.1 presents the main characteristics of two main types of secondary data.

In addition to the two main types of RWD (electronic medical records [EMRs] and administrative claims), there are other sources of data less frequently used in observational research. They include data from surveys, drug, or patient registries (registries usually collect de novo data in the prospective manner) and population-based disease registries. Fig. 6.1 presents a spectrum of data sources for observational and interventional studies used in the drug development continuum (Box 6.2).

The following part of this section aims to characterize the most common types of data sources used for conducting observational studies.

Administrative Medical Claims

When individuals covered by health insurance receive healthcare services, claims are generated and submitted to the insurer for payment or reimbursement. Claims may be submitted in electronic or paper form. Health plans generate and store data detailing services provided and the level of payment for those services. Data originating from claims also include demographic information about covered individuals, such as age, gender, or ZIP code. This information can be used for various research purposes (Fig. 6.2).[4]

Administrative claims data include inpatient and/or outpatient medical claims from a private insurance plan (e.g., UnitedHealthcare) or pharmacy claims maintained by a pharmacy benefit manager (e.g., Express Scripts). Claims submitted for services reimbursed under Medicaid or Medicare are examples of data from the public sector. Administrative claims data can

---

BOX 6.1
Real-World Data

- Real-World Data (RWD) plays a vital role in supplementing efficacy and safety findings in randomized clinical trials (RCTs)
- The use of RWD allows putting RCT findings into broader general population context.

TABLE 6.1

Characteristics of Data Sources Used for Observational Research

	Electronic Medical Records Database	Administrative Claims Database
Source	Medical records, ordering system	Health insurance claims/receipts
Population	Patients in a medical institute	Beneficiaries
Contents	In- and outpatient information, laboratory measurements	Medical and dispensing claims
Identification of disease	Medical records, indication, ICD code, disease name	ICD code, disease name
Follow-up	Within institute or network	Within health insurance network
Advantages	Amount and depth of information, linkage to disease registries	High number of patients
Example	CPRD, Kaiser Permanente, Optum-Humedica	MarketScan, Optum, Medicare

CPRD, Clinical Practice Research Datalink; *ICD*, International Classification of Diseases.
Adapted from Tanaka S, Tanaka S, Kawakami K. Methodological issues in observational studies and non-randomized controlled trials in oncology in the era of big data. *Jpn J Clin Oncol*. 2015;45(4):323–327.

include a variety of different healthcare services, including outpatient medical office visits, hospitalizations, drug prescription, and medical equipment.[4]

Using administrative claims data for observational research poses certain challenges. One of them is the turnover of individuals in health plans. If, for whatever reason, an individual changes a health plan (e.g., due to job changing or due to employer's change of a health plan), claims for that individual would no longer be captured and data collected. To deal with that challenge, a researcher may use eligibility criteria to identify people in the administrative data who were continuously eligible for benefits during the duration of the study. Another challenge can originate from changes in coding practices, particularly important when considering longitudinal studies that require several years of continuous data. These coding changes may be due to changes in reimbursement policies, changes in documentation practices, or changes in the diseased coding systems themselves (e.g., switch between ICD classification versions from ICD-9 to ICD-10)[4] (Box 6.3).

Electronic medical records/electronic health records

In contrast to administrative databases, EMRs data are recorded as part of a clinical patient's care and not for billing purposes. This type of database consists of data entered by health care professionals into electronic databases and is maintained primarily for documenting the patient's conditions and treatments.[2] Physicians maintain records of all visits and events that include information, such as the following: diagnoses (outpatient conditions diagnosed by general

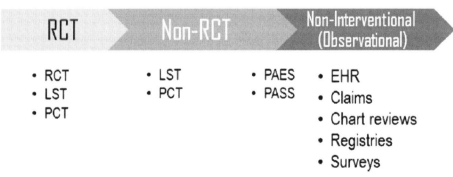

FIG.6.1 Data spectrum in relation to real-world data definition categories. *EHR*, electronic health records; *LST*, large simple trial; *PAES*, post-authorization efficacy study; *PASS*, post-authorization safety studies; *PCT*, pragmatic clinical trial; *RCT*, randomized controlled trial.

BOX 6.2
Types of Real-World Data

- There are several types of Real-World Data used in observational research
- The most commonly used are medical and pharmacy claims and electronic medical records

BOX 6.3
Administrative Medical Claims

- This type of data originates from medical or pharmacy claims
- Claims are generated and submitted to the insurer for payment or reimbursement
- Although not originally intended for research purposes, claims are valuable source of real-world data for observational research

Record Generation Process

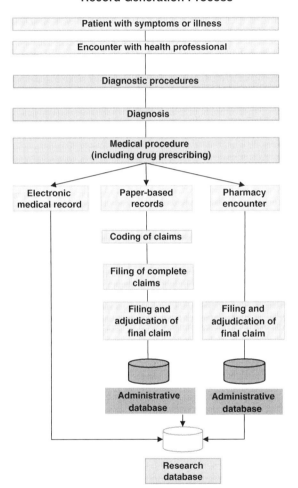

FIG. 6.2 The generation of healthcare utilization databases.

BOX 6.4
Electronic Medical Records/Electronic Health Records

- Electronic medical records/electronic health records (EMRs/EHRs) data are recorded as part of clinical patient care
- EMRs/EHRs could contain data in structured form, as well as in unstructured form (e.g., physicians notes)
- Data from the unstructured parts of EMRs could be explored via natural language processing algorithms

detailed information on patients' profiles, such as alcohol consumption, smoking, height, and weight, although this type of information may be missing for a certain proportion of patients.[2]

The data contained in EMRs are typically quite complex, given the longitudinal nature and volume of information included.[4] EMR databases may originate from one institution or be a product of an EMR data merger from multiple institutions (some commercial organizations create data warehouses containing data from multiple institutions). Databases created from several sources can offer advantages in terms of sample size, but there may be issues with data consistency and the EMR's structure itself.[4]

In contrast to administrative claims, EMRs may contain both structured data and unstructured information. The unstructured information in EMRs is available in the form of clinical notes, problem lists, or pathology reports. This information could often be extracted from unstructured text using text-mining techniques, such as natural language processing algorithms. Exploring unstructured parts of the EMRs allows enriching patients' records by adding information that is absent in the structured sections of the EMRs (e.g., results of genomic tests, histologic types of tumors with no specific ICD code, etc.) (Box 6.4).

practitioners; conditions diagnosed by outpatient specialist; information pertaining to hospital admissions, including hospital diagnoses), patient's medical history, prescriptions issued, laboratory tests ordered, as well as lab test results. In comparison to administrative databases, EMR databases usually include much more

Linkage of data sources

Sometimes the information needed to conduct studies may reside in separate databases. The process of identifying subjects across databases and consolidating their information is called data linkage.[5] A single dataset does not always contain all the information (variables) necessary to conduct a study. Integration of two or more datasets may increase usability of the combined dataset by increasing the number of variables available in the database (e.g., by adding a patient's vital status to the EMRs) or by increasing the depth of the data available (e.g., by adding lab values from EMRs to the claims database).

Record linkage refers to the linking together of data relating to the same individual from separate source files. The data linkage can be deterministic, probabilistic, or mixed (hybrid). For any record-linkage project, a few basic issues must be addressed:

- What is the best way to achieve a high linkage rate in a cost-effective manner?
- What is a feasible technical approach to linking the data?
- What is the correct linkage rate among the records that are linked?
- Is the linkage legally feasible?

Deterministic record linkage can be defined as specified attributes from dataset A that match the same specified attributes in dataset B. The attributes used to match records from two or more datasets may include social security number, ZIP code, name, gender, and birth date. This way of record matching is a subject of error due to coding errors, incorrect values, misspelled names, or duplicate use of the same value for different individuals. However, deterministic linking is characterized by high specificity, i.e., the number of true matches among the linked pairs is high, provided exactness of variables is sufficiently high and error rates are not extreme. At the same time, the deterministic process may have low sensitivity as many true matches are not found even if error rates per variable are low (Fig. 6.3).

Probabilistic record-linkage takes place when some of the attributes from dataset A match some of the attributes in dataset B, with the specification that a level of agreement surpasses a defined threshold. For all possible record pairs, the procedure assigns one of two "linkage weights" for each linking variable, depending on whether the variables in this pair agree or not. A positive weight is assigned when the variable agrees in this record and a negative weight is given when the variable disagrees. For each possible record pair, the linkage weight is assigned for each linking variable

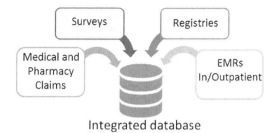

FIG. 6.3 Creating the complete patient record across the healthcare continuum. *EMRs*, electronic medical records.

BOX 6.5
Linkage of Data Sources

- Record linkage is a process of identifying subjects across databases and consolidating their information into one dataset
- Record linkage refers to the linking together of data relating to the same individual from separate source files
- There are two main methods of linking data: deterministic record linkage and probabilistic record linkage

---

and summed over all variables, where the sum reflects the probability that these two records belong to the same individual[6] (Box 6.5).

There are also limitations and challenges in linking data from a number of sources, the most prominent being (1) silos of information (different data bases structure originating from particular healthcare systems), (2) lack of standardization (no single governing body to mandate standard terminologies), (3) patient privacy and security, and (4) lack of patient overlap between systems.

Record linkage plays an important role in the area of oncology, where studies based on claims data typically lack information on cancer clinical characteristics that are strong predictors of treatment and prognosis.[7-9]

Surveys

Another source of RWD that can be used for observational research is health surveys, conducted mainly by federal agencies, such as the Centers for Medicare and Medicaid Services (CMS) or the National Center for Health Statistics (NCHS).[4]

The CMS conducts periodic surveys of Medicare beneficiaries through the Medicare Current Beneficiary Survey. This survey examines health status and functioning, sources of healthcare costs and payments, and insurance coverage among Medicare beneficiaries.

Long-Term Care Minimum Data Set data are also available for research. These data represent a broad assessment of all residents in long-term care facilities that receive Medicare and Medicaid reimbursements.[4]

The Agency for Healthcare Research and Quality (AHRQ) maintains two useful data sources: the Healthcare Cost and Utilization Project (HCUP) and the Medical Expenditure Panel Survey. The HCUP is a family of databases, software tools, and related products developed through a Federal-State-Industry partnership and sponsored by the AHRQ. HCUP databases are derived from administrative data and contain encounter-level, clinical and nonclinical information, including all listed diagnoses and procedures, discharge status, patient demographics, and charges for all patients, regardless of payer (e.g., Medicare, Medicaid, private insurance, uninsured), beginning in 1988. These databases enable research on a broad range of health policy issues, including cost and quality of health services, medical practice patterns, access to healthcare programs, and outcomes of treatments at the national, state, and local levels.

The NCHS maintains a set of health-related surveys of the US population. Two frequently used surveys are the National Ambulatory Medical Care Survey and the National Hospital Ambulatory Medical Care Survey. Both of these surveys are based on representative samples of the US population and collect data regarding the administration and prescription of drugs during the respondent's visit or as a result of the visit. Information about chief complaints, diagnoses made, and other services provided are also included in the data. Other survey databases available via the Centers for Disease Control and Prevention (CDC) include the National Health and Nutrition Examination Survey (NHANES), the National Health Interview Survey or the National Health Insurance Survey.[4,10–12] To learn more about NCHS surveys please visit the CDC website https://www.cdc.gov/nchs/surveys.htm#tabs-2-1.

Registries
Patient and drug registries
A registry is an organized system that uses observational study methods to collect uniform health-related data (clinical, demographic, laboratory, etc.) to evaluate specified outcomes for a population defined by a particular disease, condition, or exposure, and that serves one or more predetermined scientific, clinical, or policy purposes.[13] Registries are classified according to how their populations are defined. For example, drug (product) registries include patients who have been exposed to certain biopharmaceutical products or medical devices. Health services registries consist of patients who have had a common procedure, clinical encounter, or hospitalization. Disease or condition (patient) registries are defined by patients having the same diagnosis, such as cystic fibrosis or lung cancer.[13]

Registries vary in complexity from simply recording product use as a requirement for reimbursement to more systematic efforts to collect prospective data on many types of treatment, risk factors, and clinical events in a defined population. Patients' follow-up could be prospective, retrospective, or a combination of both. The mode and duration of follow-up could range from days to decades, depending on research questions and disease of interest.[14] Registries are being used to fill important gaps in evidence, put data from clinical trials into the real-world context, and help understand how trial results can be applied in practice. Data from registries are also used to support timely decisions by regulatory agencies about safety and help payers in making decisions regarding medical products coverage (payment)[14] (Box 6.6).

Population-based cancer registries
Although patients and drug registries collect data from randomly enrolled individuals from a group of patients with certain predefined characteristics, they usually cannot be extrapolated to a specific part of the general population living in a certain country or region. This is because the population covered by such registries is usually not defined in the way that allows for calculation of incidence, prevalence, or mortality rates. In contrast, this limitation does not apply to the population-based registries that cover a well-defined population of known size and age structure.

The original function of the population-based cancer registry was to calculate rates of incidence so that the risk of various cancers in different populations could be compared. Although this still remains their most basic role, the activities of cancer registries have developed far beyond this to include studies of cancer cause and prevention.[15]

BOX 6.6
Registries

- A registry is an organized system that uses observational study methods to collect uniform health-related data
- There are two main types of registries: drug (product) registry and patient registry
- Registries fill gaps in evidence, put data from clinical trials into the real-world context

Cancer registry data can be used in a wide variety of areas of cancer control ranging from etiological research to primary and secondary prevention to healthcare planning and evaluation of patient care. Although most cancer registries are not obliged to do more than provide the basis for such uses of the data, cancer registries possess the potential for developing and supporting important research programs using the information they collect.[16]

The main objective of the cancer registry is to collect and classify information on all cancer cases in order to produce statistics on the occurrence of cancer in a defined population and to provide a framework for assessing and controlling the impact of cancer on the community. The collection of information on cancer cases and the production of cancer statistics are only justified, however, if use is made of the data collected. Cancer registry information may be used in a multitude of areas, and the value of the data increases if comparability over time is maintained.[16]

There is an obvious need for additional data sources to evaluate safety of oncology treatments in postmarketing settings, where large numbers of patients are exposed to particular treatment regimens or specific drugs. Data from population-based cancer registries contain important information (such as histology, grade, stage, and behavior) necessary to analyze the safety of a particular cancer treatment in a certain group of cancer patients (e.g., toxicities may differ by different histology or disease stage); however, clinical details are usually missing. On the other hand, administrative claims and EMR datasets contain crucial clinical details (e.g., information on treatment continuum, treatment adverse reactions, or preexisting comorbidities), while they often lack cancer-specific information on the tumor itself.[17]

Data from population-based cancer registries are commonly used to assess incidence and prevalence patterns of particular tumor types. However, when linked with other data sources, they can also be used for assessing baseline safety profiles of particular treatment regimens and for prospective safety monitoring of newly approved treatments.

An example of such linkage is the US Surveillance, Epidemiology and End Results (SEER)-Medicare database that links cancer registry data from US SEER cancer registries with Medicare administrative claims. SEER registries have been the foundation for decades of population-based cancer-related research. In addition, SEER-Medicare linked databases are also widely used for cancer studies related to those 65 years of age and older. These data have been available for decades to researchers under certain data use agreements and have been used in numerous peer-reviewed studies.[18]

Currently, SEER registries cover 28% of the US population (see Fig. 6.4).

REAL-WORLD OBSERVATIONAL STUDY DESIGNS

As has been discussed previously, real-world observational studies can be an extremely valuable source of information regarding the effectiveness and safety of human therapeutics. Some real-world observational studies may seek to estimate disease or treatment prevalence, describe treatment patterns, or characterize the burden of an illness. Other times, the goal of the study is comparative—for instance to evaluate relative effectiveness or safety of a drug or other health intervention. Just like the RCT, such real-world observational studies seek to estimate the causal relationship between drug exposures and outcomes of interest. Unlike RCTs, however, in observational studies, the investigator does not assign the treatment. The implications of this are critical, as without the ability to account for reasons *why* patients may receive certain therapies (e.g., their clinical indication, economic or quality influences, etc.), the estimate of any effect of a drug on an outcome may be biased, and an incorrect and potentially harmful decision could result. This makes clear the high stakes of carefully considering for such studies, within the clinical context under investigation, the appropriate study design and analytic methods as well as how to interpret study results considering potential sources of bias. The following sections will outline, at a high level, common study design archetypes for real-world observational studies (Box 6.7), along with key strengths and limitations. A subsequent section will discuss interpretation and potential sources of bias in real-world observational studies.

Types of Studies
Cross-sectional studies
In this type of observational study, exposures and health outcomes from a study population are assessed at the same or a similar point in time.[19] Cross-sectional studies may employ primary data collection (e.g., via surveys, examinations, or testing of collected biological samples) or secondary data sources (e.g., medical charts or administrative claims) or both. Cross-sectional studies with an appropriate sampling design provide an efficient means to estimate the prevalence of health behaviors (e.g., smoking), health states (prevalence of vaccination against measles), and health outcomes, particularly chronic conditions (hypertension, diabetes). With the resulting data, associations between exposures and patient characteristics or disease prevalence (such as prevalence odds) can be estimated.

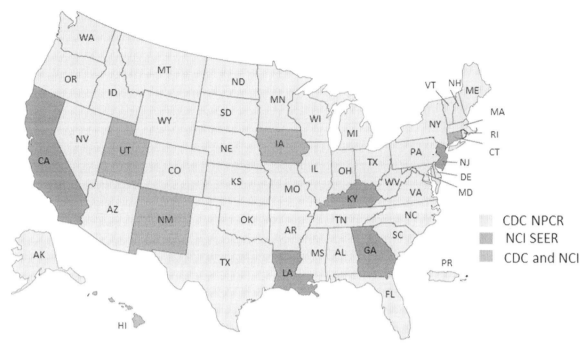

FIG. 6.4 Surveillance, Epidemiology and End Results (SEER) areas and non-SEER areas population-based cancer registries in the United States. *CDC*, Centers for Disease Control and Prevention; NCI, National Cancer Institute; NPCR, National Program of Cancer Registries. (https://commons.wikimedia.org/wiki/File: United_States_Public_Domain_Map.svg. This image is a modified work of a Unites States Department of Justice employee, taken or made as as part of that person's official duties. As a work of the US federal government, the image is in the public domain (17USC §101 and 105).)

Furthermore, repeated cross-sectional studies in the same population can be used to establish trends over time—for instance, to evaluate the effect of a public health intervention or policy change. One example is the NHANES, which has been conducting cross-sectional interviews and exams of the US population since the early 1960s in order to understand the prevalence and risk factors for disease.[20]

A principal limitation of cross-sectional studies is inherent temporal ambiguity, the inability to separate disease risk factors from disease consequences (i.e., to determine cause and effect). In addition, cross-sectional surveys often utilize self-reported health or exposure data, which suffer from potential (differential) recall bias, in which participants with certain health outcomes may be more likely to recall an exposure than those without. Lastly, prevalent patients in cross-sectional studies will be enriched for those with longer duration of disease.[21]

Cohort studies

In cohort studies, two or more groups without the outcome under study are identified based on their

> ### BOX 6.7
> ### Observational Study Design
>
> - The design of real-world observational studies depends on the type of research question and type of data available for a study
> - Real-world observational studies seek to estimate the causal relationship between drug exposures and outcomes of interest
> - Unlike RCTs, in observational studies, the investigator does not assign the treatment

different level (magnitude, presence/absence) of an exposure (e.g., a disease or treatment).[19] The exposure status may not be known at the time of study initiation, so as long as there is expected heterogeneity in exposure status, two or more cohorts can be subsequently derived. Examples include the Nurses' Health Studies,[22] which enrolled participants in the original cohort based on their profession (registered nurse), and the Framingham Heart Study,[23] which enrolled participants from one location (Framingham, MA). Many cohorts with various exposures (e.g., smoking status, oral contraceptive use, hyperlipidemia, statin use) have been derived from these study populations, enabling the identification of numerous risk factors and corresponding opportunities to intervene in public health.[24,25] In secondary data studies, exposed and unexposed cohorts are often derived from patients with a shared insurance provider (i.e., administrative claims database studies), healthcare provider (electronic health record [EHR] studies), or simply based on a set of participating sites or centers.

Generally, cohort studies are prospective (meaning that exposure information is collected prior to outcome status), which is the key to mitigating certain types of bias (e.g., recall bias and differential misclassification).[21] This definition holds whether or not a study is utilizing data from a contemporary or historical time period (e.g., a study can be historical and prospective).[21]

The "parallel group" cohort study is frequently used in real-world studies evaluating drug effectiveness and safety, whereby a cohort of new initiators of a drug are compared to new initiators of another drug with regard to subsequent clinical outcomes of interest.[26,27] In cohort studies, both absolute event rates (e.g., per 1000 person-years) as well as relative measures (e.g., relative risk, hazard ratio) can be estimated.[21] This is important as the absolute risk or rate is necessary to determine population impact, such as the number needed to harm or number of events expected to be caused by various treatments.

Case-control studies

In case-control studies, patients are selected based on the presence (cases) or absence (controls) of the outcome of interest. The prevalence of the exposure is then compared between cases and controls in order to estimate a measure of association (often, the odds ratio). In general, studies should include incident cases (or recently diagnosed cases) as prevalent patient populations will be enriched in those with longer duration of disease and if the exposure is associated with recovery or survival, bias will result.[21]

These studies are well suited for study of rare outcomes and when there is a long induction period between the exposure and outcome.[28] For instance, a case-control study was used to identify the association between maternal use of diethylstilbestrol and clear cell carcinoma among girls and young women (aged 14–22 years) who had been exposed in utero.[29] The long latency between exposure and incident cancer and rarity of the outcome made this study design appropriate. Critical to the success of a case-control study is the appropriate selection of controls.[21] Conceptually, controls should represent the population from which cases are drawn (i.e., they should reflect the

exposure prevalence in the population from which cases arose). Frequently, matching is employed to ensure cases and controls are similar on a set of known characteristics that may affect exposure prevalence. Hospital-based case-control studies are studies in which cases are identified in the hospital and their controls are selected from a pool of inpatients with other conditions. Nested case-control studies are those conducted within a cohort study; cases are those that arose during follow-up, and controls can be selected from a pool of cohort members free of the outcome (Box 6.8). Several mechanisms exist; controls can be selected at the end of the study, they can be selected at the same time a case is identified, or selected from the at-risk pool at study start (called case-cohort studies). The nested case-control makes sense particularly when additional and costly or resource intensive exposure information is needed. Rather than collecting these data (e.g., full genome sequencing) on the entire cohort, limiting to cases and a group of controls can be a more efficient use of resources.

Meta-analysis of observational studies

Meta-analysis refers to the contrasting, estimating of differences, or synthesis of results across individual studies. An initial step in this process is the conduct of a systematic literature review, which aims to apply a consistent and transparent method to the identification of, and abstraction from, in-scope literature on the study topic. The conduct of a systematic review typically entails the development of a search frame (e.g., specific databases, published vs. gray literature, etc.), one or more search algorithms (terms, keywords, and operators), a set of study inclusion/exclusion criteria, and an abstraction form to ensure consistent collection of required data elements. A key underlying meta-analytic principle is that quantitative synthesis of results across studies should only be done if one would have expected the same result in each included study.[21] In the context of observational studies, in particular, the topic of meta-analysis has

---

BOX 6.8
Types of Observational Studies

- The most frequently used study designs are cross-sectional, cohort, and case-control design
- Cross-sectional studies assess exposures and health outcomes at one (the same or similar) point in time
- Cohort studies are prospective, meaning that exposure information is collected prior to outcome status, regardless of the study utilizing data from a contemporary or a historical time period
- In case-control studies, the prevalence of the exposure is compared between cases and controls in order to estimate a measure of association (e.g., odds ratio)

been sometimes controversial. This is because of the heterogeneity of observational studies, even on the same topic, with regard to design, included populations, exposure or case definitions, analytic approach, and study quality. A rigorous evaluation of included studies is therefore warranted in order to carefully understand each study and sources of heterogeneity and determine whether an individual study analysis is more appropriate than a synthesis of results across studies. For studies determined to be homogenous enough or where meta-regression may be employed to account for heterogeneity, meta-analysis can proceed. Generally, this entails use of either a fixed or random effects model to estimate the weighted average of the effect estimate pooled across included studies. Indirect comparisons via network meta-analyses are used to make comparisons between two treatments included in different studies, although typically randomized and not observational studies are used for this application (Box 6.9).

BOX 6.9
Meta-Analysis of Observational Studies

- Meta-analysis allows for synthesis of results across several individual studies
- Meta-analysis can be performed if included studies were homogenous enough or if meta-regression was employed to account for heterogeneity

Design Considerations in Large Secondary Data Sources

The use of secondary data sources (EHR, administrative claims) is increasingly prevalent in pharmacoepidemiologic investigations. In this case, the data exist already and there is no ability to influence how or what data has been collected. Rather than study design therefore, the question relates to analytic design in the context of the clinical question and how to best address sources of bias given the strengths and limitations of the available data. As previously discussed, these data sources often include very large numbers of patients, making power or precision less of a concern. There are also frequently large amounts of data for each person, although they may have been collected for purposes other than research and so not extremely granular or specific to the study question. Given these attributes, one approach in selecting analytic design is to consider the primary source of treatment variability.[27] For instance, if a drug exposure varies over time within an individual and has a rapid wash-out, and the outcome of interest is acute at onset, a case-crossover design may be useful.[30] In this analytic design patients serve as their own cases and controls, which is useful in that stable confounding factors (e.g., gender, age, comorbidities, genetic profile) are inherently balanced (Fig. 6.5).[31] The use of an instrumental variable approach may be feasible if providers or health centers tend to utilize different treatments, for

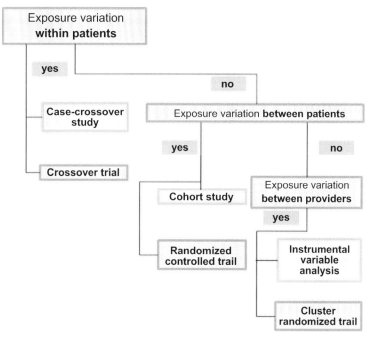

FIG. 6.5 Study design choice by source of exposure variation.

reasons other than the make-up of their patient populations (e.g., preference, formulary)[32] (Box 6.10).

SELECTED ASPECTS OF REPORTING AND INTERPRETATION OF STUDY RESULTS

There are significant environmental drivers toward more efficient and generalizable evidence generation than that derived from RCTs alone. The 21st Century Cures Act,[33] for instance, signed into law in December 2016, legislates the development of a framework to use RWD to support not only safety but also the approval of new therapeutic indications, without compromising the high standard set for evidence-based decision making. The ability to utilize real-world studies as a means for clinical, economic, and regulatory decision is predicated on the ability to generate high quality (i.e., valid) evidence in an ethical, transparent, and reproducible manner. A number of concerns have been raised, however, about the current state of real-world studies, including among them uncertainty of their internal validity, a frequent lack of clarity around methodologic and analytical decisions, the potential for "data dredging" and selective publication, and the potential for poor data quality to affect results. Even when the most rigorous scientific process is utilized, there will be limitations, uncertainty, and potential sources of bias. To this end, suggested best practices were recently published by a joint task force of the International Society for Pharmacoepidemiology and the International Society for Pharmacoeconomics and Outcomes Research with an eye toward addressing these concerns for hypothesis-evaluating studies, in particular of the type needed for such decision making[34] (Fig. 6.2). These recommendations parallel the expectations for conducting experimental studies in many ways (Fig. 6.6).

BOX 6.10
Design Considerations in Large Secondary Data Sources

When designing an observational study, it has to be remembered that the data exist already and there is no ability to influence how or what data has been collected

A priori, determine and declare that a study is a Hypothesis Evaluation Treatment Effectiveness (HETE) study or an Exploratory study based on conditions outlined below

Post a HETE study protocol and analysis plan on a public study registration site prior to conducting the study analysis

Publish HETE study results with attestation to conformance and/or deviation from the study protocol and original analysis plan. Possible sites include a medical journal, or a publicly available website

Enable opportunities to replicate HETE studies (i.e., for other researchers to be able to reproduce the same findings using the same data set and analytic approach). The ISPE companion paper lists information that should be reported in order to make the operational and design decisions behind a RWD study transparent enough for other researchers to reproduce the conduct of the study

Perform HETE studies on a different data source and population that the one used to generate the hypotheses to be tested unless it is not feasible (e.g. another data set is not included)

Authors of the original study should work to publicly address the methodological criticisms of their study once it is published

FIG. 6.6 Recommendations for good procedural practices for hypothesis evaluating treatment effectiveness studies (HETE). *RWD*, real-world data; *ISPE*, international society of pharmacoepidemiology. (Adapted from Berger ML, et al. Good practices for real-world data studies of treatment and/or comparative effectiveness: recommendations from the joint ISPOR-ISPE Special Task Force on real-world evidence in health care decision making. *Pharmacoepidemiol Drug Saf*. 2017;26(9):1033–1039. https://doi.org/10.1002/pds.4297.)

CONCLUSION

In summary, there is an increasingly strategic role for epidemiologic real-world studies throughout the product life cycle. Real-world evidence has been and will continue to be used to make decisions that impact the public health. As is the case with any rapidly evolving field, ensuring state-of-the-art scientific thinking and following good practices will ensure that the promise of efficient and valid evidence from real-world studies can be realized (Box 6.11).

REFERENCES

1. Makady A, et al. What is real-world data? A review of definitions based on literature and stakeholder interviews. *Value Health.* 2017;20(7):858–865.
2. Torre C, Martins AP. Overview of pharmacoepidemiological databases in the assessment of medicines under real-life conditions. In: Lunet N, ed. *Epidemiology - Current Perspectives on Research and Practice.* InTech; 2012:208.
3. Tanaka S, Tanaka S, Kawakami K. Methodological issues in observational studies and non-randomized controlled trials in oncology in the era of big data. *Jpn J Clin Oncol.* 2015;45(4):323–327.
4. Harpe SE. Chapter 4. Using secondary data in pharmacoepidemiology. In: Yang Y, West-Strum D, eds. *Understanding Pharmacoepidemiology.* New York, NY: The McGraw-Hill Companies; 2011.
5. Selby JV. Linking automated databases for research in managed care settings. *Ann Intern Med.* 1997;127(8 Pt 2):719–724.
6. Meray N, et al. Probabilistic record linkage is a valid and transparent tool to combine databases without a patient identification number. *J Clin Epidemiol.* 2007;60(9):883–891.
7. Dore DD, et al. Linkage of routinely collected oncology clinical data with health insurance claims data—an example with aromatase inhibitors, tamoxifen, and all-cause mortality. *Pharmacoepidemiol Drug Saf.* 2012;21(suppl 2):29–36.
8. Herk-Sukel MP, et al. Record linkage for pharmacoepidemiological studies in cancer patients. *Pharmacoepidemiol Drug Saf.* 2012;21(1):94–103.
9. van Herk-Sukel MP, et al. New opportunities for drug outcomes research in cancer patients: the linkage of the Eindhoven Cancer Registry and the PHARMO Record Linkage System. *Eur J Cancer.* 2010;46(2):395–404.
10. Parsons VL, et al. Design and estimation for the national health interview survey, 2006-2015. *Vital Health Stat.* 2014;2(165):1–53.
11. Blackwell DL, Lucas JW, Clarke TC. Summary health statistics for U.S. adults: national health interview survey, 2012. *Vital Health Stat.* 2014;10(260):1–161.
12. NCHS, Technical Notes for Summary Health Statistics Tables: National Health Interview Survey. CDC.
13. Gliklich RE, Dreyer NA. *Registries for Evaluating Patient Outcomes: A User's Guide.* 2nd ed. Rockville, MD: Agency for Healthcare Research and Quality; 2010.
14. Dreyer NA, Garner S. Registries for robust evidence. *JAMA.* 2009;302(7):790–791.
15. Parkin DM. The role of cancer registries in cancer control. *Int J Clin Oncol.* 2008;13(2):102–111.
16. Jensen OM, Storm HH. Purposes and uses of cancer registration. In: Jensen OM, et al., eds. *Cancer Registration. Principles and Methods.* Lyon: IARC; 1991:7–21.
17. Tyczynski JE. Pharmacoepidemiology and population-based cancer registries: should there be a link? In: *PharmacoEpi & Risk Management Newsletter.* 2010;3–5(6).
18. Kuo TM, Mobley LR. How generalizable are the SEER registries to the cancer populations of the USA? *Cancer Causes Control.* 2016;27(9):1117–1126.
19. Coggon D, Barker DJP, Rose G. *Epidemiology for the Uninitiated.* 5th ed. London: BMJ Books; 2003.
20. *National Health and Nutrition Examination Survey, C.f.D.C.a.P.N.H.a.N.E.;* 2017. Available from: https://www.cdc.gov/nchs/nhanes/about_nhanes.htm.
21. Rothman KJ, Greenland S, Lash TL. *Modern Epidemiology.* 3rd ed. United States: Philadelphia: Wolters Kluwer Health/Lippincott Williams & Wilkins; 2008.
22. *Nurses' Health Studies;* 2017. Available from: https://www.hsph.harvard.edu/nutritionsource/nurses-health-study/.
23. Framingham Heart Study: A Project of the National Heart, Lung, and Blood Institute and Boston University. https://www.framinghamheartstudy.org/. Accessed December 13, 2017.
24. Mendis S. The contribution of the Framingham Heart Study to the prevention of cardiovascular disease: a global perspective. *Prog Cardiovasc Dis.* 2010;53(1):10–14. https://doi.org/10.1016/j.pcad.2010.1001.1001.
25. Colditz GA, Philpott SE, Hankinson SE. The impact of the nurses' health study on population health: prevention, translation, and control. *Am J Public Health.* 2016;106(9):1540–1545. https://doi.org/10.2105/AJPH.2016.303343. Epub 2016 Jul 26.
26. Johnson ES, et al. The incident user design in comparative effectiveness research. *Pharmacoepidemiol Drug Saf.* 2013;22(1):1–6. https://doi.org/10.1002/pds. 3334. Epub 2012 Oct 1.

27. Schneeweiss S. A basic study design for expedited safety signal evaluation based on electronic healthcare data. *Pharmacoepidemiol Drug Saf.* 2010;19(8):858−868.

28. Silva IDS. *Cancer epidemiology: principles and methods.* France: International Agency for Research on Cancer; 1999.

29. Herbst AL, Ulfelder H, Poskanzer DC. Adenocarcinoma of the vagina. Association of maternal stilbestrol therapy with tumor appearance in young women. *N Engl J Med.* 1971; 284(15):878−881. https://doi.org/10.1056/NEJM19710 4222841604.

30. Kilpatrick RD, et al. The association of vitamin D use with hypercalcemia and hyperphosphatemia in hemodialysis patients: a case-crossover study. *Pharmacoepidemiol Drug Saf.* 2011;20(9):914−921.

31. Maclure M. The case-crossover design: a method for studying transient effects on the risk of acute events. *Am J Epidemiol.* 1991;133(2):144−153.

32. Streeter AJ, et al. Adjusting for unmeasured confounding in nonrandomized longitudinal studies: a methodological review. *J Clin Epidemiol.* 2017;87:23−34. https://doi.org/ 10.1016/j.jclinepi.2017.04.022. Epub 2017 Apr 28.

33. Kesselheim AS, Avorn J. New "21st century cures" legislation: speed and ease vs science. *JAMA.* 2017; 317(6):581−582. https://doi.org/10.1001/jama.2016.20 640.

34. Berger ML, et al. Good practices for real-world data studies of treatment and/or comparative effectiveness: recommendations from the joint ISPOR-ISPE Special Task Force on real-world evidence in health care decision making. *Pharmacoepidemiol Drug Saf.* 2017;26(9):1033−1039. https://doi.org/10.1002/pds.4297.

CHAPTER 7

Vaccine Pharmacovigilance

FABIO LIEVANO, MD • MARIETTA VAZQUEZ, MD, FAAP •
JEREMY D. JOKINEN, PHD, MS

INTRODUCTION

Vaccinations are one of the most effective and cost-saving cost-effective public health interventions[1] and have achieved remarkable success globally by substantially reducing morbidity and mortality to diseases that once were very common (Box 7.1).[2-5] Although vaccines are highly effective and have a favorable benefit-risk profile, all vaccines have a safety profile that needs to be monitored like any other pharmaceutical product.[6] In recent decades, the availability and use of certain vaccines has vastly increased around the world, thereby considerably reducing the incidence of vaccine-preventable disease. In some instances, the incidence of adverse events due to vaccination appears more frequently and prominently than the disease itself. In these situations, it may appear that vaccinations are no longer necessary, but it has been observed that if vaccination coverage decreases, and/or if large cohorts of unvaccinated individuals accumulate, eventually the disease may return and cause large epidemics.[7,8] In some circumstances, false claims and rumors about the safety of a vaccine may also lead to lowered vaccination coverage rates and result in

subsequent outbreaks.[9,10] These consequences have harmed global immunization efforts, as in the case of polio eradication and vaccination campaigns in West Africa in the early 2000s.[11,12]

Timely surveillance of adverse events due to vaccines is critical to make vaccination efforts effective and to prevent loss of confidence in the vaccines by the public and governments. Unfounded fears about the safety of a vaccine may have significant consequences in public health and loss of confidence among the public.[13] In addition, lawsuits, lack of funding for research and development of new vaccines, and loss of interest among vaccine manufacturers may occur.

Monitoring of vaccine safety is complicated by both the disease prevalence and epidemiology. For example, influenza vaccine is mostly used in colder seasons, cholera and dengue vaccines are used in endemic areas, and zoster vaccine is applied to seniors. In each circumstance, it is always essential to balance the risks and benefits of a determined vaccine to a specific population. Regulators ensure that research in vaccine safety is appropriately conducted from development through postmarketing. Currently, clinical trials involve tens of thousands of individuals during all phases of vaccine research and approval. However, even after vaccine licensure, vaccines continue to be monitored through large epidemiological cohort studies to identify any gap and minimize the risk of adverse events (Box 7.2).

Unlike other pharmaceutical products, the general consensus is that vaccines should provide very high efficacy against the disease and few or no adverse events. In addition, some adverse events may not be seen during the clinical development program and may only be observed after some thousands, hundreds of thousands, or millions of doses are administered. Additionally, as vaccine effectiveness results in reduced threat from the disease, the benefit-risk ratio is

> **BOX 7.1**
> **Importance of Vaccine Safety**
>
> - Vaccinations are one of the most cost-effective public health interventions.
> - The use of vaccines has vastly increased in many places of the world, reducing the incidence of vaccine-preventable disease.
> - Rumors and false claims may hinder vaccination program.
> - Surveillance of vaccines is critical to maintain public confidence.

maintained only to the extent that safety is confirmed in the broad, on-market experience.[14] Under these conditions, the identification of a safety signal would require the involvement of many thousands of patients in an epidemiological study to assess the true incidence of the adverse reaction.

In the United States, examples of large epidemiological studies conducted after vaccine licensure to better understand the relationship of vaccines to significant signals of adverse events include:

- Autism and measles, mumps, and rubella (MMR) vaccine, with over 90,000 privately insured participants in the United States demonstrated that receipt of the MMR vaccine was not associated with increased risk of autism spectrum disorders.[15]
- Increase of the incidence of febrile seizures with the quadrivalent measles, mumps, rubella, and varicella (MMRV) vaccine versus the MMR and varicella vaccines given separately. The study enrolled over 83,000 MMRV vaccine recipients compared with over 370,000 recipients of MMR and varicella vaccines. The results demonstrated that in the 12- to 23-month-olds who received their first dose of measles-containing vaccine, fever and seizure episodes were seen 7–10 days after vaccination. Vaccination with MMRV results in one additional febrile seizure for every 2300 doses given.[16]
- Surveillance for 16 prespecified autoimmune disorders observed during an observational safety study of the quadrivalent human papillomavirus vaccine (HPV4) in 189,629 women who received ≥1 dose of HPV4 and were followed for 180 days after each dose in two managed care organizations.[17]

Vaccines hold tremendous promise to continue contributing to public health. However, the nature of the disease epidemiology and intended use of vaccines—doses are traditionally administered to otherwise healthy individuals—result in a need for robust and carefully designed pharmacovigilance practices to ensure the safety of the public is maintained.

MODERN VACCINE HISTORY RELATED TO PHARMACOVIGILANCE

Rotavirus Vaccine: an Example of Safety Surveillance

In 1998, a rotavirus vaccine (RotaShield) was licensed for use in the United States. Clinical trials in the United States, Finland, and Venezuela had found it to be 80%–100% effective at preventing severe diarrhea caused by rotavirus A (Box 7.3); researchers had detected no statistically significant serious adverse effects.[18] The manufacturer of the vaccine, however, withdrew it from the market in 1999, after reports that the vaccine may have contributed to an increased risk for intussusception, or bowel obstruction, in one of every 4670–9474 vaccinated infants. After 8 years of delay, other manufacturers were able to introduce new generation rotavirus vaccines which were shown to be more safe and effective in children.[19]

Measles, Mumps, and Rubella Vaccine: Autism Controversy

In the United Kingdom, the MMR vaccine was the subject of controversy after the publication of a 1998 paper by Andrew Wakefield and others in *The Lancet* which reported case histories of 12 children mostly with autism spectrum disorders with the onset of the condition soon after administration of the vaccine.[9] At a 1998 press conference, Wakefield suggested that giving children the vaccines in three separate doses would be safer than a single vaccination. This suggestion was not supported by the paper, and multiple large subsequent peer-reviewed studies have failed to show any association between the vaccine

---

BOX 7.2
Monitoring Vaccine Safety

- Each vaccine's risks and benefits must be balanced depending on the disease prevalence and epidemiology.
- Vaccines are generally administered to healthy people and must therefore provide very high efficacy against diseases and few or no adverse effects.
- Some adverse events may not be seen during the development program and clinical trials.
- Therefore, large epidemiological studies are needed post vaccine licensure to assess the true incidence of adverse reactions.

BOX 7.3
Safety Surveillance: the Rotavirus Vaccine and Infants

- In 1998, a rotavirus vaccine was licensed after clinical trials showed it to be 80%–100% effective with no significant adverse effects.
- However, the vaccine was withdrawn in 1999 after discovering that it may have increased the risk of intussusception in one of every 4670–9474 vaccinated infants.
- Eight years later, other manufacturers were able to introduce safer, more effective vaccines.

and autism.[20] It later surfaced that Wakefield had received funding from plaintiffs against vaccine manufacturers and that he had not properly disclosed colleagues or medical authorities potential conflicts of interest[21]; if this had been known, the article may have never been accepted to The Lancet. Wakefield has been exposed on scientific grounds for influencing a decline in vaccination rates in many countries with this made-up data (vaccination rates in the United Kingdom dropped to 80% in the years following the study),[22] as well as on ethical grounds for the way the research was conducted.[23] In 2004, the MMR-and-autism interpretation of the paper was formally retracted by Wakefield's coauthors,[24] and in 2010, *The Lancet's* editors fully retracted the paper (Box 7.4).[25]

The Centers for Disease Control (CDC)[26] and the Institute of Medicine's Immunization Safety Review Committee[20] have concluded that there is no evidence of a link between the MMR vaccine and autism. Additionally, a systematic review conducted by the Cochrane Library concluded that there is no credible link between the MMR vaccine and autism.[27] The Cochrane review also recognized that the MMR vaccine has prevented diseases that still may cause complications including death; the lack of confidence in the MMR vaccine has adversely affected public health and the vaccination program.

Lawsuits against pharmaceutical companies were brought by parents who believed there may be a link between vaccination and autism, but the mounting evidence to the contrary from numerous safety surveillance efforts was conclusive. A special court convened in the United States to review claims under the National Vaccine Injury Compensation Program ruled on February 12, 2009 that parents of autistic children are not entitled to compensation in their contention that certain vaccines caused autism in their children.[28]

Polio Eradication: the Boycott in Northern Nigeria

Public trust is essential in promoting public health because such trust plays an important role in the population's compliance with the proposed public health interventions, especially vaccination programs. If public trust is eroded, as in the MMR vaccine example above, the result can be rejection of safe and effective health interventions.

In northern Nigeria in 2003, the political and religious leaders of Kano and other states brought the polio immunization campaign to a halt by calling on parents not to allow their children to be immunized.[29] These leaders argued that the polio vaccine could be contaminated with antifertility agents, HIV, and cancerous agents.

The boycotts ostensibly came about in response to rumors, endorsed by high-ranking public figures, that the polio vaccine was an American conspiracy to spread HIV and cause infertility in Muslim girls.[31] However, other complex factors were at play. The international response to these boycotts was impressive, and successful negotiations eventually restored immunization programs (Box 7.5).[32] Internal dynamics of the boycott to the vaccination campaign have not yet been thoroughly reviewed. Societal factors that enabled these rumors to spread at the grass-roots level and include the important views of several key individuals who fueled the issue at that time. The challenges of society, politics and personalities in Kano suggest further evaluations and learning that may be applied today (Fig. 7.1).[29]

MONITORING VACCINE SAFETY DURING PRELICENSURE
Clinical Trials

Vaccines, like other pharmaceutical products, undergo thorough and extensive laboratory and animal studies to assess efficacy and safety (Box 7.6). Phase I trials

---

BOX 7.4
"Vaccines Cause Autism": the Measles, Mumps, and Rubella Vaccine Controversy

- In 1998, Andrew Wakefield and others published a paper linking administration of the measles, mumps, and rubella (MMR) vaccine with the onset of autism spectrum disorders in 12 children.
- Subsequent to publication, it was discovered that Wakefield had received funding from plaintiffs against vaccine manufacturers. Subsequent peer-reviewed studies have failed to show any association between the MMR vaccine and autism.
- Despite this, vaccination rates in the United Kingdom dropped to 80% in the years following Wakefield's "study."

BOX 7.5
Boycott in Northern Nigeria: the Polio Vaccine Controversy

- In 2003, major Nigerian political and religious leaders told parents not to let their children be immunized against polio because the vaccine could be contaminated with HIV and harmful agents.
- These boycotts came in response to complex societal factors, including rumors that the polio vaccine was an American conspiracy to spread HIV.
- Successful negotiations eventually restored the immunization program.

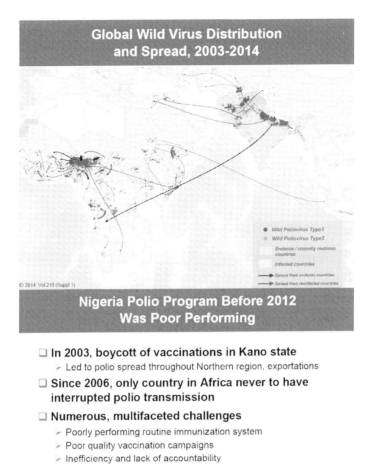

Global Wild Virus Distribution and Spread, 2003-2014

ID 2014: Vol.210 (Suppl 1)

- Wild Poliovirus Type1
- Wild Poliovirus Type3
- Endemic / recently endemic countries
- Infected countries
- Spread from endemic countries
- Spread from re-infected countries

Nigeria Polio Program Before 2012 Was Poor Performing

❑ **In 2003, boycott of vaccinations in Kano state**
  ➢ Led to polio spread throughout Northern region, exportations

❑ **Since 2006, only country in Africa never to have interrupted polio transmission**

❑ **Numerous, multifaceted challenges**
  ➢ Poorly performing routine immunization system
  ➢ Poor quality vaccination campaigns
  ➢ Inefficiency and lack of accountability

FIG. 7.1 Global re-emergence after temporary boycott of polio vaccination in Nigeria, 2003.[30]

BOX 7.6
Three Phases of Clinical Trials

- Phase 1: few participants; antibody production is measured; likely only common adverse events will be identified.
- Phase 2: hundreds of participants; components, formulation technique, number of doses, and the best dose are studied and identified.
- Phase 3: number of participants (often thousands) depends on estimated efficacy; safety data are collected as common local and systemic reactions are identified.

typically involve few participants and are likely to detect only commonly occurring adverse events; in the phase I studies, antibody production is usually measured. In phase II, hundreds of participants are enrolled, and among the studies include evaluation of different concentrations, components, formulation techniques, number of doses, and the identification of the best dose. In phase III, the sample size depends on the estimates around efficacy. In regard to safety, common local and systemic reactions are identified. Parallel to the assessment of safety and efficacy in any phase of development is ensuring the vaccines follow Good Manufacturing Practices and that sufficient lots are tested for efficacy and safety (Fig. 7.2).

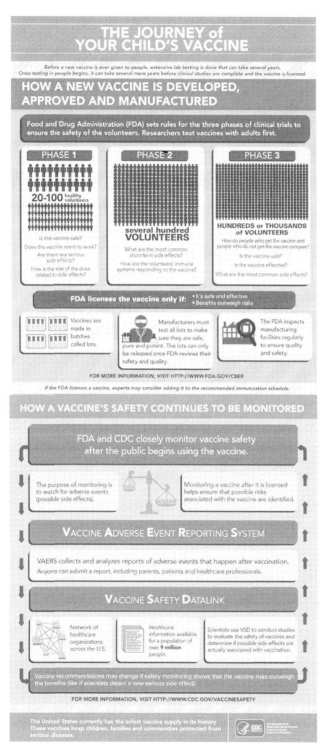

FIG. 7.2 Journey of a new vaccine: from development to license for use.[33]

Vaccine Product Approval Process

The US Food and Drug Administration's (FDA) Center for Biologics Evaluation and Research (CBER) is responsible for regulating vaccines in the United States.

Each sponsor of a new vaccine product must follow a multistep approval process, which typically includes the following:

- An Investigational New Drug (IND) application
- Prelicensure vaccine clinical trials
- A Biologics License Application (BLA)
- Inspection of the manufacturing facility
- Presentation of findings to FDA's Vaccines and Related Biological Products Advisory Committee (VRBPAC)
- Usability testing of product labeling

Vaccine clinical development follows the same general pathway as for drugs and other biologics. A sponsor who wishes to begin clinical trials with a vaccine must submit an IND application to the FDA (Box 7.7). The IND describes the vaccine, its method of manufacture, and quality control tests for its release. Also included is information about the vaccine's safety and ability to elicit a protective immune response (immunogenicity) in animal testing, as well as the proposed clinical protocol for studies in humans.

Premarketing (prelicensure) vaccine clinical trials are typically conducted in three phases, as is the case for any drug or biologic. Initial human studies, referred to as Phase 1, are safety and immunogenicity studies performed in a small number of closely monitored subjects. Phase 2 studies are dose-ranging studies and may enroll hundreds of subjects. Finally, Phase 3 trials typically enroll thousands of individuals and provide the critical documentation of effectiveness and important additional safety data required for licensing. At any stage of the clinical or animal studies, if data raise significant concerns about either safety or effectiveness, the FDA may request additional information or studies, or may halt ongoing clinical studies.

If successful, the completion of all three phases of clinical development can be followed by the submission of a BLA. To be considered, the license application must provide the multidisciplinary FDA reviewer team (medical officers, microbiologists, chemists, biostatisticians, etc.) with the efficacy and safety information necessary to make a benefit-risk assessment and recommend or oppose the approval of a vaccine. Also during this stage, the proposed manufacturing facility undergoes a preapproval inspection during which production of the vaccine as it is in progress is examined in detail.

Following the FDA's review of a license application for a new indication, the sponsor and the FDA may present their findings to the FDA's VRBPAC. This non-FDA expert committee (scientists, physicians, biostatisticians, and a consumer representative) provides advice to the agency regarding the safety and efficacy of the vaccine for the proposed indication.

Vaccine approval also requires the provision of adequate product labeling to allow healthcare providers to understand the vaccine's proper use, including its potential benefits and risks, to communicate with patients and parents, and to safely deliver the vaccine to the public.[34]

POSTLICENSURE

The FDA continues to oversee the production of vaccines after the vaccine product and the manufacturing processes are approved, in order to ensure continuing safety (Box 7.8). After licensure, monitoring of the

---

BOX 7.7
Vaccine Approval: a Multistep Process

- The sponsor of a new vaccine must submit an Investigational New Drug application, which describes the vaccine's method of production, safety, and efficacy to the US Food and Drug Administration (FDA).
- During or after clinical trials (Phases 1, 2, and 3), the FDA can halt studies or request additional information or studies.
- If all three phases are successful, the sponsor can submit a Biologics License Application which informs the FDA of the benefit-risk assessment based on safety and efficacy information. The proposed manufacturing facility must also have a preapproval inspection.
- After the FDA's review, the FDA and the sponsor must present their findings to the Vaccines and Related Biological Products Advisory Committee.
- Finally, if approved, the vaccine product must be labeled properly.

BOX 7.8
Postlicensure Requirements

- The product and manufacturing process must be monitored by the US Food and Drug Administration (FDA) for as long as the manufacturer holds a license for the product.
- Unless an alternative procedure is approved, manufacturers have to submit the results of their own vaccine lot tests (and possibly samples of each lot) to the FDA upon request.
- Even once on the market, many vaccines have Phase 4 studies in order to continue identifying adverse events.
- The Vaccine Adverse Event Reporting System helps the government identify problems.

vaccine product and of production activities, including periodic facility inspections, must continue as long as the manufacturer holds a license for the product. If requested by the FDA, manufacturers are required to submit to the FDA the results of their own tests for potency, safety, and purity for each vaccine lot. They may also require submitting samples of each vaccine lot to the FDA for testing. However, if the sponsor describes an alternative procedure which provides continued assurance of safety, purity, and potency, the CBER may determine that routine submission of lot release protocols (showing results of applicable tests) and samples is not necessary.

Until a vaccine is administered to the general population, not all potential adverse events can be anticipated. Thus, many vaccines undergo Phase 4 studies—formal, protocol-driven studies of a vaccine once it is commercially available. Furthermore, surveillance systems are in place to further detect adverse effects. The Vaccine Adverse Event Reporting System (VAERS) is a passive surveillance reporting system that is used to identify problems after marketing begins.[35]

The US FDA's CBER regulates biologic products and ensures their safety and efficacy (Box 7.9). These products include blood and blood products, vaccines, and cellular, tissue, and gene therapies. CBER evaluates safety throughout the product's life cycle and has integrated the following programs into its regulatory decision-making processes[36] (Fig. 7.3):

1. Postlicensure Rapid Immunization Safety Monitoring (PRISM)—a subcomponent of the Sentinel System focusing on vaccine safety surveillance. PRISM has been deployed for refinement and evaluation of

---

BOX 7.9
Three Surveillance Programs

- Center for Biologics Evaluation and Research 's Postlicensure Rapid Immunization Safety Monitoring helps proactively evaluate safety signals during premarket and postmarket reviews.
- Sentinel assessments use automated surveillance tools to improve patient privacy and monitoring efficacy.
- The Centers for Disease Control and Prevention's Vaccine Safety Datalink partners with large health plans to help monitor and understand rare and serious adverse events.

A variety of automated tools for active safety surveillance have been developed for FDA's use in Sentinel. These include routine querying tools such as summary tables, modular programs, and software toolkits that can be used quickly in a distributed data environment. Collectively, these tools support FDA's Active Risk Identification and Analysis (ARIA) program.

Capability	Summary Table	Level 1 Query	Level 2 Query	Level 3 Query
Descriptive Analyses				
Calculate prevalence and incidence rates	✓	✓	✓	✓
Assess exposure to a medical product and define exposed time		✓	✓	✓
Allow optional cohort inclusion and/or exclusion criteria		✓	✓	✓
Define clinical concepts using complex algorithms		✓	✓	✓
Define clinical concepts using laboratory result values		✓	✓	✓
Adjusted Analyses with Sophisticated Confounding Control				
Covariate identification and extraction			✓	✓
Propensity score estimation and matching			✓	✓
Self-controlled risk interval (SCRI) design			✓	✓
Sequential Adjusted Analyses with Sophisticated Confounding Control				
Binomial maximized sequential probability ratio testing				✓

For more information concerning ARIA and Sentinel surveillance tools, click on the links below.

- Active Risk Identification and Analysis (ARIA)
- Routine Querying Tools
- Software Toolkit Library
- Health Outcome of Interest Validations and Literature Reviews

Note that information obtained through Sentinel is intended to complement other types of data and information compiled by FDA scientists, such as adverse event reports, published study results, and clinical trials, which can be combined with Sentinel data and used by FDA to inform regulatory decisions regarding medical product safety. FDA may access the data available through Mini-Sentinel for a variety

FIG. 7.3 Surveillance tools.

Active Risk Identification and Analysis (ARIA) is FDA's active post-market risk identification and analysis system, which is comprised of pre-defined, parameterized, re-usable routine querying tools that enable safety surveillance in Sentinel. In contrast to a traditional pharmacoepidemiology study, there is no protocol and no customized programming. ARIA fulfills the FDA's Amendments Act mandate to conduct drug/medical product safety surveillance.

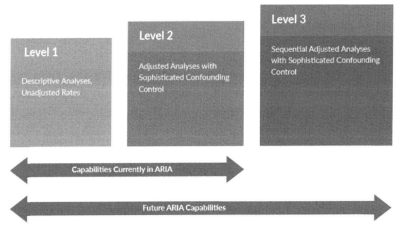

FIG. 7.4 Active risk identification and analysis (ARIA).

potential safety signals identified during premarket and postmarket reviews. One characteristic of the Sentinel System is that it enables CBER to proactively assess biologics safety, under real-world conditions, reflecting patient care in the United States. This capability enhances safety monitoring and allows CBER to systematically evaluate safety signals identified during premarket trials, as well as signals that emerge after products are released to the market.[37]

2. Sentinel assessments make use of the automated surveillance tools that support FDA's Active Risk Identification and Analysis System[38] (Fig. 7.4). This approach improves the efficiency of FDA monitoring and ensures patient privacy through the use of the Sentinel Distributed Database.

3. In addition to safety monitoring activities completed by the vaccine manufacturer and regulatory authorities, there is additional surveillance managed by the CDC. In 1990, the CDC established the Vaccine Safety Datalink (VSD) to address gaps in the scientific knowledge of rare and serious adverse events following immunizations (AEFIs). This program involves partnerships with large health plans to monitor vaccine safety.[39]

BENEFIT RISK—THE PROVIDER AND CONSUMER LEVEL

Vaccine administration differs considerably from administration of medicines because vaccines are

> ### BOX 7.10
> ### Levels of Benefit-Risk Assessments
>
> - Players involved in monitoring vaccine safety include regulatory agencies, academia, the medical community, the industry, and the general public.
> - The healthcare professional and the vaccine provider play key roles in preventing, identifying, and managing adverse events following immunization (AEFI).
> - Studies, guidelines, and algorithms can all help determine the relationship between AEFI and the vaccine.

provided to populations of children and adults that are mostly healthy. There is little or no tolerance for side effects (Box 7.10). In addition, reduction of the infectious disease as a consequence of the long-term use of a vaccine may result in complacency. This complacency may result in reoccurrence of outbreaks as demonstrated in measles outbreaks in Europe and the United States after measles elimination. The reoccurrence of disease is the result of the fall of the administration coverage.[40] Vaccine scares such as those associating the combined measles-mumps-rubella vaccine with autism, and whole-cell pertussis vaccines with encephalopathy, result in reduction of vaccination coverage, and eventually, when sufficient susceptible persons accumulate, the result is a disease resurgence.

The evaluation of the benefits and risks of vaccines should be implemented continuously and should be comprehensive. In addition to adverse event monitoring typical to medicines, the evaluation should include basic elements of purity, stability, and sterility in all phases of clinical development through postmarketing.

Safety assessments conducted by regulators, industry, and academia increase confidence in the vaccine as the amount of data of available increases and permits the identification of potential risks. Health care professionals involved with immunization and vaccine providers have a role in the prevention, early identification, investigation, and risk management of AEFIs. Health care providers should investigate AEFIs and report them in accordance with current guidelines for assessing and reporting AEFI. The ultimate objective for all involved is to ensure vaccines have a favorable benefit-risk profile.[40]

THE FUTURE
Active Surveillance

Comprehensive surveillance of AEFI is required to detect potentially serious adverse events that may not be identified in prelicensure vaccine trials. Surveillance systems, traditionally passive, relying on spontaneous reporting, now include active surveillance and supplemental strategies incorporated into vaccine safety programs. These include active screening for targeted conditions of interest (e.g., hospitalization), monitoring of new data sources, and real-time methodologies to detect changes in vaccine safety data in these sources.[41]

Real-World Evidence

Scientifically based, postmarketing safety surveillance is critical to ensure public confidence in vaccinations. Additionally, these practices ultimately reduce morbidity and mortality of vaccine-preventable diseases. The infrastructure and scientific methods for postmarketing safety surveillance have continuously improved over the last decades. Supporting and always improving this system will continue to be important as the number of people to be vaccinated continues to increase.[42]

Ongoing safety research is part of public health programs. These programs ensure regulatory agencies receive the information required to make decisions about current and future programs. Agencies require the information to address concerns and rumors when they start before they become widespread and harm immunization programs. Safety monitoring systems established in the United States and Europe, among others, with methodology that ranges from the rapid cycle analysis for expedited detection of potential safety issues to planned large observational studies have been useful to detect safety issues. However, the ultimate test depends on monitoring adverse events in large populations over several months or even years. The latter requires the link of disparate databases to make the system more efficient and enable rapid signal detection. The connection of these databases is technologically complicated, but it is necessary to avoid the same cases being reported several times and overrepresent the magnitude of the risk. As technology evolves and improves, more concerted action globally will move vaccine safety monitoring to a real-time, proactive activity.[43]

Maternal Vaccination

(Box 7.11). Maternal immunization, a public health strategy, demonstrated prevention of potentially serious disease for both mothers and their infants. The mother's antibody, transferred across the placenta, can protect babies from infections during a time when they are most needed. Although maternal vaccination can have potential benefits, many vaccines remain Category B drugs because the safety and effectiveness are not established in pregnant women or nursing mothers as part of prelicensure clinical trials.[44] Renewed efforts in evidence generation and novel pathways for approval are needed to move this strategy forward.

BOX 7.11
Vaccinations During Pregnancy

- Though maternal vaccinations can help protect infants, many vaccines are Category B drugs due to inconclusive safety and efficacy information for pregnant or nursing women.
- Pregnancy exposure registries are used to gather data on pregnancy outcomes after vaccination and the effects of drugs and vaccines given during pregnancy or while breastfeeding.
- More studies are needed.

Systems for monitoring the safety of maternal vaccination

Postlicensure vaccine safety monitoring allows for rapid identification of new adverse events as well as potential increases in known adverse events. Several methods are available to measure the postlicensure safety of vaccines given during pregnancy.

Pregnancy exposure registries collect and maintain postlicensure safety data on the effects of drugs and vaccines given during pregnancy or while breastfeeding. Sanofi Pasteur, GlaxoSmithKline, CSL Biotherapies, Merck & Co, and Novartis Vaccines and Diagnostic Research have maintained such a registry. These registries collect data on pregnancy outcomes and newborn health following vaccination.

However, with the exception of reports of incidental administration, few studies have been published using these data.

Passive systems, such as the VAERS, have been used to monitor postlicensure safety of vaccines given in the general population. These systems allow health providers, and in some cases the public, to submit reports of AEFI experienced. These systems are useful for monitoring vaccine safety across populations and for collecting information on postvaccination events.

Active surveillance systems have also been implemented as a means of directly collecting select postvaccination events from recently immunized pregnant women. Systems for performing active surveillance typically enroll pregnant women at the time of vaccination and prospectively monitor them for a defined period of time. These systems are valuable in identifying the reactogenicity of vaccines and capturing pregnancy-specific outcomes in a large sample. A recent review of 47 countries indicated that all 30 countries with a national immunization policy targeting pregnant women had a passive vaccine safety surveillance system; however, only 11 (23%) of these countries had active surveillance systems to detect serious AEFI in pregnant women and a few systems had published their findings.

Observational studies can also provide important information on the occurrence of AEFI in pregnant women (Box 7.12). For example, the VSD, established in the 1990s, is a retrospective cohort which includes health data from 9 healthcare organizations, including over 9 million US individuals each year. One of the initiatives of VSD included the establishment of a "pregnancy platform," a dataset used to monitor the safety of vaccines given in pregnancy. This dataset includes demographic information, birth information, vaccination records, hospital, emergency, and outpatient information, and other data. It also allows for

> **BOX 7.12**
> **The Future of Surveillance**
>
> - Surveillance of adverse events following immunization helps find serious adverse events that might not have been identified in prelicensure trials.
> - Active surveillance strategies are replacing passive ones that rely on spontaneous reporting.
> - Active surveillance strategies include screening for conditions of interest, monitoring new data sources, and detecting changes in vaccine safety data in real time.

the ability to conduct long-term follow-up of birth cohorts over multiple years.

Observational studies, such as the VSD, are useful as they typically include large sample sizes and are better powered to identify less common AEFI. However, they are subject to certain biases, such as confounding and misclassification.

Advances in active surveillance methods and infrastructure combined with an emphasis on maternal vaccination offer the unique opportunity to prevent vulnerable populations from potentially lethal disease. Healthcare providers play a critical role in promoting maternal vaccination. Women commonly cite concerns about the safety of a vaccination to the fetus when refusing vaccination during pregnancy; results from studies evaluating adverse pregnancy outcomes should reassure pregnant patients that maternal vaccination is safe to the fetus. Healthcare providers may find results from studies measuring the reactogenicity of vaccination during pregnancy useful when communicating to pregnant women what to expect following vaccination. To support this potentially game-changing public health strategy, continued monitoring and communication of safety information to healthcare providers and their patients is critical.

REFERENCES

1. World Bank. *World Development Report 1993. Investing in Health.* New York: Oxford University Press; 1993.
2. WHO. *Wkly Epidemiol Rec.* 1980;55:121−128.
3. Deria A, Jezek Z, Markvart K, Carrasco P, Weisfeld J. The world's last endemic case of smallpox: surveillance and containment measures. *Bull WHO.* 1980;58:279−283.
4. Progress towards regional measles elimination − worldwide, 2000-2016. *Wkly Epidemiol Rec.* 2017;92(43):649−660.
5. Surveillance systems to track progress towards polio eradication worldwide, 2015-2016. *Wkly Epidemiol Rec.* 2017;92(14):165−179.
6. Matthew M. *Biologic Development: A Regulatory Overview.* Waltham, MA: Parexel; 1993.

7. The resurgence of measles in the United States, 1989-1990. *Annu Rev Med.* 1992;43:451−463.

8. Measles outbreak—California, December 2014-February 2015. *MMWR Morb Mortal Wkly Rep.* 2015;20(64):153−154.

9. Wakefield AJ, et al. Ileal-lymphoid-nodular hyperplasia, non-specific colitis, and pervasive developmental disorder in children. *Lancet.* 1998;351:637−641.

10. Brown FK, et al. U.K. parents' decision-making about measles-mumps-rubella (MMR) vaccine 10 years after the MMR-autism controversy: a qualitative analysis. *Vaccine.* 2012;30:1855−1864.

11. Mitka M. Vaccine rumors, funding shortfall threaten to derail global polio eradication efforts. *JAMA.* 2004; 291(16):1947−1948.

12. Rey M, Girard MO. The global eradication of poliomyelitis: progress and problems. *Comp Immunol Microbiol Infect Dis.* 2008;31(2−3):317−325.

13. Khetsuriani N, et al. Impact of unfounded vaccine safety concerns on the nationwide measles-rubella immunization campaign, Georgia, 2008. *Vaccine.* 2010;28(39):6455−6462.

14. Plotkin SA. Vaccines: past, present and future. *Nat Med.* 2005;11(suppl 4):S5−S11.

15. Jain A, et al. Autism occurrence by MMR vaccine status among US children with older siblings with and without autism. *JAMA.* 2015;313(15):1534−1540.

16. Klein NP, et al. Measles-mumps-rubella-varicella combination vaccine and the risk of febrile seizures. *Pediatrics.* 2010;126(1):e1−e8.

17. Chao C, et al. Surveillance of autoimmune conditions following routine use of quadrivalent human papillomavirus vaccine. *J Intern Med.* 2012;271(2):193−203.

18. American Academy of Pediatrics. Prevention of rotavirus disease: guidelines for use of rotavirus vaccine. *Pediatrics.* 1998;102(6):1483−1491.

19. Trudy V. Intussusception among infants given an oral rotavirus vaccine. *N Engl J Med.* 2001;344:564−572.

20. Meadows M. IOM report: no link between vaccines and autism. *FDA Consum.* 2004;38(5):18−19. https://permanent. access.gpo.gov/lps1609/www.fda.gov/fdac/features/2004/504 _iom.html.

21. Deer B. Secrets of the MMR scare. How the vaccine crisis was meant to make money. *BMJ.* 2011;342:c5258.

22. Godlee F, Smith J, Marcovitch H. Wakefield's article linking MMR vaccine and autism was fraudulent. *BMJ.* 2011; 342:c7452.

23. Godlee F. Institutional research misconduct. *BMJ.* 2011; 343:d7284.

24. Murch SH. Retraction of an interpretation. *Lancet.* 2004; 363(9411):750.

25. Eggertson L. Lancet retracts 12-year-old article linking autism to MMR vaccines. *CMAJ.* 2010;182(4):E199−E200.

26. DeStefano F, Thompson WW. MMR vaccine and autism: an update of the scientific evidence. *Expert Rev Vaccines.* 2004;3(1):19−22.

27. Demicheli V, Jefferson T, Rivetti A, Price D. Vaccines for measles, mumps and rubella in children. *Cochrane Database Syst Rev.* 2005;(4):CD004407.

28. National Vaccine Information Center. *Autism & Vaccines: U.S. Court of Claims;* February 12, 2009. http://www. uscfc.uscourts.gov/omnibus-autism-proceedings.

29. Ghinai I, Willott C, Dadari I, Larsonb HJ. Listening to the rumours: what the northern Nigeria polio vaccine boycott can tell us ten years on. *Glob Public Health.* 2013;8(10): 1138−1150.

30. CDC. *Global Polio Eradication: Reaching Every Last Child;* February 17, 2015. https://www.cdc.gov/cdcgrandrounds/ pdf/archives/2015/february2015-H.pdf.

31. Raufu A. Polio cases rise in Nigeria as vaccine is shunned for fear of AIDS. *BMJ.* 2002;324(7351):1414.

32. Kaufmann JR, Feldbaum H. Diplomacy and the polio immunization boycott in Northern Nigeria. *Health Aff (Millwood).* 2009;28(4):1091−1101.

33. CDC. *The Journey of Your Child Vaccine;* 2018. https:// www.cdc.gov/vaccines/parents/infographics/journey-of-child-vaccine.html.

34. FDA. *Vaccine Product Approval Process;* 2017. https://www.fda. gov/biologicsbloodvaccines/developmentapprovalprocess/ biologicslicenseapplicationsblaprocess/ucm133096.htm.

35. HHA. *Vaccine Adverse Event Reporting System (VAERS);* 2017. https://www.fda.gov/biologicsbloodvaccines/development approvalprocess/biologicslicenseapplicationsblaprocess/ ucm133096.htm.

36. FDA. *Vaccines and Biologics;* 2017. https://www.fda.gov/ BiologicsBloodVaccines/default.htm.

37. FDA. *Post-Licensure Rapid Immunization Safety Monitoring (PRISM);* 2017. https://www.fda.gov/downloads/biolo gicsbloodvaccines/newsevents/workshopsmeetingsconf-erences/ucm544856.pdf.

38. Sentinel. *Active Risk Identification and Analysis System (ARIA);* 2017. https://www.sentinelinitiative.org/active-risk-identification-and-analysis-aria.

39. CDC. *Vaccine Safety Datalink;* 2017. https://www.cdc.gov/ vaccinesafety/ensuringsafety/monitoring/vsd/index.html.

40. Di Pasquale A. Vaccine safety evaluation: practical aspects in assessing benefits and risks. *Vaccine.* 2016;34:6672−6680.

41. Crawford N, et al. Active surveillance for adverse events following immunization. *Expert Rev Vaccines.* 2014;13: 265−276.

42. Ball R. Perspective on the future of postmarket vaccine safety surveillance and evaluation. *Expert Rev Vaccines.* 2014;13(4):455−462.

43. Bonhoeffer J, Black S, Izurieta H, Zuber P, Sturkenboom M. Current status and future directions of post-marketing vaccine safety monitoring with focus on USA and Europe. *Biologicals.* 2012;40(5):393−397.

44. Regan AK. The safety of maternal immunization. *Hum Vaccines Immunother.* 2016;12(12):3132−3136.

CHAPTER 8

Pharmacovigilance in Pregnancy

GWENETH LEVY, MD

INTRODUCTION

Teratogenic agents may affect development of the embryo and fetus and upon exposure by a pregnant woman can cause birth defects, fetal loss or abnormal growth and development. A teratogenic agent can be a medicinal product or other chemical agent (i.e., alcohol, nicotine), an infectious agent (i.e., rubella, cytomegalovirus), a medical condition (i.e., diabetes), an environmental toxin or genetic disorder. Teratogens cause about 10% of all birth defects (Box 8.1).[1] This chapter will primarily focus on drug exposure in pregnancy and assessing risk of congenital malformations; however, other adverse pregnancy outcomes that are of interest to physicians include spontaneous abortions, stillbirths, preterm births, and small for gestational age (SGA) births.

The majority of prescription medications available have not been adequately evaluated to determine risks during pregnancy in humans.[2] Preclinical developmental and reproductive toxicity studies in animal species are conducted; however, the results from these studies may not always be predictive of human risk. Thus, upon marketing approval of a medicinal product, human data is often lacking in respect to in utero drug exposure during pregnancy. Upon approval of a new drug, companies may be required to perform enhanced postmarketing surveillance, a pregnancy registry or another well-designed study to assess teratogenic drug effects and other adverse pregnancy outcomes.

MEDICATION USE IN PREGNANT WOMEN

Many women enter pregnancy with a previous medical condition, and some may develop new medical conditions during pregnancy (Box 8.2). At some point during pregnancy, approximately 90% of women in the United States have taken at least one medication while about 70% of medications are taken during the first trimester.[3] Approximately half of all pregnancies in the United States are unplanned.[4] Thus, a woman may have taken a medication during her first trimester, the most critical time period of embryo-fetal development, before knowing she was pregnant.

Despite the relatively widespread use of medicinal products during pregnancy, there is a paucity of human data regarding the reproductive risk of medications in women of childbearing potential (WOCBP) and the impact on the developing fetus.[5] When a medicinal product is first marketed, generally the only data in the label informing patients and healthcare professionals of reproductive risk is the preclinical reproductive safety data from testing in animals. The burden of risk assessment of medication use in pregnancy is then placed on the patient and healthcare provider or prescriber. This underscores the importance of understanding the effects of medications on the developing fetus and the pregnant woman.

BOX 8.1
Introduction

- Congenital anomalies may be the result of teratogenic agents.
- The majority of prescription medications in pregnant women have not been adequately evaluated.

BOX 8.2
Medication Use in Pregnant Women

- Approximately half of all pregnancies in the United States are unplanned. Thus, a woman may have taken a medication during her first trimester, the most critical time period of embryo-fetal development, before knowing she was pregnant.
- Understanding the effects of medication on the developing fetus and the pregnant woman is important.

STAGES OF EMBRYO-FETAL DEVELOPMENT

Susceptibility to teratogenic agents varies with the developmental stage at the time of fetal exposure (Box 8.3). The most vulnerable time period by which the fetus is exposed to a teratogenic agent is the third through the eighth week of the first trimester, also known as the period of organogenesis, or embryonic period. Most birth defects in the fetus are known to be caused by exposure to a teratogenic agent during the period of organogenesis. Within this time of rapidly dividing cells, there are critical time periods of development for each organ, during which an exposure to a

teratogenic agent can cause major malformations (i.e., neural tube defects, cleft lip) (see Figs. 8.1 and 8.2).

Effects of teratogens through the second week after conception are not known to cause birth defects but often result in an "all or none effect," meaning that exposure at this preembryonic phase (cleavage and implantation) either results in death of the embryo or complete recovery of the conceptus. Exposure to a teratogen during the fetal period (week 9 through birth) may result in minor malformations (i.e., clinodactyly) or functional defects such as growth retardation.

THALIDOMIDE AND HISTORY OF REGULATIONS

Thalidomide was the first drug recognized to cause birth defects in humans (Box 8.4). In the late 1950s, thalidomide was used in the treatment of morning sickness in pregnant women. In Europe, Australia, and Japan, approximately 10,000 children were born with limb reduction defects, or phocomelia, after a few years of use in pregnant women.[6] Consequently, after proof by

---

BOX 8.3
Stages of Embryo-Fetal Development

- Most birth defects in the fetus are known to be caused by exposure to a teratogenic agent during the period of organogenesis.

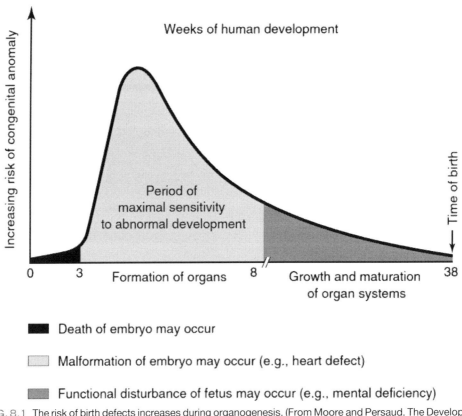

FIG. 8.1 The risk of birth defects increases during organogenesis. (From Moore and Persaud. The Developing Human 10th edition. Chapter 20 Page 474.)

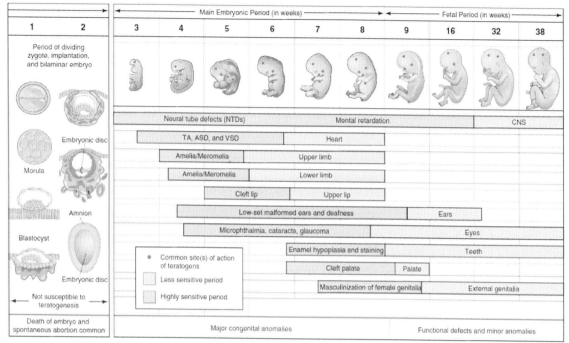

FIG. 8.2 Critical periods in human prenatal development. During the first 2 weeks of development, the embryo is usually not susceptible to teratogens; a teratogen damages all or most of the cells, resulting in death of the embryo, or damages only a few cells, allowing the conceptus to recover and the embryo to develop without birth defects. During highly sensitive periods (*mauve*), major birth defects may be produced (e.g., amelia, the absence of limbs, neural tube defects, spina bifida cystica). During stages that are less sensitive to teratogens (*green*), minor defects may be included (e.g., hypoplastic thumbs). *ASD*, artial septal defect; *CNS*, central nervous system; *TA*, truncus arteriosus; *VSD*, ventricular septal defect. (From Moore and Persaud. The Developing Human 10th edition. Chapter 20 Page 474.)

> **BOX 8.4**
> **Thalidomide and the History of Regulations**
>
> - Thalidomide was the first drug recognized to cause birth defects in humans.
> - As a result of the thalidomide tragedy, regulatory agencies developed a systematic approach to reproductive toxicity testing.

scientists that in utero exposure to thalidomide caused phocomelia, thalidomide was banned in most countries in 1961. Thalidomide was also found to cause congenital heart, ear, and ocular malformations. The US Food and Drug Administration's (FDA) Dr Frances Oldham Kelsey prevented the approval of thalidomide in 1960 in the United States because of her concerns about the drug causing peripheral neuropathy. Numerous teratogenic agents have since been identified to cause birth defects in humans[6] (see Table 8.1).

The thalidomide tragedy heightened awareness of the importance of rigorous testing of the safety of pharmaceutical products prior to marketing approval and ignited the significance of assessing drugs in the context of benefit and risk. Reproductive risk became a focal point of new commissions, societies, and regulations that were imposed regarding testing of drugs. It was recognized that there were differences in sensitivity between animal species and that developmental toxicity testing should be conducted in two different species. As a result, the United States and international regulatory agencies developed a systematic approach to reproductive toxicity testing for pharmaceuticals.

DEVELOPMENTAL AND REPRODUCTIVE TOXICOLOGY

Developmental and Reproductive Toxicology (DART) studies in animals are performed according to

TABLE 8.1
Teratogens That Cause Human Birth Defects

Agents	Most Common Birth Defects
DRUGS	
Alcohol	Fetal alcohol syndrome: IUGR, mental deficiency, microcephaly, ocular anomalies, joint abnormalities, short palpebral fissures
Androgens and high doses of progestogens	Various degrees of masculinization of female fetuses: ambiguous external genitalia resulting in labial fusion and clitoral hypertrophy
Aminopterin	IUGR; skeletal defects; CNS malformations, notably meroencephaly (most of the brain is absent)
Carbamazepine	NTD, craniofacial defects, developmental retardation
Cocaine	IUGR, prematurity, microcephaly, cerebral infarction, urogenital defects, neurobehavioral disturbances
Diethylstilbestrol	Abnormalities of uterus and vagina, cervical erosion and ridges
Isotretinoin (13-*cis*-retinoic acid)	Craniofacial abnormalities; NTDs such as spina bifida cystica; cardiovascular defects; cleft palate; thymic aplasia
Lithium carbonate	Various defects, usually involving the heart and great vessels
Methotrexate	Multiple defects, especially skeletal, involving the face, cranium, limbs, and vertebral column
Misoprostol	Limb abnormalities, ocular and cranial nerve defects, autism spectrum disorder
Phenytoin	Fetal hydantoin syndrome: IUGR, microcephaly, mental deficiency, ridged frontal suture, inner epicanthal folds, eyelid ptosis, broad and depressed nasal bridge, phalangeal hypoplasia
Tetracycline	Stained teeth, hypoplasia of enamel
Thalidomide	Abnormal development of limbs such as meromelia (partial absence) and amelia (complete absence); facial defects; systemic anomalies such as cardiac, kidney, and ocular defects
Trimethadione	Development delay, V-shaped eyebrows, low-set ears, cleft lip and/or palate
Valproic acid	Craniofacial anomalies, NTDs, cognitive abnormalities, often hydrocephalus, heart, and skeletal defects
Warfarin	Nasal hypoplasia, stippled epiphyses, hypoplastic phalanges, eye anomalies, mental deficiency
CHEMICALS	
Methylmercury	Cerebral atrophy, spasticity, seizures, mental deficiency
Polychlorinated biphenyls	IUGR, skin discoloration
INFECTIONS	
Cytomegalovirus	Microcephaly, chorioretinitis, sensorineural hearing loss, delayed psychomotor/mental development, hepatosplenomegaly, hydrocephaly, cerebral palsy, brain (periventricular) calcification
Hepatitis B virus	Preterm birth, low birth weight, fetal macrosomia
Herpes simplex virus	Skin vesicles and scarring, chorioretinitis, hepatomegaly, thrombocytopenia, petechiae, hemolytic anemia, hydranencephaly
Human parvovirus B19	Fetal anemia, nonimmune hydrops fetalis, fetal death
Rubella virus	IUGR, postnatal growth retardation, cardiac and great vessel abnormalities, microcephaly, sensorineural deafness, cataract, microphthalmos, glaucoma, pigmented retinopathy, mental deficiency, neonate bleeding, hepatosplenomegaly, osteopathy, tooth defects

TABLE 8.1 Teratogens That Cause Human Birth Defects—cont'd	
Agents	**Most Common Birth Defects**
Toxoplasma gondii	Microcephaly, mental deficiency, microphthalmia, hydrocephaly, chorioretinitis, cerebral calcifications, hearing loss, neurologic disturbance
Treponema pallidum	Hydrocephalus, congenital deafness, mental deficiency, abnormal teeth and bones
Venezuelan equine encephalitis virus	Microcephaly, microphthalmia, cerebral agenesis, CNS necrosis, hydrocephalus
Varicella virus	Cutaneous scars (dermatome distribution), neurologic defects (e.g., limb paresis [incomplete paralysis]), hydrocephaly, seizures, cataracts, microphthalmia, Horner syndrome, optic atrophy, nystagmus, chorioretinitis, microcephaly, mental deficiency, skeletal anomalies (e.g., hypoplasia of limbs, fingers, toes), urogenital anomalies
RADIATION	
High levels of ionizing radiation	Microcephaly, mental deficiency, skeletal anomalies, growth retardation, cataracts

CNS, Central nervous system; *IUGR*, intrauterine growth restriction; *NTD*, neural tube defect.
From Moore and Persaud. The Developing Human 10th edition. Chapter 20 Page 473. Table 20-6.

International Council of Harmonization guidelines (Box 8.5). The purpose of the DART studies is to identify safety hazards and potential adverse effects in the animal's reproductive system, fetal development, and peri-/postnatal effects of the offspring after the exposure to a drug through the placenta and lactation. Performing animal studies is essential to assess the relevance to humans.

For medicinal products that are small molecules, there are three studies in animals that will suffice to test reproductive toxicity. Since susceptibility to teratogenic agents varies with the developmental stage at the time of exposure, testing is continued during all stages of the reproductive process. The three studies are described below:[7,8]

1. Fertility and Early Embryo Development Study: This study is designed to detect effects of a medicinal product on folliculogenesis and sperm development, mating performance, and development of the fertilized ova through the implantation stage. The fertility study is generally performed in the rodent or rabbit.[7,8]

2. Embryo-Fetal Development: This study is designed to evaluate effects of a medicinal product on fetal development through the period of organogenesis (embryogenesis). The Embryo-Fetal Development study is conducted in two species, one rodent (preferably rat) and one non-rodent (preferably rabbit).[7,8]

3. Peri-/Postnatal Evaluation: This study is designed to evaluate the effects of a medicinal product on mother and offspring when exposure occurs from

> **BOX 8.5**
> **Developmental and Reproductive Toxicology**
>
> - The purpose of the developmental and reproductive toxicology (DART) studies is to identify safety hazards and potential adverse effects in the animal's reproductive system, fetal development, and peri-/postnatal effects of the offspring after the exposure to a drug through placenta and lactation.
> - Performing animal studies is essential to assess the relevance to humans.
> - DART studies in large molecules (i.e., immunoglobulins) differ from small molecules in that there is limited cross-reactivity in rats and rabbits.
> - Immunoglobulin placental transfer is low during the first trimester.
> - Determination of the dose to be tested is a critical step.

implantation through the late stages of gestation, birth, lactation, weaning of the pregnant or lactating female, and development of the offspring. The Peri-/Postnatal Evaluation is conducted in one species, preferably rat.[7,8]

The appropriate animal species must be chosen for DART studies. The species used should be well characterized with respect to fertility and background rates of malformation and embryo-fetal death.[8] The medicinal product being tested should be pharmacologically active in the animal species used. When the medicinal product (i.e., small molecule) is pharmacologically active in rodents and rabbits, both species should be used for Embryo-Fetal Development (EFD) studies, unless embryo-fetal death or teratogenicity has already been identified in one species.

DART studies in large molecules (i.e., immunoglobulins) differ from small molecules in that there is limited cross-reactivity in rats and rabbits. Immunoglobulins are often only pharmacologically active in nonhuman primates (NHPs). Several study designs can be considered for medicinal products pharmacologically active only in NHPs. The sponsor can justify performing separate EFD and/or Peri-/Postnatal Evaluation (PPND) studies, if there is a concern that the mechanism of action might lead to an adverse effect on embryo-fetal development or pregnancy loss.[9] However, one well-designed study in NHPs called an enhanced PPND (ePPND) which includes dosing from day 20 of gestation (day of implantation) through birth is often performed.[9] The ePPND generally tests fewer monkeys than performing separate EFD and PPND studies, and thus is generally preferred, if appropriate. Timing of these studies during clinical development varies depending on species used and whether pregnancy prevention can be managed during clinical trials that include WOCBP.[9]

Embryo-fetal exposure during gestation should also be taken into consideration. High-molecular-weight proteins (>5000 Da), such as immunoglobulins, do not cross the placenta by simple diffusion.[9] Immunoglobulins require the neonatal Fc receptor (FcRn) to be transported across the placenta. The timing of immunoglobulin transport via this receptor varies across species.[10] In humans, since the FcRn on the placental syncytiotrophoblast is barely detectable before gestational week 14, IgG placental transfer is minimal in the first trimester in humans (and NHPs),[10] hence limiting large molecule drug transfer to the fetus during the period of organogenesis. IgG placental transfer increases early in the second trimester, reaching the highest levels late in the third trimester.[10]

In addition, determination of the dose is a critical step in performing DART studies. The highest dose and subsequent intervals of lower dosages chosen should be based on previously performed pharmacokinetic and toxicology studies, preferably in the same species. For the EFD studies, difficulty in interpretation may arise when fetal toxicity is observed at dose levels that were also toxic for the mother, as often it cannot be assumed that fetal toxicity was secondary to maternal toxicity.[8]

Genotoxicity

Genotoxicity testing is performed on medicinal products to detect the potential to induce genetic damage, which can affect germ cells. (Box 8.6). Damage to DNA may result in gene mutations, recombination of chromosomes, or larger scale chromosomal damage. If a medicinal product is genotoxic and targets rapidly dividing cells, then the product is presumed to cause teratogenicity or embryo-fetal lethality. In the case of a drug with proven genotoxicity, EFD studies may not be needed. Genotoxicity studies routinely performed for small molecules are not needed for biologics, as these medicines are not expected to interact directly with DNA or other chromosomal material.[11]

If a product is genotoxic, irreversible alterations to DNA can take place in the germ cells that are undergoing or completing meiosis (spermatocytes, preovulatory oocytes). In females, genotoxic pharmaceuticals may cause DNA damage to the oocytes or directly affect the embryo or fetus. In males, a genotoxic pharmaceutical may cause DNA damage in the sperm, potentially resulting in adverse effects in the conceptus of a female sexual partner.

Adverse reproductive outcomes have been seen in animals when males treated with genotoxic pharmaceuticals were mated with untreated females.[12] Mating male rats that were exposed to chronic low-dose cyclophosphamide with untreated female rats resulted in increases in pre- and postimplantation loss and growth-retarded fetuses.[12] Given these data, it is prudent to prevent pregnancy when the use of genotoxic drugs is unavoidable. For male and female subjects and female partners of male subjects in clinical trials, contraceptive measures are recommended for studies involving genotoxic products. This will minimize the risk of potential adverse embryo-fetal effects for geno-

---

BOX 8.6
Genotoxicity

- Preclinical genotoxicity testing is essential for a small-molecule medicinal product.
- In females, genotoxic pharmaceuticals may cause DNA damage to the oocytes or directly affect the embryo or fetus.
- In males, a genotoxic pharmaceutical may cause DNA damage in the sperm, potentially resulting in adverse effects in the conceptus of a female sexual partner.

toxic pharmaceuticals. Such contraceptive guidance is likely to be included in product labeling.

CONTRACEPTIVE MEASURES IN CLINICAL TRIALS

The general recommendation[13] is that "all female reproduction toxicity studies and the standard battery of genotoxicity tests should be completed prior to the inclusion, in any clinical trial, of WOCBP not using highly effective birth control or whose pregnancy status is unknown" (Box 8.7). In September 2014, Clinical Trials Facilitation Group (CTFG) guidance[14] was published entitled "Recommendations related to contraception and pregnancy testing" and the aim was to provide practical guidance on contraception use and pregnancy testing in clinical trials, focusing on the early stages of pregnancy concerning teratogenicity and fetotoxicity.

The CTFG guidance[14] presents three reproductive risk categories for female subjects of childbearing potential and the requirements for contraception use in clinical trials (refer to guidance for definitions and specific methods of birth control):

- Demonstrated or suspected human teratogenicity/fetotoxicity in early pregnancy
  - WOCBP should use one *highly effective method* of birth control throughout the clinical trial and until the end of relevant systemic exposure (additional five half-lives after cessation of study drug). The timeframe of five half-lives sufficiently allows for the elimination of approximately 97% of a pharmaceutical from circulation before fertilization could occur.[15]
  - Highly effective methods are defined as methods that can achieve a failure rate of less than 1% per year when used consistently and correctly.[4,14] Although not part of CTFG

guidance, some regulatory authorities may require an additional method of contraception.
  - Pregnancy testing should be monthly throughout clinical trial.
- Possible human teratogenicity/fetotoxicity in early pregnancy
  - WOCBP should use one *highly effective method* of birth control throughout the clinical trial and until the end of systemic exposure.
  - Pregnancy testing should be at least at the end of relevant exposure, and additional testing should be considered depending on the length of the clinical trial.
- Unlikely human teratogenicity/fetotoxicity in early pregnancy
  - WOCBP should use at least an *acceptable effective method* of contraception and at a minimum throughout the study.
  - Additional pregnancy testing during the clinical trial is not necessary unless a woman has a suspected pregnancy

CTFG guidance[14] provides the recommendation that no male contraception is required in clinical trials for products which are not genotoxic and have no teratogenicity/fetotoxicity at subtherapeutic systemic exposure levels. Male contraception is recommended for male subjects with a pregnant or nonpregnant WOCBP partner and should use condoms in a clinical trial until the end of relevant systemic exposure in order to avoid potential exposure to an embryo or fetus, in the following situations:

- For nongenotoxic investigational products which have demonstrated or suspected human teratogenicity/fetotoxicity in early pregnancy at subtherapeutic systemic exposure levels, where it is theoretically possible that relevant systemic concentrations may be achieved in WOCBP from exposure to seminal fluid (i.e., some small molecules): consideration should be taken for the male subject to use condoms throughout the study and until the end of systemic exposure (additional five half-lives after cessation of study drug).
- For genotoxic investigational products, the male subject should use condoms during the study and for an additional 90 days after cessation of study drug to cover the spermatogenic cycle (explained below). For products with a half-life of more than 1 week, condoms should be used for 90 days plus an additional five half-lives. For his nonpregnant WOCBP partner, contraception recommendations should also be considered for the same timeframe.

BOX 8.7
Contraceptive Measures in Clinical Trials

- In the Clinical Trials Facilitation Group guidance, there are three reproductive risk categories for female subjects of childbearing potential requiring the use of contraception during clinical trials.
- Male subjects taking genotoxic products, when sexually active with a woman of childbearing potential, should use condoms in a clinical trial until the end of relevant systemic exposure in order to avoid potential exposure to an embryo or a fetus.

The spermatogenic cycle takes approximately 70 days, with 64 days for germ cells to develop from spermatogonia to spermatozoa and another 2–5 days for spermatozoa to pass through the epididymis.[12] An additional 3 weeks residence time for unejaculated sperm is included which then equals 90 days. Thus, in determining timeframe for contraceptive use in males for a genotoxic drug, the recommendation is to use condoms for an additional 90 days after systemic exposure to the medicinal product has ended (thus, 90 days + 5 half-lives).

For females taking genotoxic investigational products, the CTFG recommendation is to use contraception during the study and for an additional 30 days after cessation of study drug to cover the ovulatory cycle. For products with a half-life of more than 1 week, contraception should be used for 30 days plus an additional five half-lives after discontinuation of the study drug. For females using genotoxic anticancer pharmaceuticals, regulatory authorities may require much longer periods of contraception use after cessation of study drug in order to cover the period of folliculogenesis.

Seminal Fluid Exposure During Pregnancy

Since humans may have intercourse during pregnancy, seminal fluid could enter the female reproductive tract and be absorbed, and hence the theoretical possibility that the conceptus may be exposed to drugs in seminal fluid. Certain antimicrobials have been shown to have more than 10 fold higher seminal fluid concentrations in comparison to blood.[16] Assuming 100% vaginal absorption of a seminal dose of a medicinal product with a high semen–blood concentration ratio, exposure levels in the female sexual partner have been predicted to be three or more orders of magnitude lower than the plasma concentrations in the male who was administered the drug.[17] Many drugs have been shown to be

present in the seminal fluid, although most are present at such low concentrations that there would be little concern to a pregnant partner and fetus.[12] Moreover, the author was unable to find any documented report of teratogenic findings via seminal transfer in humans.

There have been some conflicting reports in animals regarding seminal transfer. Lutwak-Mann (1964)[18] had shown that the presence of thalidomide in semen in rabbits when mated with untreated females can cause malformations in the offspring. However, recent studies performed by the Health and Environmental Sciences Institute (HESI), Developmental and Reproductive Toxicology (DART) Technical Committee, addressed risk to the female partner and developing conceptus from seminal drug transfer of both small and large molecules.[16] Data generated from the experimental animal models suggest that chemical transmission in semen will not produce clinically meaningful exposures to the conceptus.[19] In a study performed by Hui et al., in pregnant rabbits, it was found that thalidomide concentrations in maternal plasma, yolk sac cavity fluid, and embryo following intravaginal administration of thalidomide were two- to sevenfold lower than their respective levels after oral administration.[20] In a consequent EFD study in rabbits administered oral and intravaginal thalidomide at doses greater than 10,000-fold higher than the expected amount of thalidomide in human semen, no developmental abnormalities in the fetuses of the pregnant rabbits were found.[20] These data demonstrated no preferred mechanism of transfer of thalidomide from vagina to conceptus, and thus, no developmental toxicity risks were evident with thalidomide exposure via the vaginal route.[20]

For biologics, a study in cynomolgus monkeys showed that monoclonal antibodies (immunoglobulins or large molecule therapeutics) transferred via seminal fluid does not reach pharmacologically relevant plasma levels in the mother or fetus.[21] This was further elucidated in a study in healthy human male subjects to evaluate the risk of seminal fluid transmission of an immunoglobulin product to pregnant partners. The study showed that levels of the immunoglobulin in seminal fluid were low, indicating a negligible risk to a fetus exposed via seminal fluid transfer to a pregnant partner.[22] In addition, there is a lack of a placental receptor for immunoglobulin transfer during the first trimester of pregnancy,[10] thus precluding large molecule drug transfer to the fetus during the period of organogenesis.

BOX 8.8
Seminal Fluid Exposure During Pregnancy

- Many drugs have been shown to be present in the seminal fluid, although most are present at very low concentrations.
- Monoclonal antibodies (immunoglobulins or large molecule therapeutics) transferred via seminal fluid do not reach pharmacologically relevant plasma levels in the mother or fetus.

Collection of Pregnancy Information in the Clinical Trial Setting

Pregnant women are typically actively excluded from clinical trials (Box 8.9). Despite strict contraception requirements to prevent pregnancy during clinical trials, there may be women who become pregnant. Since the usual procedure is to discontinue study drug treatment in pregnant women from the trial immediately, drug exposure is usually limited to only the first trimester. The pregnancy should be followed to term and the outcome obtained.

Data collection in postmarketing surveillance

The European Medicines Agency (EMA), Committee for Medicinal Products for Human Use guidance entitled "Guideline on the exposure to medicinal products during pregnancy: need for post-authorization data" (May 2006)[23] provides guidance on how to monitor drug exposure during pregnancy, requirements for reporting pregnancy outcomes, and recommendations regarding presentation of data collected. Postmarketing surveillance is a means of collecting information on pregnancy and includes spontaneous reports, case reports or literature, reports from health authorities or other pharmaceutical companies, pregnancy exposure registries (PERs), healthcare database studies, and case-control studies.

For all methods of postmarketing surveillance, a woman should be monitored for adverse effects throughout the entire pregnancy. Every effort should be made to collect the pregnancy outcome and gestational age at birth in order to assess preterm and postterm births. Both normal and abnormal pregnancy outcomes are important. Outcomes collected will include live births with or without congenital anomalies, spontaneous abortions (fetal loss before 20 weeks of gestation), stillbirths with and without fetal defects (fetal loss after 20 weeks of gestation), elective terminations with and without fetal defects, and ectopic pregnancies.

Congenital malformations should be fully described, including the severity and whether any interventions, including surgery, are planned. Attempts should be made to obtain records from the pediatrician or teratologist. A major congenital abnormality is a life-threatening structural anomaly or one likely to cause significant impairment of health or functional capacity and which requires medical or surgical intervention.[23] A minor congenital anomaly is a structural anomaly not likely to cause functional or cosmetic problems.[23] Conditions that qualify as major and minor birth defects can be found on the Metropolitan Atlanta Congenital Defects Program (MACDP) code defect list. The MACDP uses active tracking methods to detect and follow birth defects among infants and children born to mothers living in metropolitan Atlanta.[24] The MACDP code defect list includes major and minor birth defects that are tracked by MACDP, as well as conditions that are not considered birth defects (exclusion list) and those conditions that are considered birth defects only under certain circumstances.[24] Major and minor defects can be adjudicated by the sponsor, along with individual case review to determine if clusters of two or more minor abnormalities might in combination constitute a syndrome or constellation of findings.

For cases of spontaneous abortion and stillbirth, information on the time of occurrence and any previous history of miscarriage is important. Attempts should be made to collect information on any fetal defects that occurred with stillbirths or elective terminations. Given spontaneous abortions often occur before the end of the first trimester (prior to 13 weeks), information regarding fetal or chromosomal abnormalities can be difficult to obtain.

Collection of exposure timing, dose, and duration of the medicinal product is of utmost importance and should be recorded as accurately as possible. Collection of preconception exposure timing is also important for those medicinal products that are genotoxic or have long half-lives. To evaluate exposure timing, it is imperative to obtain the last menstrual period and/or date of conception as well as the accurate dates of drug therapy. In addition, a detailed maternal and infant history is prudent for analysis and understanding of pregnancy

---

BOX 8.9
Data Collection in Post-Marketing Surveillance

- Pregnant women are typically actively excluded from clinical trials.
- Postmarketing surveillance is a means of collecting information on pregnancy.
- All efforts should be made to collect the pregnancy outcome in postmarketing surveillance.
- Congenital malformations should be fully described in postmarketing surveillance.
- Collection of exposure timing, dose, and duration of the medicinal product should be collected in post-marketing surveillance.

cases. If paternal exposure cases are necessary to follow for a drug of interest, the pregnancy outcome as well as information on the biological father and the pregnant mother is also important. Often, sponsors will collect information on an infant through a certain age in an effort to understand adverse or developmental effects on a drug during infancy or childhood. This can be achieved by follow-up attempts to contact the patient or healthcare professional via phone or structured questionnaires.

METHODS OF SURVEILLANCE

Randomized controlled clinical trials are rarely performed on pregnant women, given the ethical concerns of exposure to the fetus (Box 8.10). Postmarketing safety studies are needed to assess risk in order to acquire clinically relevant human data for the label and provide useful information for treating or advising patients who are pregnant or anticipating pregnancy.[25] Common postmarketing studies include PERs, healthcare database studies, and case-control studies (see Chapter 6). Other means to collect information on teratogenic risk are through spontaneous reports, case reports, population-based surveillance methods, and Teratology Information Services. There are strengths and limitations to all of these methods.

Signal Detection by the Sponsor

Marketing authorization holders have established routine safety surveillance programs that collect and report adverse event information (see Chapter 2), including those from drug-exposed pregnancies (Box 8.11). Spontaneous reports of product pregnancy exposures may originate from various sources, including consumers, healthcare professionals, case reports in the literature, health authorities, and reports from other pharmaceutical companies. However, the data provided in spontaneous reports are often limited, as patients can have poor recall of events that have occurred or limited knowledge regarding important medical details of the case. Underreporting of events is a major issue, and the lack of a denominator (the number of pregnant women exposed to the drug) makes reporting rates difficult to calculate. Given the limitations of spontaneous reporting, additional studies are often necessary to gather more meaningful clinical data regarding pregnancy outcomes.

Pregnancy Exposure Registries

According to the FDA's Pregnancy Labeling Task Force, "a pregnancy exposure registry is a prospective observational study that actively collects information on

> **BOX 8.10**
> **Methods of Post-Marketing Surveillance**
>
> - Postmarketing safety studies are needed to assess risk in order to acquire clinically relevant human data for the label and provide useful information for treating or advising patients who are pregnant or anticipating pregnancy.
> - Common postmarketing studies include pregnancy exposure registries, healthcare database studies, and case-control studies.

> **BOX 8.11**
> **Signal Detection by the Sponsor**
>
> Marketing authorization holders have established routine safety surveillance programs that collect and report adverse events, including those from drug-exposed pregnancies.

> **BOX 8.12**
> **Pregnancy Exposure Registries**
>
> - A pregnancy exposure registry (PER) is a prospective observational study.
> - In the majority of PERs, the primary endpoint is focused on the overall incidence of major congenital malformations.
> - Internal and external comparator (or "control") groups are used.
> - Limitations in study design may exist for a PER.

medicinal product exposure during pregnancy and associated pregnancy outcomes[26]" (Box 8.12). Typically, women are enrolled prospectively, after exposure to a product but before the conduct of any prenatal tests that could provide knowledge of the outcome of pregnancy. Information is collected systematically throughout the pregnancy and infants are often monitored after birth for up to a year or longer. PERs focus on a disease, a drug, or a class of drugs used to treat certain condition(s). They can be set up by the drug manufacturer, a research group, or academic medical centers. Enrollment is voluntary, so a pregnant woman can either self-refer or enroll through her healthcare provider.

A PER collects pregnancy outcomes, including live births with and without birth defects, spontaneous abortions and stillbirths with and without birth defects, premature births, and SGA newborns. In the majority of PERs, the primary endpoint is focused on the overall incidence of major congenital malformations in the fetuses/infants of the women treated with the drug during pregnancy. A requirement for enrollment should be that the pregnant woman was exposed to a drug at the point in gestation with the highest risk of causing teratogenic or other adverse effects. For congenital anomalies, this is most often the first trimester, but there are drugs which may cause adverse effects in later trimesters. For example, angiotensin-converting-enzyme inhibitors such as captopril, when used during the second and third trimesters of pregnancy, can cause oligohydramnios associated with fetal lung hypoplasia and skeletal deformations.[27] The presence of a combination of minor and/or major defects may constitute a syndrome or pattern, which may only be recognizable by a specialist in the field. The length of follow-up of the infants varies depending on the endpoints of the study, with some PERs having longer follow-up timeframes to evaluate any association of drug exposure and infant developmental delay.

Internal and external comparator (or "control") groups are used to control for various factors and strengthen the understanding of the observed effects.[28] Internal comparison groups may include a group of patients who would have the same data collection as the patients with the focus of interest (i.e., those with specific drug exposure or particular disease in common), in comparison to another group who does not have the drug exposure or condition of interest.[28] An external (or "historical") comparison group refers to a large group of patients in the general population. Population-based registries, such as the MACDP[24] and the European Surveillance of Congenital Anomalies,[29] collect data on infants with birth defects who live in a particular region, and also help with predictions regarding the general population. Statistical analyses can be performed on outcomes with comparisons between internal or external control groups.

A well-known limitation for a PER is that it is unlikely to enroll a sufficient number of exposed pregnancies to detect a modest increase in risk (e.g., a two- to fivefold increase) for a specific defect.[26] Given the prospective nature of a PER, selection bias may also pose a problem, since the women who volunteer to participate may be in better health and more likely to follow the advice of physicians (and consequently be at lower risk of adverse pregnancy outcomes). Other biases can be introduced through inherent differences in co-variates between those exposed to the drug of interest and those who lack that exposure, sometimes limiting the conclusions that can be drawn from these investigations. Additionally, registries can have low

enrollment and the potential for a significant number of patients to be lost to follow-up, which results in a large amount of missing data. Low enrollment may delay definitive conclusions about teratogenic risk for many years after drug launch, or result in futility and closure of the PER.

The FDA Guidance (2002) "Establishing Pregnancy Exposure Registries"[30] provides methodological rigor and a more standardized approach for development of a pregnancy registry. The FDA has established a website[31] listing the pregnancy registries of which they are aware.[26]

Electronic Healthcare Databases

Another source of postauthorization data collection being used increasingly in recent years is electronic healthcare databases (Box 8.13). The Scandinavian countries (Denmark, Sweden, Finland, Norway, and Iceland) have population-based birth registries that link health-related information from mothers and infants and are supplemented by infant hospital discharge records.[28] A major advantage of this type of registry is that nearly all pregnant women attend maternity health clinics from early pregnancy until after birth, which eliminates both selection bias (given enrollment is not voluntary) and recall bias (does not require maternal recollection of past events because information is recorded by the prescriber).[28] Other advantages are the easy access to more complete information and a large number of patients (unless there are a relatively small number of pregnant women exposed to the drug of interest). Given the backgrounds of physicians entering the outcome data, there may be a need for a specialist to validate via chart review that pregnancy outcomes are accurately captured including the major and minor malformations and any patterns or syndromes.

Another example of databases that provide on-market data is administrative claims databases such as

---

BOX 8.13
Electronic Healthcare Databases

- The Scandinavian countries (Denmark, Sweden, Finland, Norway, and Iceland) have population-based birth registries that link health-related information from mothers and their infant and are supplemented by infant hospital discharge records.[28]
- Another example of databases that provide on-market data is administrative claims databases such as Optum (United Healthcare) and MarketScan.

Optum (United Healthcare) and MarketScan. These databases require linkage of mother-to-infant data to perform drug exposure pregnancy studies. A potential limitation is that the insured patients captured in these claim databases may not represent the general population, and data are only captured on individual patients while they are covered under a specific insurance company. Consequently, long-term follow-up of mother-infant pairs can be challenging.

Case-Control Studies

Case-control studies declare a specific outcome of interest (i.e., specific birth defect) and determine whether cases with the event of interest and controls had similar or different rates of exposure to a particular drug or class of drugs (Box 8.14). Case-control studies are performed retrospectively because the pregnancy outcomes are already known. Data are collected through interviews, questionnaires, or medical chart review. Often they are conducted as part of current ongoing case-control surveillance studies, such as the US National Birth Defects Prevention Study[32] or the Slone Epidemiology Center Birth Defects Study.[33] An example of two large case-control studies that supported product labeling showed that maternal use of paroxetine during the first trimester of pregnancy was associated with a two- to threefold increased risk of right ventricular outflow tract obstructions.[34,35]

Labeling

The product label is a means to communicate prescribing information of medications to healthcare professionals and patients (Box 8.15). In addition to other aspects of drug information, the label informs healthcare professionals and patients of the risks associated with reproduction and pregnancy.

In December 2014, the FDA published guidance ("the final rule") called the Pregnancy and Lactation Labeling Rule (PLLR).[36] The PLLR requires changes to the content and format of the pregnancy and lactation sections of the product label and supersedes other previous labeling guidance in the United States. One of the biggest changes with the PLLR format is the removal of the pregnancy letter categories (A, B, C, D, and X). The system of assigning a pregnancy letter category to each medication was established in the United States in 1979 to communicate risk of drug-related fetal effects; however, the letter categories had issues related to interpretation, in that using one letter to designate risk may not provide an accurate or comprehensive view. Consequently, the PLLR labeling guidance now allows for

> ### BOX 8.14
> ### Case-Control Studies
>
> - Case-control studies declare a specific outcome of interest (i.e., specific birth defect) and determine whether cases with the event of interest and controls had similar or different rates of exposure to a particular drug or class of drugs.

> ### BOX 8.15
> ### Product Labeling
>
> - The product label is a means to communicate prescribing information of medications to healthcare professionals and patients.
> - One of the biggest changes with the pregnancy and lactation labeling rule (PLLR) format is the removal of the pregnancy letter categories (A, B, C, D, and X).
> - PLLR guidance now allows for more prescriptive and detailed language.
> - Europe's product label, the summary of product characteristics, has its own format for pregnancy labeling.

more prescriptive and detailed language, including sections for risk summary, human data, and clinical considerations. There is a new subsection of the label called "Females and Males of Reproductive Potential." This section includes information on male and female contraception requirements, frequency of pregnancy testing, and any data suggesting effects on fertility or preimplantation loss. The pregnancy section of the label also contains contact information for any ongoing PER.

Europe's product label, the Summary of Product Characteristics, has its own format for pregnancy labeling. EMA guidance entitled "Guideline on Risk Assessment of Medicinal Products on Human Reproduction and Lactation: From Data to Labeling" states that integration of the assessments of human and animal data is essential for labeling of a medicinal product.[37] The label should include information on fertility, human experience in pregnancy, nonclinical animal studies on reproductive and developmental toxicity, genotoxicity, contraception requirements, and whether the product is contraindicated in pregnancy. The guidance provides a table to apply consistency across products in order to integrate human and nonclinical data. The table is presented by steps that reflect a gradient in level of concern with corresponding wording choices that reflect level of risk.

Risk Minimization

Human teratogens in humans have risk minimization programs associated with their use (Box 8.16). The risk minimization program includes steps which should be taken to reduce the risks associated with WOCBP being prescribed a known teratogen. For example, the product label would note the importance of avoiding pregnancy by emphasizing the need for effective contraception and recommending that patients have a negative pregnancy test before each prescription.[38] An additional risk minimization activity might be to develop educational tools to provide information to the patients on the teratogenic risks of the medicine and the importance of contraception.[38] Another example is the risk evaluation and mitigation strategy (REMS) called iPLEDGE,[39] required by the FDA to eliminate fetal exposure to isotretinoin (Accutane), a potent teratogen, through a restricted distribution program. This program includes all isotretinoin compounds, including the generic versions.[40] This REMS program requires that patients complete an informed consent form, comply with monthly pregnancy tests (including two negative tests prior to the start of drug use), and document that two methods of birth control are being used during treatment. The program also requires documentation of a negative pregnancy test before the pharmacy can release medication refills to the patient.

Pregnancy data from the iPLEDGE program over several years past have shown that failure to comply with the contraception requirements (e.g., did not use two forms of birth control, did not use contraception on the date of conception, unsuccessful at abstinence) was the most common reason for a pregnancy to result.[41] Prescriber counseling on proper contraceptive use and patient education to reinforce the risks of pregnancy are prudent to further the public health goal of avoiding fetal exposure to this high-risk teratogen. However, in a survey of internal medicine physicians, only 65% of participating physicians appeared to have an understanding of failure rates of various contraceptive agents.[42] In addition to improving patient compliance, specialists and primary care physicians prescribing Accutane or other teratogens may need continuing medical education on counseling patients about potential teratogens and contraception.

CONCLUSIONS

When a drug is first marketed, often the only available data is from animal reproductive toxicology studies which can be difficult for prescribers to translate into the potential risk for human teratogenicity (Box 8.17). Despite the lack of human safety data, WOCBP can be treated with medications before pregnancy is known, given over half of all pregnancies are unplanned.[4] Pregnant women are often exposed during the first trimester, which is the period critical for organogenesis with the highest risk of having an abnormal outcome, if a drug has potential teratogenic effects.

Given the lack of human experience upon initial marketing of a drug, postmarketing surveillance of drug use in pregnancy is of utmost importance in an effort to detect teratogenic effects. Although the sponsor is obligated to collect and analyze spontaneous reports, the passive mechanism of spontaneous reporting may be considered inadequate to routinely detect drug-induced adverse fetal outcomes or birth defects. Therefore, it is important to develop other methods of proactive surveillance to obtain human data to sufficiently detect a risk or provide reassurance of the lack of risk. The ultimate goal is to provide relevant human data on reproductive drug effects in the prescribing label in order to better inform patients and healthcare professionals of the safety or risks of medicinal products.

Obtaining human data on the safety of drug use during pregnancy is a significant public health need in order for physicians and other healthcare provides to better counsel patients about risks to the fetus. Numerous regulations and guidance have been put forth in order to more adequately assess the use of prescription medications during pregnancy and promote the presentation of more useful clinical information in labels.

BOX 8.16
Risk Minimization Programs

- Teratogens known to cause birth defects in humans have risk minimization programs associated with their use.
- The risk minimization program includes steps which should be taken to reduce the risks associated with women of childbearing potential being prescribed a known teratogen.

BOX 8.17
Conclusions

- The goal is to provide relevant human data on reproductive drug effects in the prescribing label in order to better inform patients and healthcare professionals of the safety or risks of medicinal products.
- Proper labeling of safety of drug use during pregnancy is a significant public health need in order for physicians and other healthcare provides to better counsel patients about risks to the fetus.

REFERENCES

1. Banholzer M, Buergin H, et al. Clinical trial considerations on male contraception and collection of pregnancy information from female partners. *J Transl Med.* 2012;10:129.
2. Chambers C. Over-the-counter medications: risk and safety in pregnancy. *Semin Perinatol.* 2015;39:541–544.
3. Sinclair S, Miller R, Chambers C, Cooper E. Medication safety during pregnancy: improving evidence-based practice. *J Midwifery & Womens Health.* 2016;61:52–67.
4. Trussell J, Wynn LL. Reducing unintended pregnancy in the United States. Editorial *Contraception.* 2008;77:1–5.
5. Mazer-Amirshahi M, Samiee-Zafarghandy S, Gray G, et al. Trends in pregnancy labeling and data quality for US-approved pharmaceuticals. *Am J Obstet Gynecol.* 2014;211:690.e1–e11.
6. Kim JH, Scialli AR. Thalidomide: the tragedy of birth defects and the effective treatment of disease. *Toxicol Sci.* 2011;122(1):1–6.
7. Garg R, Bracken W, Hoberman A, Enright B, Tornesi B. In: Gupta R, ed. *Reproductive and Developmental Toxicology.* 2nd ed. Elsevier; 2017. Chapter 6: Reproductive and Developmental Safety Evaluation of New Pharmaceutical Compounds. 101–127.
8. ICH S5 (R3). *Detection of Toxicity to Reproduction for Human Pharmaceuticals;* 2017. http://www.ich.org/products/guidelines/safety/article/safety-guidelines.html.
9. Food and Drug Administration (FDA). *Guidance for Industry: ICH S6 Addendum to Preclinical Safety Evaluation of Biotechnology-Derived Pharmaceuticals.* May 2012. https://www.fda.gov/downloads/Drugs/GuidanceComplianceRegulatoryInformation/Guidances/UCM194490.pdf.
10. Pentsuk N, van der Laan JW. An interspecies comparison of placental antibody transfer: new insights into developmental toxicity testing of monoclonal antibodies. *Birth Defects Res (Part B).* 2009;86:328–344.
11. ICH S6 (R1). *Preclinical Safety Evaluation of Biotechnology Derived Pharmaceuticals;* 2011. http://www.ich.org/products/guidelines/safety/article/safety-guidelines.html.
12. Trasler J, Doerksen T. Teratogen update: paternal exposures—reproductive risks. *Teratology.* 1999;60:161–172.
13. ICH M3 (R2). *Guidance on Nonclinical Safety Studies for the Conduct of Human Clinical Trials and Marketing Authorization for Pharmaceuticals;* 2009. http://www.ich.org/products/guidelines/multidisciplinary/article/multidisciplinary-guidelines.html.
14. Clinical Trials Facilitation Group. *Recommendations Related to Contraception and Pregnancy Testing in Clinical Trials.* September 2014.
15. Byers J, Sarver J. *Pharmacology Principles and Practice.* Academic Press; 2009 [chapter 10] http://www.sciencedirect.com/science/article/pii/B9780123695215000105.
16. Chen C, Beyer B, Breslin W, et al. Introduction to the HESI DART drugs in semen consortium. *Reprod Toxicol.* 2014;48:113–114.
17. Klemmt L, Scialli A. The transport of chemicals in semen. *Birth Defects Res.* 2005;74:119–131.
18. Lutwak-Mann. Observations of progeny or thalidomide treated male rabbits. *Br Med J;* 1964:1090–1091. http://europepmc.org/articles/PMC1814448.
19. Scialli A, Bailey G, Beyer B, et al. Potential seminal transport of pharmaceuticals to the conceptus. *Reprod Toxicol.* 2015;58:213–221.
20. Hui JY, Hoffmann M, Kumar G. Embryo-fetal exposure and developmental outcome of thalidomide following oral and intravaginal administration to pregnant rabbits. *Reprod Toxicol.* 2014;48:115–123.
21. Moffat G, Davies R, Kwon G, et al. Investigation of maternal and fetal exposure to an IgG2 monoclonal antibody following biweekly intravaginal administration to cynomolgus monkeys throughout pregnancy. *Reprod Toxicol.* 2014;48:132–137.
22. Sohn W, Lee E, Kankam M, et al. An open-label study in healthy men to evaluate the risk of seminal fluid transmission of denosumab to pregnant partners. *Br J Clin Pharmacol.* 2015:1–8.
23. *Guideline on the Exposure to Medicinal Products During Pregnancy: Need for Post-Authorisation Data.* European Medicines Agency (EMA), Committee for Medicinal Products for Human Use (CHMP); 2006. http://www.ema.europa.eu/docs/en_GB/document_library/Regulatory_and_procedural_guideline/2009/11/WC500011303.pdf.
24. https://www.cdc.gov/ncbddd/birthdefects/macdp.html.
25. Howard TB, Tassinari MS, Feibus KB, Mathis LL. Monitoring for teratogenic signals: pregnancy registries and surveillance methods. *Am J Med Genet C Semin Med Genet.* 2011;157:209–214.
26. Kennedy D, Uhl K, Kweder S. Pregnancy exposure registries. *Drug Saf.* 2004;27(4):215–228.
27. *Captopril Prescribing Information;* 2017. https://www.drugs.com/pro/captopril-tablets.html.
28. Wyszynski D. Pregnancy exposure registries: academic opportunities and industry responsibility. *Birth Defects Res (Part A) Clin Mol Teratol.* 2009;85:93–101.
29. http://www.eurocat-network.eu/aboutus/whatiseurocat/whatiseurocat.
30. Food and Drug Administration (FDA). *Guidance for Industry: Establishing Pregnancy Exposure Registries;* 2002. www.fda.gov/downloads/drugs/guidancecomplianceregulatoryinformation/guidances/ucm071639.pdf.
31. https://www.fda.gov/ScienceResearch/SpecialTopics/WomensHealthResearch/ucm251314.htm.
32. http://nbdps.org/.
33. http://www.bu.edu/slone/research/studies/phis/.
34. Alwan S, Reefhuis J, Rasmussen S, Olney R, Friedman J. Use of selective serotonin-reuptake inhibitors in pregnancy and the risk of birth defects. *N Engl J Med.* 2007;356:2684–2692.
35. Louik C, Lin A, Werler M, Hernández-Díaz S, Mitchell A. First-trimester use of selective serotonin-reuptake inhibitors and the risk of birth defects. *N Engl J Med.* 2007;356:2675–2683.
36. https://www.fda.gov/biologicsbloodvaccines/guidancecomplianceregulatoryinformation/actsrulesregulations/ucm445102.htm.

37. *Guideline on Risk Assessment of Medicinal Products on Human Reproduction and Lactation: From Data to Labeling.* European Medicines Agency (EMA), Committee for Medicinal Products for Human Use (CHMP); 2009. http://www.ema.europa.eu/docs/en_GB/document_library/Scientific_guideline/2009/09/WC500003307.pdf.

38. *EMA Guideline on Risk Management Systems for Medicinal Products for Human Use.* November 2005.

39. https://www.ipledgeprogram.com/.

40. Berard A, Axoulay L, Koren G, Blais L, Perreault S, Oraichi D. Isotretinoin, pregnancies, abortions and birth defects: a population-based perspective. *Br J Clin Pharmacol.* 2007;63(2):196–205.

41. https://www.ipledgeprogram.com/documents/BC%20Lessons%20Learned%2006.13.2013.pdf.

42. Choi JS, Koren G, Nulman I. Pregnancy and isotretinoin therapy. *CMAJ.* 2013. https://doi.org/10.1503/cmaj.120729.

CHAPTER 9

Pharmacovigilance in Pediatrics

ARIEL RAMIREZ PORCALLA, MD, MPH

INTRODUCTION

The appropriate use of medications in the pediatric age group, which encompasses newborns to individuals 18 years of age, is challenging because of limited drug development within this population (Box 9.1). At the time of approval, the majority of medications have not been evaluated appropriately for use in children with a dedicated pediatric study, resulting in the lack of sufficient metabolic, safety, efficacy, and dosing information for children for most medications approved in adults. A review of drug product labeling listed in the electronic Physicians' Desk Reference showed that only 46% of products had some information on pediatric use in labeling.[1] The lack of pediatric specific information in product labels can lead to "off-label use" of medications in the pediatric population. This becomes a significant issue in specific populations of children, including preterm infants and newborns, and in children with chronic or rare diseases.[2]

In the absence of information on the optimal dose for children, off-label prescribing may put children at risk for treatment failure as medications may be given at doses that are not efficacious or safe for children. When relatively higher doses of medications are given to children, higher drug exposures may occur when compared to adults, resulting in adverse drug reactions. According to the Substance Abuse and Mental Health Services Administration, an estimated 211,209 children aged 12 years and younger visited the emergency room in 2008 due to adverse reactions to medications or nutritional products.[3]

Prior to current pediatric legislation, several inherent factors were responsible for the lack of drug development activities for the pediatric population, despite high pediatric disease burden. These include the lower prevalence of diseases for which new drugs have been evaluated for an adult indication, resulting in recruitment and feasibility challenges, ethical challenges for pediatric clinical studies, and trial complexity. In addition, depending on the disease state, there can be a low return on investment for pediatric medications. Together, these factors have led to a low number of pediatric clinical trials, even in medical conditions with high pediatric disease burden.[4]

In the context of limited clinical development, the conduct of pharmacovigilance to monitor the use of medications in the pediatric population and to identify pediatric-specific safety concerns becomes more important. Various stakeholders are involved in the impetus to encourage pharmaceutical companies to proactively plan to conduct dedicated pediatric clinical trials earlier in the drug's clinical development and to implement robust pharmacovigilance processes relevant to the pediatric population. Stakeholders include the pediatric population and their parents/caregivers, regulatory authorities, healthcare providers and their organizations, the pharmaceutical industry, and national and commercial healthcare systems, among others.

BOX 9.1
Use of Medications in Children

- Because of limited drug development for the pediatric age group, sufficient safety, efficacy, and dosing information for children is lacking in labels of numerous medicinal products.
- This predisposes children to off-label use of these medications.

LEGISLATION FOR PEDIATRIC DRUG DEVELOPMENT

To encourage pediatric drug development, regulatory authorities such as the US Food and Drug Administration (USFDA) and the European Medicines Agency (EMA) have implemented incentive-driven legislation that require pharmaceutical companies to provide a formal strategy to evaluate new medications in children (Box 9.2).

The United States

The US Congress passed the Best Pharmaceuticals for Children Act (BPCA) in 2002[3] and the Pediatric Research Equity Act (PREA) in 2003.[3] The BPCA reauthorized a provision that was originally contained in the Food and Drug Administration (FDA) Modernization Act of 1997 in 1997.[3]

The PREA requires pharmaceutical companies to submit a pediatric assessment that provides pediatric safety and efficacy data with dosing recommendations with a new drug or biologic agent application. The PREA was permanently reauthorized in the Prescription Drug User Fee Act of 2012, also known as the FDA Safety and Innovation Act. However, this requirement can be waived or deferred so that a majority of the drugs approved in the United States are granted initial approval without pediatric data, provided that a Pediatric Study Plan (PSP) has been agreed on by the pharmaceutical company and the FDA. The PSP is provided to the FDA by a pharmaceutical company planning to submit a marketing application for a drug or biological product that includes a new active ingredient, new indication, new dosage form, new dosing regimen, or new route of administration. It includes background pediatric information for the drug or biological product's proposed indication along with a proposal and timelines for pediatric studies. The intent of the PSP is to identify the need for pediatric studies so that pharmaceutical companies can initiate planning for these studies early in drug development.

Another piece of legislation addressing pediatric drug development in the United States is the BPCA which provides a 6-month patent extension for the entire moiety when a pharmaceutical company voluntarily conducts a pediatric study for an indication that the FDA may deem to have a significant public health impact for the pediatric population.[5]

These two legislations complement each other. BPCA (often called the "carrot"), provides a financial incentive in the form of 6-month pediatric exclusivity with the remaining drug patent to pharmaceutical companies that evaluate drugs in pediatric patients. In addition, this Act creates a process by which the FDA and the National Institutes of Health (NIH) can partner to obtain studies of off-patent drugs in pediatric patients. PREA (the "stick") requires pediatric assessments of new drug and biologic licensing applications for all new active ingredients, indications, dosage forms, dosing regimens, and routes of administration. The pediatric assessment must contain sufficient data to support the pediatric drug labeling.[3]

These legislations encourage the pharmaceutical industry to initiate pediatric drug development early during drug development. Twenty-one percent (21.7%) of new drugs approved by the FDA from December 2003 to July 2012 had completed pediatric assessments at the time of approval. Of those approved without pediatric assessments, only 35% were eventually evaluated for a pediatric indication, with a mean time of completion from approval of 6.5 years, suggesting that most companies were not able to meet the deadlines agreed on with the FDA.[6] Despite this, as a result of pediatric exclusivity, most drugs (92%) granted exclusivity from 1998 to 2012 by the USFDA added pediatric information to their labeling, with the majority (57%) receiving a new or expanded indication, demonstrating the legislations' positive impact in pediatric drug development in the United States.[7]

European Union

The European Union (EU) Paediatric Regulation[8] was adopted by the European Parliament and the European Council in December 2006 to establish regulatory requirements for pharmaceutical companies to develop medicines for pediatric use. The Paediatric Regulation intends to improve the health of children by facilitating the development and availability of medications for children from birth to 18 years of age. This is done by ensuring that medications used by children are of high quality, ethically researched, and authorized appropriately and by improving the availability of pediatric information to help use these medications.

Specifically, the Paediatric Regulation requires companies to submit a Paediatric Investigation Plan (PIP) prior to the submission of the marketing authorization application of a new medication, to be mutually agreed on by the Paediatric Committee (PDCO) of the EMA. The PIP provides the timing and measures being proposed by a pharmaceutical company to generate data for a pediatric indication. In particular, the PIP describes studies planned to establish safety and efficacy of the new drug in the pediatric population, including the development of an age-appropriate formulation for use in relevant pediatric age groups.[9] Once the medication is authorized in all member states of the EU and the pediatric study results are incorporated in the European label, as a reward, the medication becomes eligible for 6 months extension of the product's supplementary protection certificate, which provides a company with an additional period of market exclusivity.[10]

The PDCO, a multidisciplinary scientific committee established under the Paediatric Regulation, is responsible for the assessment and agreement of PIPs and waivers and interacts with other Agency committees, such as the Committee for Medicinal Products of Human Use and the Pharmacovigilance Risk Assessment Committee (PRAC).

The Paediatric Regulation was noted to have a considerable impact on the development of pediatric medications in the EU as it ensured that pediatric drug development is initiated early during drug development. To strengthen the Regulation's effectiveness over time, the EMA recognizes that its implementation needs to continually be improved.[11]

A summary of the legislative strategies used by the United States and the EU to ensure that companies include the evaluation of the safety and efficacy of new drug products in the pediatric population as part of the medication's overall development strategy is shown in Table 9.1.[5] Given the parallel efforts by both the FDA and the EMA to foster pediatric drug development, both have agreed to collaborate and ensure interaction and exchange of information on pediatric issues.[12]

Despite these legislations, limited information on dosing, safety, and efficacy of drugs is being generated from dedicated pediatric trials. Therefore, it is important to monitor the appropriate use of medications in children once they are on market.

UNIQUE CONSIDERATIONS IN THE PEDIATRIC POPULATION

The evaluation of safety in clinical trials and the conduct of pharmacovigilance in both pre- and postauthorization settings in children are different from those in adults and require the recognition of unique pediatric characteristics and medical conditions specific to children in general or to specific age groups (Box 9.3). These reflect the long-held principle in clinical pediatrics that "children are not just little adults".[3] Pediatric age groupings utilized for healthcare and research are based on the evolving physiologic, morphologic, and neurocognitive changes that occur during these periods. These age groupings account for age-related changes and promote consistency in reporting data. Age-appropriate

evaluations then translate to optimal dosing regimens, distinctive responses to treatment, and potential safety concerns specific for each age group. Below is a pediatric age grouping (Table 9.2) developed by the National Institute of Child Health and Human Development of the US NIH recommended for use with study inclusion and subgroup analyses in randomized clinical trials.[13]

In view of these, the evaluation of safety in children during clinical development and postauthorization require consideration of the following unique pediatric characteristics[14]:

- The types and disease burden of pediatric illnesses and medical conditions differ from adults. With potential differences in treatment response and the safety risks, the benefit-risk profile of a drug could differ between children and adults.

- Certain medical conditions only occur in the pediatric population. Examples of these include rare metabolic or genetic diseases and neonatal respiratory distress syndrome from prematurity. The evaluation of therapies for these pediatric-specific conditions are especially challenging because the entire development program will be conducted in the pediatric population, including the initial pharmacokinetic, safety, and tolerability studies. In addition, the rarity of these metabolic or genetic diseases provide greater challenges for development of their specific therapies in terms of study conduct and low commercial incentive. As a result, both the USFDA and the EMA have instituted several programs to foster the evaluation and development of medicinal products for the diagnosis and/or treatment of these rare diseases or conditions. These include the USFDA's Orphan Drug programs such as the Orphan Drug Designation Program and the Rare Pediatric Disease Priority Review Voucher Program[15,16]

- The vulnerability of children to develop adverse drug reactions and/or toxicities changes depending on the patient's age and stage of growth and development.[17]
  - Preterm newborn infants
    These infants are a heterogeneous group, from a 25-week gestation preterm low-birth weight infant to a 30-week gestation newborn, with differing characteristics and vulnerabilities. Important considerations when evaluating risk for toxicities include: (1) gestational age at birth and adjusted age (age after birth); (2) immaturity of renal and hepatic clearance mechanisms; (3) protein binding and displacement issues (e.g., bilirubin); (4) penetration of medications

TABLE 9.1
Comparison of Similarities and Differences Between US and EU Pediatric Legislation

	USFDA BPCA/FDASIA 2012	USFDA PREA/FDASIA 2012	EU-EMA Paediatric Regulation
Applies to	Incentive	Requirement	Incentive and requirement (obligations)
Scope of pediatric development	Any indication in the pediatric population where potential exists for therapeutic benefit	Same as adult indication	Derived from adult indication, within the same condition
Types of products	All medicinal products	New medicinal products and biosimilars	New medicinal products; authorized products under patent/SPC if applying for new indication/route/form
Orphan-designated products	Included from obligations	Excluded from obligations	Included from obligations
Products excluded from scope of obligations	N/A	Homeopathic, generic and traditional herbal products	Homeopathic, generic, hybrid, well-established use, traditional herbal, biosimilar medicinal products
Pediatric development	Optional	Mandatory unless waived	Mandatory unless waived
Instrument	Written Request	Pediatric Study Plan	Paediatric Investigation Plan
Waiver	N/A	4 grounds	3 grounds
Timing of plan/waiver submission	Anytime adequate data are available	End of Phase 2 studies in adults	End of Phase 1 studies in adults (during Phase 2 if justified)
Main reward	6-month patent extension on the moiety	None	6-month SPC extension (patent); 2-year extension for orphan medicinal products
Decision	FDA Review Division (PeRC with advisory role)	FDA Review Division (PeRC with advisory role)	EMA after Opinion from PDCO
18-month pediatric safety assessment by the Pediatric Advisory Committee	Yes	Yes	No
Scientific advice from regulatory authority	Typically included in global licensing fee	Typically included in global licensing fee	No cost for paediatric development

BPCA, Best Pharmaceuticals for Children Act; *EMA*, European Medicines Agency; *EU-EMA*, European Union–European Medicines Agency; *FDA*, Food and Drug Administration; *FDASIA*, Food and Drug Administration Safety and Innovation Act; *N/A*, not applicable; *PDCO*, Paediatric Committee; *PeRC*, Pediatric Review Committee; *PREA*, Pediatric Research Equity Act; *SPC*, supplementary protection certificate; *USFDA*, US Food and Drug Administration.
Penkov D, Tomasi P, Eichler I, Murphy D, Yao LP, Temeck J. Pediatric medicine development: an overview and comparison of regulatory processes in the European Union and United States. *Ther Innov Regul Sci*. 2017; 51(3):360–371.

into the central nervous system (CNS); (5) disease states unique to the neonatal period including respiratory distress syndrome and congenital heart defects such as patent ductus arteriosus; (6) unique susceptibilities of the preterm newborn such as necrotizing enterocolitis, intraventricular hemorrhage, retinopathy of prematurity, etc.; (7) rapid and variable maturation of all physiologic and pharmacologic processes leading to different dosing

- Inherent physiologic and developmental characteristics and medical conditions unique for specific pediatric age groups exist.
- These evolving characteristics make the evaluation of safety and efficacy in children in clinical trials and in post-authorization settings different from and more challenging when compared to adults.

TABLE 9.2
Pediatric Age Groupings

Stage	Definitions (Release Date July 6, 2011)
Preterm neonatal	The period at birth when a newborn is born before the full gestational period
Term neonatal	Birth–27 days
Infancy	28 days–12 months
Toddler	13 months–2 years
Early childhood	2–5 years
Middle childhood	6–11 years
Early adolescence	12–18 years
Late adolescence	19–21 years

Williams K, Thomson D, Seto I, et al. Standard 6: age groups for pediatric trials. *Pediatrics*. 2012;129(suppl 3): S153–S160.

regimens with chronic exposure; and (8) transdermal absorption of medications.

- Term newborn infants

    Although more developmentally mature than preterm newborn infants, many of the physiologic and pharmacologic issues discussed above apply to this subgroup of children. The blood-brain barrier is still not fully developed and medications and endogenous substances (such as bilirubin) could gain access to the CNS and cause toxicity. Oral absorption of medications may be less predictable. Increased susceptibility to toxicities of medications from limited clearance (e.g., chloramphenicol gray baby syndrome) can also occur in this age group. On the other hand, term newborns may be less susceptible to some types of adverse effects (e.g., aminoglycoside toxicity) than patients in older groups.

- Infants and toddlers (28 days–23 months)

    Rapid CNS maturation, immune system development, and total body growth occur during this period. Oral absorption becomes reliable. Hepatic and renal clearance pathways continue to mature. At 1–2 years of age, clearance of many drugs may exceed adult values, resulting in the need for higher efficacious doses relative to the adult doses.

- Children (2–11 years)

    Most pathways of drug clearance mature, with clearance exceeding adult values. During this period, the impact of medications on growth and development should be considered, particularly because children achieve several important milestones of psychomotor development, which can be adversely affected by CNS-active drugs. At this time, the effects of a medication on skeletal growth, weight gain, school attendance, and school performance should be determined. Recruitment in pediatric trials should ensure adequate representation across age ranges in this subgroup. Finally, the effect of a medication on puberty and the effect of puberty on the metabolism of medications should be determined.

- Adolescents (12–18 years)

    Because this is a period of sexual maturation, the effect of medications on the actions of sex hormones should be determined. The potential for pregnancy should be considered. During this time, illnesses are also influenced by pubertal hormonal and growth changes. These include insulin resistance in diabetes mellitus, recurrence of seizures around menarche, and changes in the frequency and severity of migraine attacks and asthma exacerbations. Lastly, the impact of medications on this period of rapid growth and neurocognitive development should be determined. Given that adolescents begin to assume responsibility for their own health and medications, compliance is another factor to consider.

- In chronic childhood diseases where prolonged treatment durations are needed, children are at increased risk of developing toxicities due to the longer exposure to treatment. Furthermore, the impact of medications given chronically on a child's growth and physical and cognitive development has to be evaluated through long-term studies. Some examples of chronic diseases where exposure to treatment could be prolonged include steroids for asthma, antiretroviral in HIV-infected children, and immunotherapy and immunomodulators for rheumatologic diseases.

- Because of the rapidly evolving changes in body mass, physiology, morphology, and composition in a growing child, the identification and selection of the optimal dosing regimen in children is challenging; this could result either in underdosing and treatment failure or overdosing and adverse reactions. This situation is exacerbated by the lack of pediatric pharmacokinetic (PK) and pharmacodynamic (PD) information specific to children.

- Fortunately, the efficacy and treatment response of a medication in the pediatric population can be extrapolated from the same indications as those studied and approved in adults, in situations where the pathophysiology of the illness is similar between children and adults and where drug exposures equivalent to those in adults can be achieved using appropriate pediatric dosing regimens. When extrapolation is used to estimate pediatric efficacy, pharmacokinetic studies in the relevant age groups that are likely to receive the medication, together with pediatric safety studies, will still be necessary, since the pharmacokinetic and safety profile of a drug in children cannot necessarily be extrapolated from adult clinical trials.[17] The vulnerability of children to develop toxicities depends on the maturation of organ systems such as the skin, lungs, kidney, liver, and the blood-brain barrier.

- The evaluation of formulations such as liquids, suspensions, and chewable tablets that are appropriate for pediatric patients of different age groups is paramount to ensure accurate dosing and enhance patient compliance. In addition, specific flavors and colors may encourage effective administration, and therefore compliance, of oral medications and should also be considered.[17]

Furthermore, because of the immaturity of organ systems and of metabolic processes for drugs and excipients, younger children are more susceptible to toxicities and adverse reactions. Examples of severe outcomes include respiratory depression, renal failure, metabolic acidosis, and changes in sensorium observed when drug products with excipients (such as propylene glycol and alcohol) are given to newborns, who have limited abilities to metabolize these excipients expediently.

UNIQUE PHARMACOVIGILANCE CHALLENGES FOR CHILDREN

The importance of a thorough and robust pharmacovigilance process as well as methodologies specific to the needs of the pediatric population cannot be overemphasized. Several important challenges in monitoring the safety of drugs used in children exist and are summarized in Table 9.3.

SAFETY DATA COLLECTION TO IMPROVE CHARACTERIZATION OF THE SAFETY PROFILE OF MEDICATIONS USED IN THE PEDIATRIC POPULATION

The lack of sufficient metabolic (PK/PD), safety, efficacy, and dosing information for children for most medications approved in adults puts the pediatric population at risk for "off-label use" (Box 9.4). Outcomes of off-label use include treatment failure from underdosing and increased risk for adverse reactions and toxicities from overdosing.

There is an impetus to conduct clinical trials dedicated to the pediatric population. The conduct of pediatric PK/PD studies and pediatric clinical trials is a major source of pediatric safety and efficacy information. With incentives and requirements for conducting pediatric clinical trials early on during the clinical development of a drug, the conduct of these trials are specified in both the PSP as agreed with the FDA and the Pediatric Investigation Plan as agreed with the EMA.

In the postauthorization stage, with the limitations of the pediatric clinical trial from a small sample size, safety information from clinical trials is augmented by spontaneous adverse event reports from healthcare professionals and consumers of the approved medicinal product. In addition, the required postauthorization safety studies and postmarketing requirements provide additional safety information for specific safety issues that the PRAC of the EMA (see Chapter 1) and the FDA, respectively, deem necessary to evaluate.

Surveillance of safety information from real-world evidence sources, such as patient registries and pediatric clinical trial networks established to monitor specific safety issues, provide additional safety information postauthorization (see Chapter 5). An example of a cohort used in targeted surveillance of pediatric patients is the European Pregnancy and Paediatric Cohort Collaboration, which is an international network of cohort studies coordinated by the Paediatric European Network for Treatment of AIDS, which conducts epidemiological research on HIV-infected pregnant women,

TABLE 9.3
Pharmacovigilance Pediatric Challenges

Challenge	Basis for Challenge	Implications and Other Comments
Serious and rare ADRs may be difficult to identify and monitor	Typical small sample size for pediatric clinical trials, especially for rare medical conditions	Identification and evaluation of causality will rely on evidence of association between the ADR and the drug. Stakeholders should be encouraged to report pediatric adverse events
Long-term safety outcomes such as effect on the growth and neurocognitive development of children and on the durability of response may be challenging to identify and monitor	Study design of pediatric clinical trial have typically shorter follow-up periods	Effect on growth and development and on durability of response will require longer follow-up periods
ADRs or toxicities related to "off-label use" may be underreported because of caregiver and healthcare provider legal and liability concerns	Off-label use in the pediatric population may have legal and liability concerns	The risk of "off-label use," which is common in the pediatric population may be underestimated
Underreporting of ADRs/toxicities, especially in the younger age groups as they are nonverbal, and caregivers may not fully be able to characterize the ADR/toxicity		Underestimation of ADRs in the younger age-group
Premature babies and neonates, who are at greater risk for more severe outcomes (ADRs and toxicities) may not be well represented	Small number of premature babies and neonates in clinical studies and in postauthorization exposure rates	The safety profile of a drug may be difficult to characterize in these vulnerable subpopulations, so that only serious and severe outcomes associated with a drug may be recognized

ADRs, adverse drug reactions.
Based on: CHMP. *Guideline on Conduct of Pharmacovigilance for Medicines Used by the Paediatric Population*. 2006.

BOX 9.4
Safety Surveillance in Children

- There are several sources of pediatric safety information:
  - Clinical Development: Dedicated clinical trials
  - Post-approval stage: Spontaneous adverse event reports from consumers, Pediatric cohort registries, Real-world experience [RWE] sources
- These should be utilized to optimize surveillance and evaluation of pediatric safety information to determine the evolving safety profile of medicinal products in children.

children, and children exposed to HIV in utero (including safety surveillance of HIV-infected individuals receiving a particular drug therapy). Lastly, the development of periodic regulatory safety documents, such as the Periodic Adverse Drug Experience Reports submitted to the USFDA, the Periodic Safety Update Reports submitted to the EMA, and the Developmental Safety Update Reports enable pharmaceutical companies to provide an integrated evaluation of the evolving safety profile of an approved medicinal product using safety information from these multiple data sources.

As the pediatric safety database is limited at the time of approval, safety information obtained from postmarketing sources is particularly important, especially when long-term outcomes such as the effects of a medication on a child's growth and development are of particular concern. Postmarketing surveillance and/or long-term follow-up studies can therefore provide relevant pediatric safety and/or efficacy information.

CONCLUSION

The importance of a thorough and robust pharmacovigilance process specific to the pediatric population cannot be overemphasized. Dedicated pediatric PK/PD studies and clinical trials are major sources of metabolic, safety, efficacy, and dosing information for this population. While challenges in developing and evaluating drugs for children remain, legislations have been enacted to specify regulatory requirements and provide incentives for the pharmaceutical industry, encouraging pediatric drug development to generate sufficient information for pediatric labeling. Proactive surveillance of safety information in children from a variety of sources, including pediatric clinical trials, registries, and adverse event reports from consumers, provide relevant pediatric safety and/or efficacy information. All these ensure that children are able to use medications safely and effectively.

REFERENCES

1. Sachs AN, Avant D, Lee CS, Rodriguez W, Murphy MD. Pediatric information in drug product labeling. *JAMA*. 2012; 307(18):1914–1915.
2. American Academy of Pediatrics. *Use of Off-Label Drugs for Children*; 2018. https://www.aap.org/en-us/about-the-aap/aap-press-room/pages/AAP-Makes-Recommendations-On-Use-of-Off-Label-Drugs-for-Children.aspx.
3. U.S. Food and Drug Administration. *FDA Encourages Pediatric Information on Drug Labeling*; 2016. https://www.fda.gov/Drugs/ResourcesForYou/SpecialFeatures/ucm254072.htm.
4. Bourgeois FT, Murthy S, Pinto C, Olson KL, Ioannidis JP, Mandl KD. Pediatric versus adult drug trials for conditions with high pediatric disease burden. *Pediatrics*. 2012; 130(2):285–292.
5. Penkov D, Tomasi P, Eichler I, Murphy D, Yao LP, Temeck J. Pediatric medicine development: an overview and comparison of regulatory processes in the European Union and United States. *Ther Innov Regul Sci*. 2017; 51(3):360–371.
6. Hudgins JD, Bacho MA, Olsen KL, Bourgeois FT. Pediatric drug information available at the time of new drug approvals: a cross-sectional analysis. *Pharmacoepidemiol Drug Saf*. November 2017. https://doi.org/10.1002/pds.4351 [Epub ahead of print].
7. Wharton GT, Murphy D, Avant D, et al. Impact of pediatric exclusivity on drug labeling and demonstrations of efficacy. *Pediatrics*. 2014;134:e512–e518.
8. The European Parliament and of the Council. *Regulation (EC) No. 1901/2006*; 2006. https://ec.europa.eu/health//sites/health/files/files/eudralex/vol-1/reg_2006_1901/reg_2006_1901_en.pdf.
9. Tomasi PA, Egger GF, Pallidis C, Saint-Raymond A. Enabling development of paediatric medicines in Europe: 10 years of the EU paediatric regulation. *Paediatr Drugs*. 2017;19(6):505–513.
10. The European Parliament and of the Council. *Regulation (EC) No. 469/2009*; 2009. https://ec.europa.eu/health/sites/health/files/files/eudralex/vol-1/reg_469_2009/reg_469_2009_en.pdf.
11. *Report from the Commission to the European Parliament and the Council. State of Paediatric Medicines in the EU: 10 Years of the EU Paediatric Regulation*; 2017. https://ec.europa.eu/health/sites/health/files/files/paediatrics/docs/2017_childrensmedicines_report_en.pdf.
12. European Medicines Agency. *Better Medicines for Children*; 2015. http://www.ema.europa.eu/docs/en_GB/document_library/Leaflet/2009/12/WC500026493.pdf.
13. Williams K, Thomson D, Seto I, et al. Standard 6: age groups for pediatric trials. *Pediatrics*. 2012;129(suppl 3): S153–S160.
14. Committee for Medicinal Products for Human Use (CHMP). *Guideline on Conduct of Pharmacovigilance for Medicines Used by the Paediatric Population*; 2007. http://www.ema.europa.eu/docs/en_GB/document_library/Scientific_guideline/2009/09/WC500003764.pdf.
15. U.S. Food and Drug Administration. *Developing Products for Rare Diseases and Conditions*; 2018. https://www.fda.gov/ForIndustry/DevelopingProductsforRareDiseasesConditions/default.htm.
16. U.S. Food and Drug Administration. *Clarification of Orphan Designation of Drugs and Biologics for Pediatric Subpopulations of Common Diseases — Draft Guidance for Industry*; December 2017. https://www.fda.gov/downloads/RegulatoryInformation/Guidances/UCM589710.pdf.
17. European Medicines Agency. *ICH Topic E11: Clinical Investigation of Medicinal Products in the Paediatric Population*; 2001. http://www.ema.europa.eu/docs/en_GB/document_library/Scientific_guideline/2009/09/WC500002926.pdf.

CHAPTER 10

Pharmacovigilance in Special Populations: Elderly

ANTHONY G. OLADIPO, PHARMD, MPH, BCPS • CHERYL RENZ, MS, MD

INTRODUCTION

The elderly are prone to multiple medical conditions due to changes in biological processes associated with aging. This leads to the use of multiple medications and increased risk for drug–drug interactions (DDIs), drug–disease interactions (DDis), medication errors, and adverse drug reactions (ADRs). This chapter highlights several important factors to consider when conducting safety evaluations for medicinal products used by elderly patients. These include age-related changes in pharmacokinetic and pharmacodynamic effects and the need for specialized data collection and analysis of elderly patient cohorts throughout the product life cycle. This chapter also addresses the importance of communicating risks and measures to minimize the risks to the growing elderly population.

The Growing Elderly Population

The number of the elderly is increasing (Box 10.1) worldwide. In 2017, the number of the elderly (people aged 65 years and older) was approximately 657.2 million; this number is projected to increase to 996.7 million in 2030 and 1.56 billion in 2050.[1] Projections for the size of the elderly population by region (using 65 years as the cutoff) for 2030 and 2050 are shown in Fig. 10.1.

While the number of the elderly is increasing, so is the proportion of the elderly. This is primarily due to a decline in fertility (number of live births) and decrease in mortality driven by improvements in overall health status, medical breakthroughs, and better access to healthcare services. This is reflected in the increase in average life expectancy globally by 13.8 years since 1960.[2] In 2017, approximately 8.8% of the world population was the elderly[1]; this proportion is projected to increase to 12% by 2030 and 16% by 2050.[3] The increasing proportion of the elderly worldwide will impact both healthcare needs and pharmacovigilance efforts.

Disease Burden in the Elderly

Health status in the elderly is the result of complex multifactorial biological processes dependent on physiologic, structural, and functional changes with aging (Box 10.2).[4,5] Alterations in these biological processes can increase susceptibility to diseases. Prevalence of multimorbidity (two or more chronic conditions) among the elderly ranged from 62% to 81%.[6] In addition, comorbidity increases with age[7,8] and is associated with increased risk of premature death, hospitalization, loss of physical functioning, depression, and polypharmacy.[8,9]

The most common medical conditions in the elderly population include heart disease, cancer, chronic bronchitis or emphysema, stroke, diabetes mellitus, Alzheimer disease, and arthritis.[7,8,9] Another factor is the immune response decline with age, which increases susceptibility to infection. Drugs that further alter immune function may increase the risk for infections in the elderly. Metabolic disorders can worsen with age, such as insulin resistance or diabetes. Aging leads to changes in cardiovascular function, such as decreases in cardiac output, heart rate, and vasculature elasticity, and impaired baroreflex responsiveness. Elderly patients are more susceptible to drug

---

BOX 10.1
Growing Elderly Population

The elderly population is projected to increase worldwide to
- 1 billion in 2030
- 1.56 billion in 2050

The proportion of elderly worldwide is expected to increase from 8.8% (in 2017) to 12% by 2030.

The increasing proportion of elderly worldwide will impact both healthcare needs and pharmacovigilance efforts.

Elderly Population Projections by Region: 2015-2050
(values in millions of people)

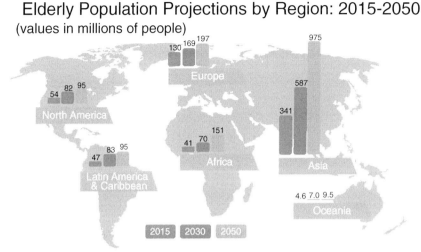

FIG. 10.1 Elderly population projections by region: 2015–50 (values in millions of people). (An Aging World. *International Population Reports. US Census Bureau, Issue March 2016*. 2015. Available at: https://www. census.gov/content/dam/Census/library/publications/2016/demo/p95–16–1.pdf.)

BOX 10.2
Age Related Physiologic or Biologic Changes Linked to Adverse Outcomes

In the elderly, multiple chronic diseases, cognitive impairment, polypharmacy, and age-related changes in biological processes increase the likelihood of drug–drug interactions, drug–disease interactions, medication errors, and adverse drug reactions.

effects that impact the cardiovascular system. For example, drugs that lower blood pressure (such as diuretics, angiotensin-converting enzyme inhibitors, or β-blockers) may increase the risk for orthostatic effects, such as syncope leading to falls. Elderly patients may also experience changes in their pulmonary status, such as reduced vital capacity, respiratory muscle weakness, decreased alveoli gas exchange, and diminished response to hypoxia and hypercapnia, which increase the risk for developing pneumonia, chronic obstructive pulmonary disease, and sleep apnea. In addition, elderly patients are more susceptible to pulmonary ADRs.

The increased prevalence of multiple chronic diseases in the elderly population[9,10] has been linked to the use of multiple medications, including prescriptions, over-the-counter medicines, and herbal remedies. The combination of advanced age, polypharmacy, and

multiple morbidities is related to DDIs,[11] DDis,[12,13] medication errors,[14] and ADRs; these are especially problematic for the elderly who reside in nursing homes.[15,16]

The elderly also experience cognitive impairment that typically manifests as problems with memory, attention, problem solving, learning, and decreased motor speed and reaction times.[17] Cognitive impairment can result from neurodegenerative diseases (especially dementia and Alzheimer disease), cardiovascular disorders, depression, stroke, and traumatic brain injury. Cognitive impairment can impede an elderly patient's ability to follow instructions on how to use a medication or remember which products to avoid (including herbal or other medicines) when taking it. Overall, due to diminishing cognition, elderly patients are prone to poor medication adherence, medication errors, and ADRs.

Medication Use in the Elderly

The elderly population has a high rate of medication usage; approximately 87%–90% use at least one medication[18,19] while 65% use three or more medications.[20] Among the elderly in nursing homes, 62% of the residents used six to eight medicines.[21] The use of multiple medications increases the risk for DDIs, noncompliance, medication errors, and ADRs. In a US-based study, the elderly were six times more likely to be hospitalized for an ADR than younger patients.[14]

Altered Pharmacokinetic and Pharmacodynamic Effects

Age-related physiologic changes, especially at the organ level, can affect both (Box 10.3) the pharmacokinetics and pharmacodynamics of medicines in the elderly. These effects are also influenced by age-related diseases, nutritional status, smoking status, and polypharmacy. In addition, elderly patients frequently take medications with narrow therapeutic indexes (where small differences in dose or blood concentration may lead to ADRs). All these factors predispose the elderly to ADRs and variability in drug response.

Absorption

Physiologic changes with aging in the gastrointestinal tract that can impact the absorption of medicinal products include increased gastric pH, reduced splanchnic blood flow, decreased gastric motility, delayed gastric emptying, and slow intestinal transit.[5] The bioavailability of drugs absorbed by passive diffusion is usually not affected by these changes from aging.[22] Impaired active transport processes along the gastrointestinal tract can decrease drug adsorption in the elderly.[23]

Reduced first-pass effect via reduced hepatic and/or gut wall metabolism occurs in the elderly. This can increase a drug's area under the curve and plasma concentration.[24] Research is required to better understand the effect of aging on the absorption of modified-release formulations or special-formulation drugs. For drugs administered intravascularly, there is no age-related effect on absorption.

Distribution

Age-related changes in body composition, protein binding, and blood flow (hepatic and renal) can affect the distribution of drugs and increase vulnerability to ADRs in the elderly. With aging, the body fat mass increases by 20%–40% and total body water and lean body mass decrease by 10%–15%.[25,26] The changes can affect a drug's volume of distribution (Vd) and half-life. In the elderly, lipophilic drugs (e.g., diazepam, verapamil, and metronidazole) have increased Vd and prolonged half-life,[27,28] which can result in drug accumulation with continued use, whereas hydrophilic drugs (e.g., edrophonium, famotidine, lithium, and digoxin) have reduced Vd, which leads to an increase in plasma concentration;[29,30] in both circumstances, there is an increased likelihood of drug-related toxicities. Age-related decreases in serum albumin concentrations or increases in α1-acid glycoprotein can affect the distribution of drugs that are highly protein bound.[27,29,31]

> ### BOX 10.3
> ### Age Related Pharamcokinetic and Pharmacodynamic Effects
>
> Age-related physiologic changes can affect both the pharmacokinetics and pharmacodynamics of medicines in the elderly.
>
> Aging does not appear to effect cytochrome (CYP) P450 enzymes (such as CYP3A4, CYP2D6, and CYP1A2). Clinically important DDIs from CYP enzymes in the elderly are not due to age per se, but due to polypharmacy and comorbidities.

The function of cerebrovascular P-glycoprotein (P-gp) decreases with aging.[32] A reduction or loss of P-gp efflux activities across the blood–brain barrier may lead to a higher concentration of the drugs and toxic metabolites, resulting in deleterious effects in the elderly.[33]

Metabolism

The aging process reduces protein binding,[29] hepatic perfusion by 40%–50%,[34] and capacity and liver size by 25%–35%.[35] Other age-related changes include the decreased ability of the liver to withstand stress and to repair damaged liver cells.[36] Generally, medications are detoxified through phases of drug metabolism in the liver. Phase I metabolism involves reduction, oxidation (via cytochrome [CYP] P 450), and hydroxylation; these metabolic processes are affected by advancing age. Phase II metabolism involves conjugation, acetylation, and glucuronidation processes; these processes are not typically impacted in the elderly[35] unless there is a downregulation of related enzymes.[37]

Age-related decline in hemoperfusion of the liver can impair hepatic drug clearance.

Drugs with a high hepatic extraction ratio (meaning a high ratio of hepatic drug clearance relative to hemoperfusion of the liver), such as propranolol, amitriptyline, diltiazem, metoprolol, and morphine, can be impacted by age-related decline in hepatic blood flow.[34,38] Drugs with low hepatic extraction ratio, such as warfarin and phenytoin, are slowly metabolized by hepatic enzymes and less impacted by age-related hepatic changes.[28,30] There is no evidence that age affects hepatocyte volume or liver chemistries.[34,39] Current evidence also suggests that aging has no effect on CYP enzymes (such as CYP3A4, CYP2D6, and CYP1A2).[40] Clinically important DDIs from CYP enzymes in the elderly are not due to age per se, but due to polypharmacy and comorbidities.

Excretion

Age-related renal function changes can adversely impact excretion of drugs and toxic metabolites leading to an increase in ADRs, especially in the setting of renal diseases associated with aging (such as hypertension, vascular disorders, and diabetes) and polypharmacy. With advancing age, renal changes include loss of renal mass by about 20%–25%,[41] a loss of glomeruli by 20%–30%, increased interstitial fibrosis, tubular atrophy, and arteriosclerosis.[42,43] As a result of age-related renal structural and functional changes, the glomerular filtration rate declines by 20%–50%. Reduced clearance of drugs excreted predominately via the kidney can result in the accumulation of drug and toxic metabolites, leading to an increased incidence of ADRs.[44]

Pharmacodynamics

The physiologic and/or biochemical response to drugs can change with advancing age because of the changes in receptor number, receptor affinity, second-messenger response, signal transduction and cellular response, and homeostatic regulation.[30,45] In the elderly, physiologic counterregulatory processes are slowed, which can increase vulnerability to ADRs. For example, benzodiazepines, anesthetic agents, opioid analgesics, antipsychotics, lithium, and anticholinergic medications can have pronounced CNS effects in elderly patients. These effects have resulted in increased frequency and severity of ADRs such as sedation, extrapyramidal symptoms, confusion, constipation, falls, and fractures.[46–49] Similarly, elderly patients taking tricyclic antidepressants, antipsychotics, diuretics, vasodilators, angiotensin-converting enzyme inhibitors, and opioids are at an increased risk of orthostatic hypotension[50] due to an age-related decline in arterial compliance and baroreceptor reflex.[51]

Pharmacovigilance in the Elderly Throughout the Product Life Cycle

Considerations during clinical development

During clinical development, the determination of efficacy and safety of medicinal products in elderly patients as part of a special population assessment is required if the product will primarily be indicated to treat a disease of the elderly (e.g., Alzheimer disease) or targets a disease that affects a sizable number of elderly patients (e.g., hypertension) (Box 10.4). The preapproval approach to geriatric assessment is consistent among most of the health authorities' requirements, worldwide.

Protocol study design for the investigation of efficacy and safety of products for use by the elderly should take into account specific age-related factors, including

> **BOX 10.4**
> **Drug Development Considerations for Elderly Patients**
>
> Both pharmaceutical companies and regulatory agencies recognize the importance of studying the efficacy and safety of medicinal products in elderly patients during product development, especially if the product will primarily be indicated to treat a disease of the elderly (e.g., Alzheimer disease) or targets a disease that affects a sizable number of elderly patients (e.g., hypertension).

cognitive functions, balance and falls, urinary incontinence, weight loss, quality of life, functional capacities, and symptoms.[52] Current guidances for clinical development[52–54] recommend having an adequate number of elderly patients in the development program to ensure adequate representation and data to assess the drug's benefit and risk in the elderly population. An appropriate size for different elderly age cohorts (65–74 years and ≥75 years) can be estimated based on the epidemiology of the intended target population. Elderly patients should be included in the same trials as younger patients unless this is not feasible. This approach allows for direct comparison of patient cohorts in the same studies.

The International Conference on Harmonisation (ICH) E7 guidance states "for drugs used in diseases not unique to, but present in the elderly, a minimum of 100 patients would usually allow detection of clinically important differences".[52] ICH E7 further recommends the sponsor to estimate the prevalence of the disease to be treated by age or examine age distribution of usage for other drugs of the same class (to ascertain the actual number of elderly patients appropriate for regulatory submission). Additional details are available in the FDA[53,54] and the ICH E7[52] guidances on the elderly.

The major health authorities will also consider patient perspective data during the drug approval process. Patient-reported outcome (PRO) measures can be incorporated into clinical trials to better understand the patient's experience with aspects of treatment, including symptom relief, ease of administration, and factors affecting adherence. Including PROs in clinical trials requires the use of validated instruments with sensitive and/or specific measurements to collect outcomes meaningful to the elderly. Alternatively a patient preference study can be conducted to elicit elderly patient preferences for treatment options in rare diseases or interventions that may be lifesaving despite substantial risks.

Pharmacokinetic studies in the elderly

The age-related effects on a drug's pharmacokinetics should be investigated, especially the dose-response effects for drugs or active metabolites with renal excretion as a major route of elimination. Standard methodological approaches include formal pharmacokinetic studies, dose-response studies, and population pharmacokinetics.[53–55] Pharmacokinetic studies may directly compare subject populations (elderly vs. younger patients, if feasible) or evaluate drug–disease interaction studies in the elderly.[53,54] Population pharmacokinetic analyses seek to identify the sources and correlation of variability in drug concentrations among the target patient population, such as associations with age or changes in renal function.[54] Additionally, relationships between drug exposures determined from population pharmacokinetic approaches and safety/efficacy outcomes in the elderly population can be explored. These analyses provide critical evidence to support dose selection during the drug approval process and may impact regulatory decisions and labeling information of the drug.[55]

Data analysis and assessment of safety in the elderly

The safety analysis of pooled data across studies by age groups (e.g., <65, 65–74, 75–84, >85 years) is recommended to assess age-related differences with respect to safety, dose response, blood level response, or other appropriate covariates (such as concomitant disease or concomitant medication use) (Box 10.5). If possible, safety data for the elderly cohorts should be compared with that of the younger age groups. When significant differences are detected, a formal pharmacokinetic study may be considered to better understand the effect of age or age-related factors on the pharmacokinetics and pharmacodynamics of the drug. These evaluations will provide clinical and scientific information for benefit-risk considerations in elderly patients.

Labeling and the elderly

Product labeling provides crucial information to healthcare providers to make benefit-risk decisions on the use of a medicinal product in their elderly patients. To do this, health authorities worldwide require that professional labeling of drugs include safety and efficacy information for the elderly. This information is usually provided under relevant sections of the label (Box 10.6). For example, the FDA guidance for geriatric labeling[55] requires information about differences in clinical data on safety and efficacy between the elderly and younger populations, pharmacokinetics or pharmacodynamics studies performed on the elderly, and specific hazards with use of the drug in the elderly.

> **BOX 10.5**
> **Approaches to Evaluations of Safety Data from Elderly Patients**
>
> Safety data from elderly patients can be assessed by age group cohorts (e.g., <65, 65–74, 75–84, >85 years) to detect age-related differences in ADRs, dose response, or other appropriate covariates (such as concomitant disease or concomitant medication use).

> **BOX 10.6**
> **Product Labeling for Elderly Patients**
>
> Product labels include important information for elderly patients regarding
> - differences in clinical data on safety and efficacy or pharmacokinetics and pharmacodynamics between elderly and younger populations
> - dose adjustment
> - special monitoring
> - DDIs

Also, the European Medicines Agency labeling guidance requires that the Summary of Product Characteristics[56] and the Patient Information Leaflet[57] contain specific instructions regarding dosage adjustment if necessary, the nature of risks (i.e., frequency, seriousness, or reversibility of the adverse reactions), or the need for monitoring in the elderly.[58] Any DDI effect specific to the elderly should also be stated in the label.

Risk communication to the elderly

The goal of risk communication to the elderly is to increase awareness or educate about potential risks and approaches to minimize the risks (see Chapter 13). This information may impact the patient's decision to use a medication or their behavior when using it. With advancing age, memory, cognition, and attention are affected, all of which impact effective risk communication to the elderly.[59] Thus health literacy factors should be considered when risk communication materials are developed.

Postapproval safety evaluation in the elderly

A robust pharmacovigilance system provides an effective framework for processes, tools, technology, and experts to perform product safety surveillance including the collection, assessment, and monitoring of ADRs from medicines used by the elderly throughout the product's life cycle. During postmarketing surveillance, new and/or serious safety risks may be detected, especially in a setting of age-related physiologic changes in elderly patients with comorbidity and polypharmacy. A product's risk management plan (RMP) (see Chapter 13) describes the pharmaceutical company's understanding of safety concerns in the elderly and captures their approach to conduct safety assessments along with the risk minimization efforts to reduce the frequency or severity of risks in the elderly population. A comprehensive analysis of risks regarding the elderly is also provided in the periodic benefit-risk evaluation report (see Chapter 13). Important safety risks with significant impact on the product's benefit-risk balance in the elderly may warrant changes to the RMP, product label, and risk communication materials directed to elderly patients.

CONCLUSION

The increasing proportion of elderly worldwide is impacting healthcare needs and pharmacovigilance efforts. In the elderly, multiple chronic diseases, cognitive impairment, polypharmacy, and age-related changes in biological processes increase the likelihood of DDIs, DDis, medication errors, and ADRs. Both pharmaceutical companies and regulatory agencies recognize the importance of studying the efficacy and safety of medicinal products in elderly patients during product development, especially when the product is intended to treat a disease of the elderly (e.g., Alzheimer disease) or a disease that affects a sizable number of elderly patients (e.g., hypertension). Safety data from elderly patients can be assessed by age group cohorts to detect age-related differences in ADRs, dose response, comorbidities, and concomitant medication use. Globally, product labels include benefit-risk information and messages regarding dose adjustments or specialized monitoring targeted at elderly patients as a means to optimize use of new medications in the growing elderly population.

REFERENCES

1. World Population Prospects. The 2017 Revision https://www.un.org/development/desa/publications/world-population-prospects-the-2017-revision.html.
2. Life Expectancy at Birth, Total (Years), World Bank. https://data.worldbank.org/indicator/SP.DYN.LE00.IN?end=2015&start=1960.
3. World Population Ageing — United Nations. 2015. www.un.org/en/development/desa/population/publications/.../WPA2015_Report.pdf.
4. Pal S, Tyler JK. Epigenetics and aging. Sci Adv. 2016;2: e1600584.
5. Cefalu CA. Theories and mechanisms of aging. Clin Geriatr Med. 2011;27:491—506.
6. Steinman MA, Lee SJ, Boscardin JW, Miao Y, et al. Patterns of multimorbidity in elderly veterans. J Am Geriatr Soc. 2012;60:1872—1880.
7. Violan C, Foguet-Boreu Q, Flores-Mateo G, et al. Prevalence, determinants and patterns of multimorbidity in primary care: a systematic review of observational studies. PLoS One. 2014;9:e102149. https://doi.org/10.1371/journal.pone.0102149.
8. Barnett K, Mercer SW, Norbury M, Watt G, et al. Epidemiology of multimorbidity and implications for health care, research, and medical education: a cross sectional study. Lancet. 2012;380:37—43.
9. Marcel ES. Multimorbidity in older adults. Epidemiol Rev. 2013;35:75—83.
10. Kennedy BK, Berger SL, et al. Geroscience: linking aging to chronic disease. Cell. 2014;159:709—713.
11. Hanlon JT, Schmader KE. How important are drug—drug interactions to the health of older adults? Am J Geriatr Pharmacother. 2011;9:361—363.
12. Mand P, Roth K, Biertz F, et al. Drug-disease interaction in elderly patients in family practice. Int J Clin Pharmacol Ther. 2014;52:337—345.
13. Dedhiya SD, Hancock E, Craig BA, Doebbeling CC, Thomas III J. Incident use and outcomes associated with potentially inappropriate medication use in older adults. Am J Geriatr Pharmacother. 2010;8:562—570.
14. Budnitz DS, Pollock DA, Weidenbach KN, Mendelsohn AB, Schroeder TJ, Annest JL. National surveillance of emergency department visits for outpatient adverse drug events. JAMA. 2006;296:1858—1866.
15. Picone DM, Titler MG, Dochterman J, et al. Predictors of medication errors among elderly hospitalized patients. Am J Med Qual. 2008;23:115—127.
16. McLean AJ, Le Couter DG. Aging biology and geriatric clinical pharmacology. Pharmacol Rev. 2004;56: 163—184.
17. Sauve MJ, Lewis WR, Blankenbiller M, Rickabaugh B, Pressler SJ. Cognitive impairments in chronic heart failure: a case controlled. J Card Fail. 2009;15:1—10.
18. Kaufman DW, Kelly JP, Rosenberg L, et al. Recent patterns of medication use in the ambulatory adult population of the United States the Slone survey. JAMA. 2002;287: 337—344.
19. Qato DM, Wilder J, Schumm LP, Gillet V, Alexander GC. Changes in prescription and over-the-counter medication and dietary supplement use among older adults in the United States, 2005 vs 2011. JAMA Intern Med. 2016; 176:473—482.
20. Patterns of Medication Use in the United States; 2006. https://www.bu.edu/slone/files/2012/11/SloneSurveyReport2006.pdf.
21. Tobias DE, Sey M. General and psychotherapeutic medication use in 328 nursing facilities: a year 2000 national survey. Consult Pharm. 2001;16:54—64, 98.
22. Corsonello A, Pedone C, Incalzi RA. Age-related pharmacokinetic and pharmacodynamic changes and related risk of adverse drug reactions. Curr Med Chem. 2010;17: 571—584.

23. Hilmer SN. ADME-tox issues for the elderly. *Expert Opin Drug Metab Toxicol.* 2008;4:1321—1323.

24. Shi S, Klotz U. Age-related changes in pharmacokinetics. *Curr Drug Metab.* 2011;12:601—610.

25. Forbes GB, Reina JC. Adult lean body mass declines with age: some longitudinal observations. *Metabolism.* 1970; 19:653—663.

26. Chutka DS, Evans JM, Fleming KC, Mikkelson KG. Drug prescribing for elderly patients. *Mayo Clin Proc.* 1995;70: 685—693.

27. Sera LC, McPherson ML. Pharmacokinetics and pharmacodynamic changes associated with aging and implications for drug therapy. *Clin Geriatr Med.* 2012;28: 273—286.

28. Turnheim K. Drug dosage in the elderly. Is it rational? *Drugs Aging.* 1998;13:357—379.

29. Onder G, Pedone C, Landi F, et al. Adverse drug reactions as cause of hospital admissions: results from the Italian Group of Pharmacoepidemiology in the Elderly (GIFA). *J Am Geriatr Soc.* 2002;50:1962—1968.

30. Greenblatt DJ, Allen MD, Shader RI. Toxicity of high-dose flurazepam in the elderly. *Clin Pharmacol Ther.* 1977;21: 355—361.

31. Bartels AL, Kortekaas R, Bart J, et al. Bloodbrain barrier P-glycoprotein function decreases in specific brain regions with aging: a possible role in progressive neurodegeneration. *Neurobiol Aging.* 2009;30:1818—1824.

32. Zeevi N, Pachter J, McCulough LD, Wolfson L, Kuchel GA. The blood-brain barrier: geriatric relevance of a critical brain-body interface. *J Am Geriatr Soc.* 2010;58:1749—1757.

33. Schmucker DL. Liver function and phase I drug metabolism in the elderly: a paradox. *Drugs Aging.* 2001;18: 837—851.

34. Le Couter DG, McLean AJ. The aging liver: drug clearance and oxygen diffusion barrier hypothesis. *Clin Pharmacokinet.* 1998;34:359—373.

35. McLachlan AJ, Pont LG. Drug metabolism in older people—a key consideration in achieving optimal outcomes with medicines. *J Gerontol A Biol Sci Med Sci.* 2012;67:175—180.

36. Kim H, Kisseleva T, Brennerb DA. Aging and liver disease. *Curr Opin Gastroenterol.* 2015;31:184—191.

37. Hubbard RE, O'Mahoney MS, Woodhouse KW. Medication prescribing in frail older people. *Eur J Clin Pharmacol.* 2013;69:319—326.

38. Schmucker DL, Sanchez H. Liver regeneration and aging: a current perspective. *Curr Gerontol Geriatr Res.* 2011;2011: 1—8.

39. Wynne H. Drug metabolism and ageing. *J Br Menopause Soc.* 2005;11:51—56.

40. Kinirons MT, O'Mahony MS. Drug metabolism and ageing. *Br J Clin Pharmacol.* 2004;57:540—544.

41. Miletic D, Fuckar Z, Sustic A, Mozetic V, Stimac D, Zauhar G. Sonographic measurement of absolute and relative renal length in adults. *J Clin Ultrasound.* 1998;26: 185—189.

42. Musso CG, Oreopoulos DG. Aging and physiological changes of the kidneys including changes in glomerular filtration rate. *Nephron Physiol.* 2011;119:1—5.

43. Mühlberg W, Platt D. Age-dependent changes of the kidneys: pharmacological implications. *Gerontology.* 1999; 45:243—253.

44. Bowie MW, Slattum PW. Pharmacodynamics in older adults: a review. *Am J Geriatr Pharmacother.* 2007;5: 263—303.

45. Turnheim K. When drug therapy gets old: pharmacokinetics and pharmacodynamics in the elderly. *Exp Gerontol.* 2003;38:843—853.

46. Mangoni AA, Jackson SH. Age-related changes in pharmacokinetics and pharmacodynamics: basic principles and practical applications. *Br J Clin Pharmacol.* 2004; 57:6—14.

47. Maxiner SM, Mellow AM, Tandon R. The efficacy, safety, and tolerability of antipsychotics in the elderly. *J Clin Psychiatr.* 1999;60:29—41.

48. Cepeda MS, Farrar JT, Baumgarten M, Boston R, Carr DB, Strom BL. Side effects of opioids during short-term administration: effect of age, gender, and race. *Clin Pharmacol Ther.* 2003;74:102—112.

49. Hutchison LC, O'Brien CE. Changes in pharmacokinetics and pharmacodynamics in the elderly patient. *J Pharm Practice.* 2007;20(1):4—12.

50. Phillips PA, Hodsman GP, Johnston Cl. Neuroendocrine mechanisms and cardiovascular homeostasis in the elderly. *Cardiovasc Drugs Ther.* 1991;4:1209—1213.

51. Mukker JK, Shankar R, Singh P, Derendorf H. AAPS advances in the pharmaceutical sciences Developing Drug Products in an Aging Society from Concept to Prescribing Sven Stegemann Editor Chapter: Pharmacokinetic and Pharmacodynamic Considerations in Elderly Population. Vol. 24; 139—151

52. ICH Harmonized Guideline. Studies in Support of Special Population: Geriatrics E7 Current Step 4 Version 1993. http://www.ich.org/fileadmin/Public_Web_Site/ICH_Products/Guidelines/Efficacy/E7/Step4/E7_Guideline.pdf.

53. ICH Harmonized Guideline. *Guidance for Industry E7 Studies in Support of Special Populations: Geriatrics Questions and Answers.* 2012. https://www.fda.gov/downloads/Drugs/GuidanceComplianceRegulatoryInformation/Guidances/UCM189544.pdf.

54. *FDA Guidance for Industry Population Pharmacokinetics;* 1999. https://www.fda.gov/downloads/drugs/guidances/UCM072137.pdf.

55. *Guidance for Industry Content and Format for Geriatric Labeling*; 2017. https://www.fda.gov/downloads/Drugs/GuidanceComplianceRegulatoryInformation/Guidances/UCM075062.pdf.

56. *A Guideline on Summary of Product Characteristics (SmPC)*; 2009. https://ec.europa.eu/health/sites/health/files/files/eudralex/vol-/c/smpc_guideline_rev2_en.pdf.

57. *Best Practice Guidance on Patient Information Leaflets*; 2017. https://www.gov.uk/government/uploads/system/uploads/attachment_data/file/328405/Best_practice_guidance_on_patient_information_leaflets.pdf.

58. Training – SmPC and Older People. http://www.ema.europa.eu/docs/en_GB/document_library/Presentation/2013/01/WC500137033.pdf.

59. Harada CN, Natelson Love MC, Triebel KL. Normal cognitive aging. *Clin Geriatr Med*. 2013;29(4):737–752.

CHAPTER 11

Medical Device Vigilance and Postmarket Surveillance

MURRAY MALIN, MD, MBA • CARL FISCHER, PHD

INTRODUCTION

Medical device vigilance and postmarket surveillance (PMS) are critical to patient safety, product improvement, and regulatory compliance. During medical device development, a manufacturer frequently performs some form of failure mode analysis. This is typically based on testing, research, or previous experience with a similar device. This analysis identifies, or anticipates, ways a device might fail, the risk of the failure, the patient impact (referred to as harm) from the failure, and the expected frequency of the failure once it is placed on the market. The manufacturer determines the acceptable level of failures based on the particular risk and the particular benefit of the device. When the premarket analysis identifies a particular unacceptable harm and frequency, the manufacturer modifies the product in order to bring the particular harm and frequency to acceptable levels.

Medical devices are very diverse in technologies, complexity, materials, and purpose. While pharmaceutical products typically are provided in a relatively limited number of forms (e.g., tablets, liquid), medical devices are not bounded so clearly. For example, the variety of medical devices include implantable cardiac pacing systems, artificial joints, hospital beds, infusion pumps, diagnostic imaging equipment, injectable dermal fillers, surgical gowns, and diagnostic test kits. While there are some general similarities between device and pharmaceutical regulation (Current Good Manufacturing Practice [CGMP] obligations, some premarket notification), there tends to be a broader spectrum of regulatory options for devices, and in some cases, regulatory obligations for devices may be considerably less rigorous than for pharmaceuticals.

Unlike the premarket process for many drugs, the vast majority of medical devices enter the market without clinical trial data to support a favorable benefit-risk ratio or the safety and effectiveness of the

specific device. Typically, manufacturers only need to demonstrate that the device is comparable to a currently marketed product. This implies that the device is as safe and effective as products currently marketed. In the United States, some devices are exempt from any premarket Food and Drug Administration (FDA) notification (e.g., exempt devices); some low risk devices are even exempt from design controls and many CGMP requirements. Thus, PMS is of great importance for devices. It is critical that a manufacturer has a system in place to assess how the product performs in real-world environments. Similar to pharmaceuticals, devices can be used under conditions or in ways that are unexpected, both within the labeled conditions and off label. Knowledge gained from user or patient feedback can be the key to identify new opportunities for using a device or recognize ways that a device may not be performing as expected.

The concept of PMS is embraced globally, including requirements set out in European Directives, Regulations and the International Organization for Standardization Quality Management and Risk Management Standards. As part of the PMS, many regulatory agencies have requirements that manufacturers, and other entities in the device manufacturing process, submit information when the entities become aware of events that may have led to patient harm. Since 1984, under FDA regulations, medical device manufacturers and importers have been required to report device-related deaths, serious injuries, and certain malfunctions. Similar reporting requirements began in Europe in 1995 under the European Medical Device Directives; these directives were updated in 2017. Additionally, some regulatory agencies require that information be submitted for some device malfunctions even in the absence of patient harm.

Data sources required for effective device vigilance include complaint and service records, which are not typically required for pharmacovigilance. Another difference between device and drug vigilance systems is the approach to risk mitigation. For devices, postmarket safety issues may be resolved through design changes, labeling changes, or some other field corrections (allowing the product to stay on the market with an in-place mitigation). In comparison for medicinal products, postmarket safety issues are typically addressed with labeling and, if necessary, implementation of additional risk minimization measures (See Chapter 13).

OVERVIEW OF POSTMARKET SURVEILLANCE AND DEVICE VIGILANCE

The performance of medical devices is dependent on the device itself, the environment it is used in, and how the device is used. In general, premarket review of medical devices, by the regulatory authority or some other entity, determines if a device meets some level of safety and effectiveness. While premarket review is important in evaluating compliance with regulatory requirements, it does not guarantee that the device is safe or would remain safe and effective on market. PMS and device vigilance are intended to ensure that marketed medical devices are, and remain, safe and effective during actual use.

In the United States, many medical devices can enter the US market through 510(k) clearance (from section 510(k) of the Food, Drug, and Cosmetic Act, which simply requires manufacturers to demonstrate that the medical device is "substantially equivalent" to a medical device that is already on the US market). Demonstration of substantial equivalence is typically done without the need for a structured clinical trial or other significant datasets to support safe and effective use. A minority of medical devices are considered to be high risk or novel and will typically require structured clinical trials and data to support safety and effective use of the device. However, the majority of devices are considered lower risk and may rely on other methods, such as bench testing and human factors studies (See Chapter 12), to demonstrate they will likely be safe. Regardless of the device type, manufacturers rely on a quality system (QS) with an effective vigilance system in place to assure continued device safety.

A similar paradigm exists in the European Union (EU), where a Conformité Européene (CE) mark is required to market medical devices. To receive a CE mark, manufacturers must submit a Declaration of Conformity, which assures that the device satisfies all requirements for CE marking (see EU Device Vigilance section for details). Controlled clinical trials are not typically required to demonstrate safety and efficacy to market a

> ## BOX 11.1
> ## Device Vigilance
>
> Device vigilance:
> - United States: a broad term that covers monitoring activities for medical devices in use.
> - European Union: concerns the responsibility of the manufacturer to inform the competent authority of incidents according to national/European legislation.
>
> Device postmarket surveillance:
> - Activities to collect and review experience gained from devices placed in the market for the purpose of identifying a need for action to minimize risk.

device in the EU, placing importance on human factors studies and PMS data to demonstrate safety and efficacy.

In vitro diagnostic devices (IVDs) and companion diagnostics are medical devices that typically do not come into contact with patients. For the majority of these products, there is no direct harm to patients from the device itself when the product fails. Rather, the risk of the diagnostic test producing false-positive or false-negative results must be adequately managed. As such, IVD manufacturers and regulators rely on robust PMS and vigilance systems to assure their safety and performance.

The fact that most devices enter the market with limited clinical data supporting safety explains why manufacturers and regulators alike recognize the importance of robust medical device vigilance and PMS systems (Box 11.1).

WHAT ARE POSTMARKET SURVEILLANCE AND DEVICE VIGILANCE?

Although there are different requirements globally, the concepts of PMS and device vigilance are embraced by regulators worldwide. In general, device PMS is a broad term that encompasses all monitoring activities and associated data to assess and mitigate risk associated with medical devices while in actual use. Device vigilance encompasses reporting of adverse events and PMS studies to regulatory authorities. Device PMS can be thought of as a collection of activities that are proactive or reactive. Proactive activities may include customer surveys, postmarketing safety studies, user feedback via training programs, registries, or information about experience with similar devices. Reactive activities may include complaints and complaint trending, assessment of service records, reports of compatibility with other devices, reports of device misuse, and customer satisfaction. Some activities, such as monitoring manufacturing processes may be either proactive or reactive (Box 11.2).

Device PMS incorporates the collection and analysis of different types of data or information from various sources. Unlike drugs and biologicals, medical devices are often mechanical, physical, or software-based products with many electronic and mechanical components that can fail and impact other devices or medicinal products. Medical devices may have long life spans and may encounter aging issues. Additionally, many medical devices are not intended to treat a specific medical condition, rather they may support the treatment of multiple medical conditions and patient populations. For example, infusion pumps are used to administer different medicinal products to patients with different medical conditions, so an infusion pump failure may affect multiple patient populations with different medical conditions and risk profiles, complicating overall benefit-risk assessment of the device.

THE VALUE OF POSTMARKET SURVEILLANCE AND MEDICAL DEVICE VIGILANCE

PMS and device vigilance can and should impact safety and new device development; examples include:

- **Product concept, requirements, and development**: PMS and device vigilance may provide useful input to new device design and user requirements (e.g., updates to design documents, such as product's failure mode and effects analysis).
- **Manufacturing**: service records and complaint trending data may help to identify problems related to the manufacturing process.
- **Sales/marketing**: PMS and device vigilance data may provide information related to off-label or unexpected product use, customer satisfaction, and patient preferences.
- **Device use**: use errors data may provide insight into potential concerns related to adequacy of medical device design, instructions for use, labeling, and/or user training.

- **Service records and complaints**: may provide information on the short- and long-term performance of the device, which may be useful throughout the product life cycle to inform the appropriate timeframe for servicing and end of life of the device.
- **Risk Management and Benefit-Risk Assessment**: PMS and device vigilance should provide information about the overall benefits and risks of the device in target populations, which can be documented in a Clinical Evaluation Report or Periodic Safety Update Report (PSUR).

US DEVICE VIGILANCE

Under the US/FDA regulatory system, device PMS and vigilance requirements are described in the QS regulation (21 Code of Federal Regulations [CFR] 820[1]) and the Medical Device Reporting (MDR) regulation (21 CFR 803[1]). There is considerable interplay between the two. For example, under the QS regulation, there is an explicit provision that complaints be evaluated "to determine whether the complaint represents an event which is required to be reported to the FDA under part 803, Medical Device Reporting," (see 21 CFR 820.198(d)[1]). This requirement partners with the required elements, under part 803, for developing, maintaining, and implementing written MDR procedures (see 21 CFR 803.17[1]) (Box 11.2).

Complaint handling is the key to any PMS or vigilance system. Although there are other means (e.g., literature review), complaints typically represent the primary means a manufacturer has to become aware of adverse events associated with a device. External complaints may also be the primary means a manufacturer has to obtain information regarding postmarket device function, even in the absence of adverse events. PMS may uncover favorable information relating to device performance or use. While this information may be informative for product development and marketing, US regulatory requirements typically do not focus on this information. This section will focus on negative postmarket information.

US requirements for complaint evaluation generally include the need for procedures dealing with complaint intake, complaint review, and complaint follow-up. Complaint procedures must ensure that "All complaints are processed in a uniform and timely manner and oral complaints are documented upon receipt" (21 CFR 820.198(a)[1]). Once received, all complaints must be reviewed to determine if an investigation is necessary (21 CFR 820.198(b)[1]). Note that, if there is a determination that no investigation is necessary, there must be a record of how that determination was reached and who made that determination. If the complaint includes "the possible failure of a device, labeling, or packaging to meet any of its specifications," the complaint must be "reviewed, evaluated, and investigated, unless such investigation has already been performed for a similar complaint and another investigation is not necessary" (21 CFR 820.198(c)[1]). The QS regulation also requires that, when an investigation is conducted, records must be maintained. There are several mandatory elements that must be documented, including the device name, complaint date, specifics of the complaint, details of any investigation, and follow-up actions (21 CFR 820.198(e)[1]).

Complaints, regardless of their source, feed into the manufacturer's Corrective and Preventive Action system (CAPA). Aside from vigilance requirements, it is through a CAPA system that complaints are analyzed. In association with other sources of quality data (e.g., quality records, service records), complaints are evaluated to identify "existing and potential causes of nonconforming product or other quality problems (21 CFR 820.100(a)[1])." The CAPA analysis process may include evaluation of postmarket complaints against anticipated (or previously observed) rates of postmarket events. This analysis may result in the need to perform some design or manufacturing modification. Depending on evaluation of risk, including severity and frequency, this may also lead to field correction (a correction done without removing product from the market) or product removal.

Under the US (FDA) regulatory system, one of the primary ways postmarket events are communicated to the FDA is through reports filed under the MDR regulations (21 CFR 803[1]). The reports themselves are also commonly referred to as MDRs. The regulation requires medical device reporting by several entities including manufacturers and importers of medical devices. The regulation also allows for voluntary reporting. Voluntary reports may be provided to the FDA by any stakeholder. The FDA typically provides some information in a voluntary report back to the manufacturer.

Mandatory MDRs are required to be submitted when the manufacturer reviews an event and determines that it falls into one of two reportable (Box 11.3) categories: "May have caused or contributed to a death or serious injury," or "malfunctioned and that the device or a similar device marketed by the manufacturer or importer would be likely to cause or contribute to a death or serious injury if the malfunction were to recur" (21 CFR 803.3[1]). No definitive determination of causality or device contribution to an event needs to have been established for an MDR to be required. Frequently,

---

BOX 11.3
Medical Device Reports

Manufactures must submit Medical Device Reports to the Food and Drug Administration when:
- A device may have caused or contributed to a death or serious injury.
- A device malfunctioned in such a way that would be likely to cause or contribute to death or serious injury.

---

a device adverse event involves many devices, confounding factors, pharmacological contribution, and user actions. It may be difficult to make a definitive determination regarding the complicity of the device in the event, much less in a short amount of time. Therefore, the "may have contributed" threshold can be quite low and may result in reporting of events when there is only unsubstantiated or modest indication of device responsibility.

Mandatory MDRs have different time frames associated with them, depending on the nature of the adverse event. Generally MDRs are required to be reported to the FDA within 30 calendar days of the manufacturer becoming aware of the event. There are some situations when an MDR must be submitted within five working days. These include when the manufacturer has determined that the event requires "remedial action to prevent an unreasonable risk of substantial harm to public health" (21 CFR 803.50[1]) or when the FDA requests that a 5-day report be submitted. Note that a manufacturer is "considered to have become aware of an event when any of its employees becomes aware of a reportable event" (21 CFR 803.3b(2)[1]). Even after an MDR is submitted, additional information may have to be provided to the FDA. When a manufacturer becomes aware of new information that augments the MDR or changes the conclusion of an MDR, the manufacturer files a "supplemental report" (21 CFR 802.52[1]) (Box 11.4, Table 11.1).

BOX 11.4
FDA MDR Database

- Some information in a Medical Device Report is made public and can be searched through the Manufacturer and User Facility Device Experience Database.
- This is similar to the Food and Drug Administration Adverse Event Reporting System for pharmaceutical products.

TABLE 11.1
Select Global Medical Device Reporting (MDR) Timelines[5,7-11]

Jurisdiction	Timescale
UNITED STATES	
5-day MDR	Manufacturer becomes aware of a report that requires remedial action to prevent an unreasonable risk to health of the general public or the Food and Drug Administration makes a written request.
30-day MDR	1. As specified in device regulations, for initial reports of a device that may have caused or contributed to a death or serious injury for a device malfunction that would be likely to contribute to a death or serious injury if it were to recur, 2. If an evaluation is pending additional information, the report still shall be filed within the required reportability timeframe using the information available at the time.
MDR follow-ups	A follow-up report is to be submitted within 30 days of receipt of additional information. This includes the results of device evaluation.
HEALTH CANADA	
48 h—reporting a foreign incident	When the decision has been made to report a foreign incident to Health Canada, a preliminary report must be submitted as soon as possible (48 h) after the manufacturer has informed the foreign regulatory agency of the intention to take corrective action or as soon as the foreign regulatory agency has required the manufacturer to take corrective action.
10 days—death or serious deterioration in state of health	If death or serious deterioration in health of the patient, user, or other person has occurred, a report must be submitted to Health Canada within 10 calendar days.
30 days—near incident	If death or serious deterioration in health did not occur as a result of the incident, but might if the incident were to recur, then the report must be submitted to Health Canada within 30 calendar days.
Follow-up reports	A follow-up report is to be submitted within 30 days of receipt of additional information.
Final reports	A final report is to be submitted within 30 days of the completion of manufacturer's investigation of the event. This includes results of returned sample investigations.
EUROPE	
2 days—serious public health threat	Report should be submitted to the appropriate NCA immediately (without delay that could not be justified) but not later than 2 calendar days after awareness by the manufacturer of this threat.
10 days—death or unanticipated serious deterioration in state of health	Report should be submitted to the appropriate NCA immediately (without delay that could not be justified) after the manufacturer established a link between the device and the event but not later than 10 elapsed calendar days (or other timeliness as required) following the date of awareness of the event.
30 days—others	Report should be submitted to the appropriate NCA immediately (without delay that could not be justified) after the manufacturer established a link between the device and the event but not later than 30 elapsed calendar days (or other timeliness as required) following the date of awareness of the event.
Follow-up reports	1. The manufacturer shall provide a follow-up report to the NCA if the investigation time reaches the time line given to the NCA within the initial report; 2. A follow-up report is to be submitted within 30 days of receipt of additional relevant information.
Final reports	A final report is to be submitted within 30 days of the completion of manufacturer's investigation of the event. This includes results of the device evaluation.
AUSTRALIA	
48 h	Report should be submitted if the information relates to an event or other occurrence that represents a serious threat to public health.

Continued

TABLE 11.1
Select Global Medical Device Reporting (MDR) Timelines[5,7–11]—cont'd

Jurisdiction	Timescale
10 days	Report should be submitted if the information relates to an event or other occurrence that led to the death, or a serious deterioration in the state of health of a patient, a user of the device, or another person.
30 days	Report should be submitted if the information relates to an event or other occurrence or recurrence of which might lead to the death or a serious deterioration in the state of health of a patient, a user of the device, or another person.
JAPAN	
15 days	When the following events related to the device are unlabeled or incidents of defects are higher than expected: deaths (domestic and overseas); disability, cases at risk of death or disability; cases that require admission or prolongation of the period of admission to a hospital or clinic for treatment; congenital diseases or anomalies in the next generation; research reports showing the possibility of the onset of cancer or other serious diseases, disabilities, or death.
30 days	Report should be submitted if the information relates to an event or other occurrence or recurrence of which might lead to the death or a serious deterioration in the state of health of a patient, a user of the device, or another person.
NEW ZEALAND	
7 calendar days	Death (actual or potential); serious injury (actual or potential).
30 calendar days	Injury (actual or potential); no injury.

NCA, National Competent Authority.

When designing a procedure to evaluate events for the FDA, it is very important that the procedure meets all the requirements specified in 21 CFR 803.[1] This regulation explicitly requires that a manufacturer "must develop, maintain, and implement written MDR procedures for timely and effective review of information, a standard review process for determining reportability, timely notification to the FDA, and recordkeeping" (21 CFR 803.17[1]). Additionally, there are specific requirements that a manufacturer must meet for establishing and maintaining MDR files. These include requirements for identifying "MDR event files" for events that are reviewed for MDR reportability as well as recordkeeping requirements (21 CFR 803.18[1]).

The FDA has published guidance relating to MDR reporting. This guidance provides much more detail regarding nuances of evaluation and reporting as well as information about variances, quarterly reporting, and engaging with the FDA (see "Medical Device Reporting for Manufacturers: Guidance for Industry and Food and Drug Administration Staff" issued November 8, 2016).

Combination Products

In the United States, combination products are any combination of a drug, biologic, and/or device. Combination products represent special challenges under the FDA regulatory system. Finished combination products are typically subject to the full CGMP requirements for the constituent parts. For example, a drug-device combination product is subject to the drug CGMP requirements (21 CFR 211[1]) and the device CGMP requirements (21 CFR 820[1]). Generally, the product as a whole (not just a particular constituent part) is subject to both requirements. Note that this requirement is independent of whether a constituent part is (or is not) legally marketable on its own. As a result, meeting regulatory requirements for PMS and vigilance includes meeting the requirements of two different regulatory systems (drugs and devices). In order to facilitate demonstrating compliance with applicable regulations, 21 CFR part 4[1] describes a streamlined way of demonstrating compliance.

For the combination product manufacturer, a system must be established to ensure that postmarket information feeds back to the appropriate unit for entry and evaluation. Also, when different contract manufactures or business units are involved in manufacturing drug and device constituent parts, there may be challenges in disseminating and reviewing postmarket information. When evaluating postmarket signals, the particular involvement of each constituent part may not always be clear.

The obligation to report MDRs still exists for combination products with device constituent parts. This obligation may be in parallel to the adverse event reporting under drug regulations. As a result, multiple adverse event reports to the FDA may be required for a single event. Given the "cause or contribute" threshold associated with MDRs, even if the event is suspected of being due purely to a drug constituent, a device MDR may still be required.

The FDA has published guidance regarding manufacturing of combination products (see "Guidance for Industry and FDA Staff: Current Good Manufacturing Practice Requirements for Combination Product" issued January 2017).

EUROPEAN UNION DEVICE VIGILANCE

In 2017, the EU updated regulations regarding medical devices and in vitro diagnostic medical devices, which are entitled Regulation (EU) 2017/745, or the EU Medical Device Regulation (EU MDR)[2] (Box 11.5), and Regulation 2017/746, or the In Vitro Diagnostic Medical Device Regulation (IVDR).[3] These Directives provide the technical and procedural obligations that manufacturers must follow prior to affixing a CE mark on the product. Manufacturers have until May 26, 2020 to implement EU MDR and until May 26, 2022 to implement IVDR; however, the requirements of the EU MDR related to PMS and device vigilance are applicable immediately and replace the corresponding requirements in previous Directives.

The European Commission supplement Directive with legally nonbinding guidelines, referred to as "MEDDEVs," which are intended to provide guidance to manufacturers related to the application of the Medical Device Directives. Although MEDDEVs are not legally binding, these guidance's (MEDDEV 2.12/1 rev 8 and MEDDEV 2.7.1 rev 4) provide greater detail on device vigilance and benefit-risk requirements specified in the EU MDR.

A CE mark must be affixed to medical devices (other than custom medical devices [Box 11.6]) to indicate conformity assessment with the EU MDR and to legally

enter the market in the EU. The EU MDR provides vigilance-related capabilities and processes required to pass "conformity assessment" for CE marking, which include[4]:

- Establishment of a systematic proactive process to collect information to accurately characterize the performance of the devices, allowing for a comparison to be made between the device and similar marketed products;
- Establishment of suitable indicators and threshold values to support continuous reassessment of the product benefit-risk analysis;
- Effective and appropriate methods and tools to investigate complaints and analyze market-related experience collected in the field;
- Methods and protocols to manage the events subject to the trend report, including the methods and protocols to be used to establish any statistically significant increase in the frequency or severity of incidents as well as the observation period;
- Methods and protocols to communicate effectively with competent authorities, notified bodies, economic operators, and users;
- Systematic procedures to identify and initiate appropriate measures, including corrective actions;
- Effective tools to trace and identify devices for which corrective actions might be necessary; and
- A postmarket clinical follow-up plan or a justification as to why one is not applicable.

In the EU,[5] a device-related event that meets all of the following criteria is considered an "incident" and should be reported to the appropriate regulatory authority:

- An event has occurred,
- The manufacturer's device is suspected to be a contributory cause of the incident, and
- The event led, or might have led, to one of the following outcomes:
  - death of a patient, a user, or another person
  - serious deterioration in the health of a patient, a user, or another person (Box 11.7)

Similar to reporting requirements in the United States, the nonoccurrence of a death or serious deterioration in health does not remove the obligation to report; the incident should be reported if it was possible that death/serious injury could have occurred under less fortunate circumstances, or if death or serious injury might occur if the incident were to occur again.

Upon becoming aware that an event has occurred, the manufacturer must assess whether the event is an incident; if so, an initial incident report must be provided in the following time lines:

- Serious public health threat: Immediately (without any delay that could not be justified), but not later than 2 calendar days after awareness by the manufacturer of this threat.
- Death or unanticipated serious deterioration in state of health: Immediately (without any delay that could not be justified) after the manufacturer established a link between the device and the event but not later than 10 elapsed calendar days following the date of awareness of the event.
- Others: Immediately (without any delay that could not be justified) after the manufacturer established a link between the device and the event but not later than 30 elapsed calendar days following the date of awareness of the event (Box 11.8).

Typically, the report is submitted to the regulatory authority in the country of occurrence of the incident.

The EU regulations require manufacturers to implement a robust incident reporting system, in addition to a system supporting clinical evaluation reports, benefit-risk assessments and aggregate reporting (i.e., PSURs). A manufacturer should also have a system in place to proactively review, analyze, and identify significant increases

or decreases in trends in complaints and incidents. A trend report should be provided to the Competent Authorities (CAs) if there is an increase in the rate of already reportable incidents, incidents that are exempt from reporting, and events not usually reportable.

In the EU, a National CA (NCA) may accept a periodic summary or trend report in lieu of individual incident reports after one or more of the initial reports have been provided to the NCA. When a manufacturer has received agreement from the NCA to switch to periodic summary reporting, they need to inform other concerned CAs of the agreement; periodic summary reporting cannot be extended to other CAs without their agreement.

There are conditions specified in the EU regulations in which device deficiencies do not need to be reported under a manufacturer's vigilance system:

- Device deficiencies that are always detected by the user prior its use (e.g., a diagnostic test that does not contain the test kit),
- Events in which the root cause was determined to be due to a patient condition (i.e., the device performed as intended and did not cause or contribute to death or serious injury),
- Events caused because the device has exceeded its service life or shelf life,
- Events not resulting in serious injury or death because a design feature in the device protected the user against the fault becoming a hazard (e.g., infusion pump alarm prevents injury to user),
- Expected and foreseeable events if the event meets all of the following criterion: the event was clearly identified in product labeling, the event is clinically well known as being foreseeable and predictable, the event is documented in the device master record with an appropriate risk assessment prior to the incident, and the side effects are acceptable in terms of patient benefit,
- There is negligible likelihood of death or serious deterioration in health from the event.

The EU regulations[6] place emphasis on the performance of clinical evaluations. A clinical evaluation is described as "a methodologically sound ongoing procedure to collect, appraise and analyze clinical data pertaining to a medical device and to evaluate whether there is sufficient clinical evidence to confirm compliance with relevant essential requirements for safety and performance when using the device according to the manufacturer's instructions for use" (MEDDEV 2.7.1 rev4). An important objective of the clinical evaluation is to provide the outcome of the product's benefit-risk assessment, including issues impacting benefit and risk profile. In the EU, clinical evaluations are needed for all classes of medical devices, and the level of clinical evidence should be appropriate for the characteristics and intended purpose of the device. Clinical evaluation is an ongoing process and should be done throughout the product life cycle. The initial clinical evaluation should be conducted during device development in order to identify data needed for initial CE marking. The initial clinical evaluation should inform of the need and nature of premarket research and design of clinical evaluations, if necessary, along with potential issues that need to be systematically addressed during PMS.

Clinical evaluations should be updated when new information from PMS impacts the current clinical evaluation and benefit-risk assessment. However, even if no such information is determined, the clinical evaluation should be updated at least annually if the device carries significant risk or the risk is not fully established, and every 2–5 years if the device does not have significant risks and the risk is well established. Updates to a clinical evaluation should specifically verify that the benefit-risk profile has remained favorable based on data obtained from PMS and whether there is a need for additional clinical data and/or clinical studies. If the regulators decide that the clinical evidence is insufficient, the manufacturer will need to stop the distribution of the affected device(s) and take appropriate corrective and preventative action to resolve it (Box 11.9).

A clinical evaluation is performed in five distinct "stages." An overview of each stage is provided below:
- Stage 0: In this stage, the scope of the clinical evaluation is defined. Manufacturers should consider the intended use(s) of the device, design features, or high-risk populations that require mitigation, current risk management documents addressing clinical risk, the current knowledge or state of the art related to the medical condition or

device technology, and an analysis of the output required from PMS/vigilance systems.
- Stage 1: In this stage, the manufacturer identifies data available to demonstrate conformity and a favorable benefit-risk ratio, in addition to data that will need to be generated or identified and summarized. Data sources may include premarket investigations, PMS and vigilance reports, device registries, incident reports, trends, complaints, analysis of returned devices, field safety corrective actions, CAPAs, literature searches, and other available data.
- Stage 2: The manufacturer provides a plan to determine scientific validity of the data, confounding influences, bias, and other factors impacting data, including issues related to adequacy of endpoints, inclusion/exclusion criteria, sample size, adequacy of follow-up period, recording of serious adverse events, and adequacy of information and procedures related to PMS and vigilance systems.
- Stage 3: An analysis of the clinical datasets is required to determine if the device demonstrates compliance with essential safety and performance requirements when used according to its intended use. Other information required includes residual risks and uncertainties, confirmation that the device achieves its intended use, plans for monitoring of adverse events, nature of the condition being treated and current standards of care and availability of other devices and treatments. The need for additional clinical data, risk of use error, adequacy of instructions for use, and the benefit-risk profile of the device should be described. If the clinical data are insufficient to demonstrate conformity with essential requirements, justification must be provided.
- Stage 4: A Clinical Evaluation Report (CER) needs to be generated and provided to the notified body to document the clinical evaluation, including all conclusions of the clinical evaluation and the benefit-risk assessment. The CER must outline and explain outputs from each stage of the clinical evaluation, and the evaluator of the clinical evaluation should verify the information is accurate and provide their resume. The clinical evaluation must demonstrate that all risks associated with use of the device for the intended purpose are acceptable and minimized when compared to the benefits provided.

When evaluating whether the benefit-risk profile is acceptable, it is important to consider if the clinical data are sufficient for all medical conditions and populations covered by the intended purpose of the device.

Combination Products

Unlike the United States, in the EU, there is no legal definition for a product where a medicinal product and a medical device are presented together (either as an integral combination or presented separately for use together). If a device is intended to administer a medicinal product, and the medicinal product is placed on the market in such a way that they form a single integral product which is intended exclusively for use in the given combination and which is not reusable, that single integral product is considered a medicinal product and is governed by Directive 2001/83/EC or Regulation (EC) No 726/2004, as applicable. In that case, the relevant general safety and performance requirements set out in Annex I of the MDR shall apply as far as the safety and performance of the device part of the single integral product are concerned.

CONCLUSION

Device PMS provides valuable information that is critical to patient safety and product improvement. PMS also provides important information that is the key to fulfilling vigilance obligations. There are many similarities in approach to PMS and vigilance for drug products and devices. Due to reduced regulatory premarket scrutiny for many devices, attention to postmarket device information is critical. While US and EU PMS and vigilance obligations differ in specifics, there is much similarity in the general approach, including how postmarket quality information is evaluated and integrated. Likewise, the fundamental concepts of adverse event reporting to regulators and competent authorities are similar throughout the world. In addition to achieving regulatory compliance, a well-performing PMS and vigilance system aids a manufacturer throughout the life cycle of a device.

DISCLOSURE STATEMENT

This chapter reflects the views of the authors and should not be construed to represent FDA's views or policies.

REFERENCES

1. https://www.gpo.gov/fdsys/pkg/CFR-2002-title21-vol1/content-detail.html. 2002.
2. EU Regulation 2017/745 the Medical Device Regulation ("EU MDR"). 2018.
3. EU Regulation 2017/746 the In Vitro Diagnostic Medical Device Regulation ("IVDR"). 2018.
4. Regulation (EU) 2017/745 the Medical Device Regulation; Annex III, "Technical Documentation on PostMarket Surveillance". 2018.
5. EU-MEDDEV 2.12 rev 8; Sect. 5. 2013.
6. EU-MEDDEV 2.7/1 revision 4. 2016.
7. Japan Pharmaceuticals and Medical Devices Agency-Article 228-20 (Adverse Reaction Reports). 2014.
8. Quality System Regulation (21 CFR 820) and the Medical Device Reporting Regulation (21 CFR 803). 2017.
9. *Health Canada Medical Device Regulations; (Sections 59 through 61.1(2)) Concerning Mandatory Problem Reporting, and Guidance Document for Mandatory Reporting for Medical Devices.* October 2011.
10. *Australian Regulatory Guidelines for Medical Devices; Version 1.1*, May 2011.
11. New Zealand Medicines and Medical Devices Safety Authority; Medical Devices: Quality Issues and Adverse Event Reporting. http://www.medsafe.govt.nz/regulatory/DevicesNew/9AdverseEvent.asp. 2018.

FURTHER READING

1. *EMA Guideline on Good Pharmacovigilance Practices, EMA Module IX — Signal Management.* 2012.
2. *FDA Guidance for Industry: Good Pharmacovigilance Practices and Pharmacovigilant Assessment.* March 2005.
3. *CIOMS Working Group VIII. Practical Aspects of Signal Detection in Pharmacovigilance.* Geneva: CIOMS; 2010.
4. *EMA Guideline on Good Pharmacovigilance Practices, EMA Module VI — Reporting AEs.* 2014.

CHAPTER 12

Application of Human Factors and Health Literacy in Pharmacovigilance

JAMES DUHIG, PHD

INTRODUCTION

The WHO defines health literacy as "the cognitive and social skills which determine the motivation and ability of individuals to gain access to, understand and use information in ways which promote and maintain good health."[1] Limitations in cognitive and/or physical functioning are part of being human, particularly as we age; additionally, emotional distress, the stress of illness, and the complexity of many healthcare systems are all part of the patient experience in seeking medical care and taking a medication.[2–4] These factors contribute to systematic problems in medication use, including overuse, underuse, and difficulties in documentation, monitoring, and education.[5,6] The resulting suboptimal care requires robust global pharmacovigilance systems to investigate the effects of medications and identify adverse events. We need to anticipate the occurrence of adverse events and medication errors and characterize their incidence and prevalence and then work to eliminate/reduce these issues, as they impact patient safety. Moreover, we have the opportunity to apply the knowledge gained from pharmacovigilance investigations to the development of products and systems to improve health outcomes by design. Human factors engineering and health literacy are cognitive behavioral scientific disciplines applied within pharmacovigilance and patient safety to reduce harm and improve outcomes.

HUMAN FACTORS

Human factors combines aspects of anthropology, sociology, and psychology with a system's engineering focus to investigate the relationships between people, environments, products, processes, and behaviors. Human factors is a design (Box 12.1) methodology for products and processes to make it easy for people to do the right thing and hard for them to do the wrong

thing. Traditionally, human factors is strongly associated with industrial engineering but it is increasingly applied to healthcare.[7] Human factors applies the knowledge of human capabilities (physical, sensory, emotional, and intellectual) and limitation to the design and development of tools, devices, systems, environments, and organizations.[8] It is also known as human factors engineering, usability engineering, ergonomics, cognitive engineering, and user-centered design. In pharmacovigilance and healthcare we may consider users to be patients, prescribers, pharmacists, caregivers, or anybody responsible for behaviors that contribute to knowledge and health outcomes.

Human factors investigates (Box 12.2) the characteristics of people, products, the environment, and other factors that will interact and influence one another in real-world use. In this respect, human factors and pharmacovigilance are each applied to gain a better understanding of people's experience with drugs and devices. Like pharmacovigilance, human factors generates evidence to inform patient safety analysis

---

BOX 12.1
Human Factors in Healthcare

- Make it easy for people to do the right thing.
- Make it hard for them to do the wrong thing.

BOX 12.2
Human Factors Key Interactions

- Intended users
- Product
- Uses
- Use environment

---

in situations where other scientific investigations may not be possible or practical. This evidence may be used in conjunction with pharmacovigilance, epidemiology, clinical safety, efficacy, and other data sources to inform decisions for patients, caregivers, providers, manufacturers, and regulatory bodies, such as the Food and Drug Administration (FDA).[9]

For example, consider a new drug that has been on the market in the United States for less than a year. The drug fulfills an important unmet need for patients and as such was approved on an accelerated schedule from the FDA. Postmarketing pharmacovigilance efforts as described elsewhere (See Chapter 2) are vital to patient safety in these circumstances, and after several months of product use, they identify an important safety signal. The manufacturer works with the FDA and others to understand the impact of this new information on the product's benefit-risk. If the overall benefits still outweigh the risks of the drug, all parties need to figure out what to do to mitigate this risk. This is a situation where human factors, as well as health literacy, can be applied to find the best way to reduce or, in some cases, eliminate this risk. Human factors can be applied to

- identify the root cause of the issue from the perspective of the patient or provider,
- determine if the issue is likely to persist,
- inform the evaluation of risk controls,
- rapidly prototype and user-test specific risk mitigations to develop an effective control.

In this example, human factors could support pharmacovigilance and postmarketing safety by assessing if this safety issue represents new information to prescribers or existing information that may not have been sufficiently communicated previously. The most important component of human factors is that it provides the perspective of the intended user. If prescribers were aware of this safety issue but for a medically valid reason purposefully did not change their actions, then a risk mitigation to inform them of this safety issue is likely to have little real-world effect.

There are multiple distinct human factors activities that are applied individually and collectively as part of a user-centered design throughout a product life cycle (multiple resources are available that provide in-depth descriptions of these activities.[7,8]). A variety of human factors methods can be used to determine the key elements, actions, and relationships important to pharmacovigilance and patient safety. Contextual inquiry, ethnography, user profiles, task analysis, use-related risk analysis, and medical severity assessment are scientifically valid methods for answering the five W's,

---

> **BOX 12.3**
> **Usability Testing**
>
> - Formative or exploratory testing that searches through multiple iterations and rapid prototyping for the optimal design for the intended use.
> - Summative or validation testing confirms likely real—world performance of the product.

---

namely, *who, what, where, when, and why*, as they apply to the development of safe and effective products and processes. These steps as performed in the context of a pharmacovigilance investigation seek to identify a pattern that would indicate a systemic underlying patient safety issue. If such a systemic risk is determined, human factors user-testing may be employed to develop an effective risk control.

Usability testing (Box 12.3) consists of early-stage exploratory, or formative, evaluations and later-stage validation, or summative, evaluations. In both stages, human factors is driven by user evidence attained from people with the same characteristics as the intended final user of the product being developed. Fidelity to real-world situations and the ability to execute user-testing relatively quickly in comparison to other methods that rely on collecting data from individuals make human factors a particularly valuable complement to pharmacovigilance. User-testing for drugs and devices most commonly relies on simulated-use testing where participants will simulate the actions they would perform in a real-world situation, e.g., a nurse would administer an injection into a mannequin. The intended users, uses, and environment are observed and questioned to provide insights into the perception, cognition, and action of the user experience. These insights are first integrated into the design of the intended product during the first stage of user-testing called formative or exploratory evaluations. Formative user-testing includes rapid prototyping and testing of the product in a process of design iterations. When performance and subjective feedback from participants indicates a design has been optimized, summative or validation testing is performed to confirm a product's likely performance in the real world. Human factors summative simulated-use test conditions attempt to mirror real-world use on any characteristics of users, uses, product, or environment that may affect outcomes. When completed, user-testing provides investigators with data to inform decision-making about the likely usability and performance of the product.

HEALTH LITERACY

Pharmacovigilance efforts often identify systemic threats to patient safety that have root causes related to issues in communication. To be successful, health communication has to be clear between healthcare professionals, patients, and the healthcare systems they use. People have better health outcomes when they understand their discharge instructions, when they know how to take their medicines correctly, and when they know who to call if they have questions.[10] However, a systemic issue in health communication that manifests as a threat to patient safety is impaired health literacy. According to a 2013 report by the World Health Organization (Box 12.4), "Health literacy is a stronger predictor of an individual's health status than income, employment status, education level, and racial or ethnic group."[11]

Health literacy is an intersection of communication factors that affect health. Three of the key contributors are listed in the following.

- Healthcare system—factors related to the complexity of the healthcare system and the demands it places on a person, such as policies and procedures, the environment and physical space, information that constantly changes, and navigation of the system.
- Individual—factors related to a person, including reading, writing, communicating, confidence, emotions and attitudes, and knowledge of health.
- Healthcare professionals—factors related to a healthcare professional, including how they communicate information in writing and when speaking.

Impaired or limited health literacy is a significant barrier to patient safety efforts, particularly the communication of benefit and risk.[12–14] Health literacy (Box 12.5) is more than information absorption; it also entails interaction, participation, problem-solving, cultural competency, communication, beliefs, activation, decision-making, and health system awareness.[4,15,16]

More than 93 million Americans may have trouble engaging, understanding, and utilizing written medication information.[17] People in the lowest categories of health literacy comprise 34%–55% of the US adult population and are able to perform only the simplest tasks with easily identifiable information. This estimate, and comparable estimates of health literacy globally, calls into question the value of drug product information because its content typically uses medical jargon and prioritizes numeracy skills.

Numeracy (Box 12.6) refers to the ability to understand numbers and is especially relevant in

---

BOX 12.4
Health Literacy Predicts Individual's Health Status Better Than

- Income
- Employment status
- Education level
- Racial or ethnic group

BOX 12.5
Health Literacy

- Interaction
- Cultural competency
- Decision-making
- Numeracy skills
- Beliefs/attitudes/values

BOX 12.6
Numeracy

- The ability to understand numbers.
- Especially relevant in pharmacovigilance because risks and benefits may be expressed as percentages or ratios.

---

pharmacovigilance because risks and benefits may be expressed numerically as percentages or ratios.[18–20] Impaired numeracy skills limit people's ability to make informed health decisions, including negatively affecting their ability to weigh long-term versus short-term benefits.[18,21] A large number of studies have examined comprehension of health materials and found that individuals with lower health literacy were significantly less able to navigate, retrieve information, and make inferences to support the safe and appropriate use of a medicine.[15,16,22,23] Written patient information uses a specialized medical terminology that is unfamiliar to many individuals and is often composed at a reading level much more advanced than the skills of the intended audience. The elderly are especially vulnerable to medication errors derived from issues in health literacy. The implication of this to health outcomes is that the people identified through pharmacovigilance as most in need of additional resources to aid in their decision-making

> **BOX 12.7**
> **Plain Language**
>
> - Communication that the audience can understand the first time they read or hear it.

process are the people least capable of utilizing the information that is most commonly available.

In order to arrive at a solution we must reconceptualize the problem. More than a decade after its groundbreaking health literacy work, the National Academies of Sciences, Engineering, and Medicine (NASEM) Roundtable on Health Literacy revised the definition of health literacy to better capture the interplay between the factors that influence health behaviors and health outcomes:

> *While early work focused on individual skills (and deficits) and specific products (brochures and documents, for example), we, the authors, have come to a greater appreciation that health literacy is multidimensional—it includes both system demands and complexities as well as the skills and abilities of individuals.*

The system demands and complexities noted in this conceptualization are likely to be related to the root causes of patient safety issues identified in pharmacovigilance investigations. When determining how to mitigate or eliminate these items, in addition to a human factors approach, a health literacy focus on the use of plain language is strikingly useful. Plain language (Box 12.7) is communication that the audience can understand upon first exposure.[24,25] This seemingly simple consideration is a value-added challenge to the communication of benefit-risk information to the healthcare community.

CONCLUSION

Human factors and health literacy are vital disciplines to be applied in conjunction with pharmacovigilance to improve health outcomes and reduce the impact of safety-related events including medication errors. There exists significant opportunity to enhance synergy between these disciplines through the application of postmarketing learnings back into the early stages of product life cycle. Global health authorities' changes to prioritize accelerated approval for innovative products and increasing requests for real-world evidence in determining a product's benefit-risk is making this type of comprehensive pharmacovigilance necessary. These global regulatory changes have consequently increased opportunity to apply postmarketing safety information back into design and development to close the loop of patient experience.

REFERENCES

1. Sorensen K, et al. Health literacy and public health: a systematic review and integration of definitions and models. *BMC Public Health.* 2012;12(1):80.
2. Montagne M. The metaphorical nature of drugs and drug taking. *Social Sci Med.* 1988;26(4):417–424.
3. Wolf MS, et al. In search of low health literacy: threshold vs. gradient effect of literacy on health status and mortality. *Social Sci Med.* 2010;70(9):1335–1341.
4. Wolf MS, et al. To err is human: patient misinterpretations of prescription drug label instructions. *Patient Educ Couns.* 2007;67(3):293–300.
5. Shrank WH, et al. The quality of pharmacologic care for adults in the United States. *Med Care.* 2006;44(10):936–945.
6. Schroeder SR, et al. Cognitive tests predict real-world errors: the relationship between drug name confusion rates in laboratory-based memory and perception tests and corresponding error rates in large pharmacy chains. *BMJ Qual Saf.* 2017;26(5):395–407.
7. Carayon P, Wood KE. Patient safety: the role of human factors and systems engineering. *Stud Health Technol Inform.* 2010;153:23–46.
8. Carayon P, ed. *Handbook of Human Factors and Ergonomics in Health Care and Patient Safety.* 2nd ed. CRC Press; 2017:876.
9. Lievano F, et al. The future of safety science is happening now: the modernization of the benefit-risk paradigm. *Pharmacoepidemiol Drug Saf.* 2017;26(8):869–874. https://doi.org/10.1002/pds.4241. Epub 2017 Jun 8.
10. *Organizational Change to Improve Health Literacy: Workshop Summary.* 2013. Washington, DC.
11. World Health Organization, ed. *Health Literacy: The Solid Facts.* 2013:76.
12. Nielsen-Bohlman L, Institute of Medicine (U.S.). Committee on Health Literacy. *Health Literacy: A Prescription to End Confusion.* Vol. xix. Washington, DC: National Academies Press; 2004:345.
13. Zhang Y, Baicker K, Newhouse JP. Geographic variation in the quality of prescribing. *N Engl J Med.* 2010;363(21): 1985–1988. https://doi.org/10.1056/NEJMp1010220. Epub 2010 Nov 3.
14. World Health Organization; 2011. [Cited 2011 1/9/2011]. Available from: http://www.who.int/healthpromotion/conferences/7gchp/track2/en/index.html.
15. Wolf MS, et al. Literacy and learning in health care. *Pediatrics.* 2009;124(suppl 3):S275–S281.
16. Wolf MS, Gazmararian JA, Baker DW. Health literacy and health risk behaviors among older adults. *Am J Prev Med.* 2007;32(1):19–24.
17. Kutner MA, National Center for Education Statistics. *The Health Literacy of America's Adults Results from the 2003 National Assessment of Adult Literacy.* Vol. xiv. Washington, DC: U.S. Dept. of Education, National Center for Education Statistics; 2006:60.

18. Peters E, et al. Numeracy skill and the communication, comprehension, and use of risk-benefit information. *Health Aff.* 2007;26(3):741−748.
19. Gigerenzer G, Edwards A. Simple tools for understanding risks: from innumeracy to insight. *Br Med J.* 2003; 327(7417):741−744.
20. Yin HS, et al. Effect of medication label units of measure on parent choice of dosing tool: a randomized experiment. *Acad Pediatr.* 2016;16(8):734−741.
21. Tormey LK, et al. *The Impact of Medication Self-Efficacy and Health Literacy on Patient-Reported Outcomes in Inflammatory Bowel Disease.* Digestive Disease Week (DDW); 2016:S399.
22. Fiss T, et al. Cognitive impairment in primary ambulatory health care: pharmacotherapy and the use of potentially inappropriate medicine. *Int J Geriatr Psychiatry.* 2013; 28(2):173−181.
23. O'Conor R, et al. Health literacy, cognitive function, proper use, and adherence to inhaled asthma controller medications among older adults with asthma. *Chest.* 2015;147(5):1307−1315.
24. Parker RM, Wolf MS. Health literate equates to patient-centered. *J Health Commun.* 2015;20(12):1367−1368.
25. Parker RM, Wolf MS, Kirsch I. Preparing for an epidemic of limited health literacy: weathering the perfect storm. *J Gen Intern Med.* 2008;23(8):1273−1276.

CHAPTER 13

Benefit-Risk Management

CHERYL RENZ, MS, MD • MONDIRA BHATTACHARYA, MD

INTRODUCTION

Medicinal products are developed to provide therapeutic benefits (favorable effects) for patients, such as curing a disease, slowing its evolution, or alleviating its symptoms. These products can also cause risks (unfavorable or harmful effects) via adverse drug reactions (ADRs) (Chapter 4). ADRs can range from frequent and minor symptoms, such as nausea or headache, to rare but severe events such as anaphylaxis, liver failure, or cancer. The evaluation of the benefits and the risks associated with a medicinal product is called benefit-risk assessment. The product's intended indication and target population are critical to this assessment.

The regulators and pharmaceutical sponsors (industry) are responsible for ensuring that the benefit-risk balance of a product is positive for the intended patient population. Conducting a benefit-risk assessment is a complex task (Box 13.1); it involves the evaluation and integration of a large amount of data, varying in type, source, relevance, and uncertainty, which evolves throughout the life cycle of the product. The assessment can be further complicated by individual patient variability and dose-response effects. The same information about a product's benefits and risks may be interpreted differently by the developer, the regulator, the healthcare professional, and the patient. In the recent decades, the regulators and the developers have taken steps to systematize their benefit-risk decision-making through the use of structured decision analysis approaches.

HISTORICAL BACKGROUND

The field of benefit-risk assessment is rooted in several important events in pharmaceutical history (Fig. 13.1). In 1928, the bacteriologist Dr. Alexander Fleming serendipitously discovered that a substance produced by the mold *Penicillium notatum* had bactericidal properties after the mold contaminated a Petri dish of *Staphylococcus aureus*. Fleming found that his "mold juice" was capable of killing a wide range of harmful bacteria, including streptococcus, meningococcus, and the diphtheria bacillus. During his acceptance speech for the Nobel Prize in Physiology or Medicine (1945), Fleming foreshadowed the need to balance benefit and risk when he warned that the overuse of penicillin could lead to resistant bacteria.[1]

In 1938, another antibiotic, sulfanilamide, was reformulated from a tablet to a liquid as a means to remove its bitter taste. The elixir was tested for taste and smell only. Its consumption led to 107 deaths, as the elixir contained a toxic solvent (diethylene glycol). This misfortune led to the passage of the first legislation (1938 Food, Drug, and Cosmetic Act) to require pharmaceutical manufacturers to test the safety of their products.[2]

The event that has most directly impacted the current approach to benefit-risk evaluation was the thalidomide tragedy in the 1950s.[3-5] Thalidomide was a medication originally marketed in European countries as a treatment for insomnia but later was used "off-label" to alleviate morning sickness. Its toxic effects occurred to the unborn fetus resulting in birth defects characterized by deformities of the limbs from shortening or absence of the long bones. In the United States, thalidomide was never approved because the Food and Drug Administration (FDA) reviewer, Dr. Frances Kelsey, did

---

BOX 13.1
The Complexity of Assessing Benefit-Risk

- Disease state characterization
- Data integration
- Patient variability
- Dose-response effects
- Uncertainty

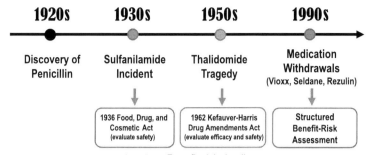

FIG. 13.1   Benefit-risk timeline.

not find the efficacy and safety information adequate to assess the product's benefits and risks. This tragic event led to the strengthening of the regulatory review process for new medicines. In the United States, Congress passed the 1962 Kefauver-Harris Drug Amendments Act requiring evidence of both safety and efficacy before a medication could be approved and sold.[6] Similar actions were taken by regulators in other countries.

Regulatory agencies worldwide have been and continue to be responsible for the review of new medicinal products on a public health basis. Sometimes different regulatory agencies reach different decisions based on the same information. During the 1990s a series of well-publicized events involving the withdrawal of high-profile medications from the world market generated considerable skepticism of the regulatory approval process. For example, the withdrawal of rofecoxib (Vioxx) for cardiovascular events and cardiovascular deaths,[7–9] cerivastatin (Baycol or Lipobay) for fatal rhabdomyolysis,[10] terfenadine (Seldane) for QT prolongation and fatal arrhythmias,[11] and troglitazone (Rezulin) for liver failure[12] drew attention to the imperfections of the regulators' benefit-risk decisions.

STRUCTURED BENEFIT-RISK ASSESSMENT

The product withdrawals in the 1990s led the public to question and scrutinize the basis for regulatory benefit-risk decision-making. The regulators also recognized the need to improve the consistency, transparency, and communication of their benefit-risk assessments, including how the evidence was weighed and balanced.[13,14] As a result, the regulators have launched structured approaches to evaluate, contextualize, and communicate their benefit-risk decisions (Box 13.2).[15–17] In addition, the regulators expect the developers to present their products' benefit-risk profiles in a similar manner, for example, in their marketing authorization applications (e.g., in Section 2.5.6 of

---

BOX 13.2
Advantages of a Structured Benefit-Risk Assessment

A structured Benefit-Risk Assessment can improve:
- consistency
- transparency
- documentation
- cross-functional understanding of the product
- communication of benefit-risk decisions

---

the Clinical Overview, the "Benefits and Risks Conclusions," of the Common Technical Document[18–20]).

To support a structured approach, various benefit-risk frameworks have been developed by the regulators, the developers, and the partnership between both to serve as platforms to guide the qualitative evaluation and the communication of benefit-risk assessments (Figs. 13.2–13.5). For example, the European Medicines Agency (EMA) sponsored the benefit-risk methodology project that included the release of the PrOACT-URL framework[16,17] and the FDA released a guidance on their structured benefit-risk framework.[15] Beginning in 2017, the FDA is using this framework in the review of all new drug and biological licensing applications.

Expert judgment has been and remains the cornerstone of benefit-risk assessments. However, a framework can provide a platform to facilitate a structured approach so that the decision-makers can discuss, synthesize, summarize, and make decisions about a product's benefit-risk profile, across the life cycle of the product. A framework can also serve as a template to structure, document, and communicate the benefit-risk decisions. While there are many different versions of benefit-risk frameworks, there are commonalities across them, which aid, not replace, expert judgment. In general a benefit-risk framework includes (Box 13.3; Fig. 13.6) the following:

Problem	1. Determine the nature of the problem and its context. 2. Frame the problem.
Objective	3. Establish objectives that indicate the overall purposes to be achieved. 4. Identify criteria for (a) favourable effects, and (b) unfavorable effects.
Alternatives	5. Identify the options to be evaluated against the criteria.
Consequences	6. Describe how the alternatives perform for each of the criteria, i.e., the magnitudes of all effects, and their desirability or severity, and the incidence of all effects.
Trade-off	7. Assess the balance between favorable and unfavorable effects.
Uncertainty	8. Report the uncertainty associated with the favorable and unfavorable effects. 9. Consider how the balance between favorable and unfavorable effects is affected by uncertainty.
Risk tolerance	10. Judge the relative importance of the decision maker's risk attitude for this product. 11. Report how this affected the balance reported in Step 9.
Linked decisions	12. Consider the consistency of this decision with similar past decisions, and assess whether taking this decision could impact future decisions.

FIG. 13.2 PrOACT-URL framework: developed by the EMA Benefit-Risk Methodology Working Group.

FDA — Benefit-Risk Integrated Assessment

Benefit-Risk Dimensions

Dimension	Evidence and Uncertainties	Conclusion and Reasons
Analysis of Condition		
Current Treatment Options		
Benefit		
Risk and Risk Management		

FIG. 13.3 The FDA benefit-risk framework.

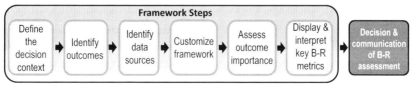

FIG. 13.4 Benefit-Risk Action Team Framework developed by the Pharmaceutical Research and Manufacturers of America. *B-R*, Benefit-Risk.

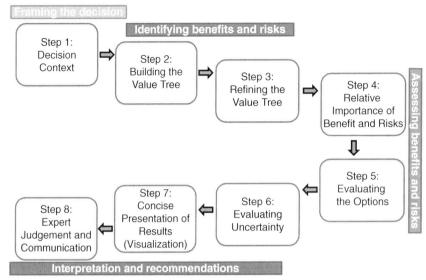

FIG. 13.5 The Unified Methodologies for Benefit-Risk Assessment framework developed by the Centre for Innovation in Regulatory Science.

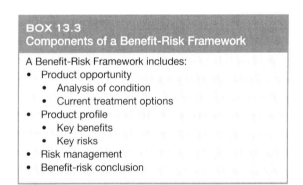

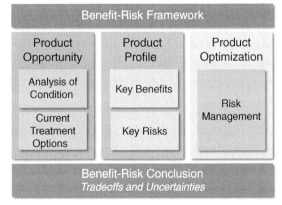

FIG. 13.6 Benefit-risk framework for medicinal products.

1. Product Opportunity—why the product is needed. This provides the clinical context for weighing the benefits and risks. Product opportunity is based on
   a. Analysis of Condition: The nature and severity of the condition the product is intended to treat or prevent.
   b. Current Treatment Options: The key benefits and risks of the most commonly available treatments for the condition and identification of unmet medical need. The background rates for the key benefits and risks of the current treatment options can be compared with those of the product of interest. This review should also include off-label therapies (if they are generally recognized as acceptable treatment options, either by endorsement from treatment guidelines or used commonly because of limited or an absence of approved treatment options) and products for the condition in late-stage development.
2. Product Profile—what the product can do. Product profile can also be thought of as describing the product's value proposition. It focuses on the key benefits and key risks of the product, based on indication. The benefits and risks may vary across different subpopulations or different dosing regimens.
3. Product optimization, also referred to as risk management, describes whether (and how) the product's risk(s) can be characterized and managed. Product optimization typically includes
   a. plans to further characterize a product's risks,

  b. interventions to minimize a product's key risks so that the product's benefits outweigh its risks.
4. Benefit-Risk Conclusion—the overall assessment summary that takes into account
  a. the therapeutic context and comparator products;
  b. the analysis of the product's specific benefits and risks, including their magnitude, tradeoffs, and clinical relevance;
  c. the risk management strategies and the expected impact on the benefit-risk balance;
  d. the acknowledgement of any limitations or uncertainties related to
    i. the selected endpoints of the clinical trials or the clinical data (of note, most studies are powered to demonstrate efficacy, not safety)
    ii. manufacturing factors
    iii. quality issues
    iv. other aspects of the benefit-risk assessment

Application of (Box 13.4) a benefit-risk framework can support industry's phase-gated decisions and discussions with the regulators. It can also be used by regulators to communicate the rationale and the basis of their decisions. Use of the abovementioned simple benefit-risk framework, which has taken into account the core elements of the FDA, EMA, and industry-based examples, can meet the needs of (and expectations of) worldwide regulatory agencies during product submission and postmarketing reviews.

INTEGRATING THE LIFE CYCLE APPROACH TO BENEFIT-RISK WITHIN A BIOPHARMACEUTICAL COMPANY

The evaluation of benefits and risks should be an ongoing process throughout the product life cycle. At the basis of this life cycle approach is the fundamental question: do the benefits outweigh the risks for the product's intended indication and expected use? This section will describe an approach to integrate benefit-risk assessments into (Box 13.5) the product life cycle and offer ways the assessment can inform and support different aspects of the drug development process.

The Benefit-Risk Assessment Team

Within a biopharmaceutical company (Box 13.6), there are many different functional representatives who can provide input into the benefit-risk assessment. Ideally one function, such as a dedicated Benefit-Risk Management group or members of the pharmacovigilance organization, can be responsible for understanding the current regulations and best practices about benefit-risk assessment and how they pertain to the company's processes and procedures. This team representative can facilitate the structured approach to benefit-risk

> **BOX 13.4**
> **Applications of Benefit-Risk Frameworks**
>
> Benefit-Risk Frameworks are used by regulatory agencies and industry to support:
> - Drug development milestone decisions
> - New product marketing applications
> - Postmarket reviews

> **BOX 13.5**
> **The Product Life Cycle and Benefit-Risk**
>
> Assessing benefit-risk should occur throughout the product life cycle.

> **BOX 13.6**
> **Benefit-Risk Management Team**
>
> A dedicated Benefit-Risk Management group can drive a company's cross-functional participation in a structured approach to benefit-risk decision-making.

decision-making by using a dedicated framework, either preexisting (Figs. 13.2—13.5) or developed in house.

Although a consultative Benefit-Risk Management group could logically reside in several different functions within a biopharmaceutical research and development organization, there are strategic advantages to placing this group within a pharmacovigilance organization. For example, the evolution of a product's benefit-risk profile after approval is primarily due to the identification of new risks or refinement of the characterization (severity or frequency) of known risks; the work to collect and analyze the emerging risk information is the primary responsibility of the pharmacovigilance organization. Placing the Benefit-Risk Management group within the pharmacovigilance organization allows members to have direct access to emerging risk information and then advise on its impact to the existing benefit-risk profile.

The company should define which functional representatives are participants in the benefit-risk decision-making team. Typically, this team includes representatives from safety/pharmacovigilance, clinical development, regulatory sector, medical affairs, epidemiology, statistics, health economics and outcomes research, and commercial and legal sectors (Table 13.1). The team may also include a project manager to facilitate meeting conduct and documentation of the discussions and decisions.

TABLE 13.1
Example of a Biopharmaceutical Company's Benefit-Risk Management Team Membership

Benefit-Risk Management Team Membership	
Facilitators	• Benefit-Risk Management or Pharmacovigilance • Project Management
Functional representatives	• Pharmacovigilance • Clinical Development • Regulatory • Medical Affairs • Epidemiology • Statistics • Health Economics and Outcomes Research • Commercial[a] • Legal

[a] The commercial representative can provide information learned from market research and the patient journey assessment regarding the patient perspective to inform the team's decision-making.

TABLE 13.2
Information Sources to Inform Benefit-Risk Decision-Making

Information Sources to Inform the Life Cycle Approach to Benefit-Risk	
• Toxicology reports • Investigator brochure • Clinical study reports • Clinical development plan/asset plan • Product safety plan/developmental RMP • Statistical analysis plan • Regulatory documents • Risk management plan • DSUR/PSUR/PBRER • Briefing books	• Disease opportunity profile • Disease treatment guidelines • Target product profile or claims • Label/company core data sheet • PROs/QoL instruments and domains • Patient journey • New drug application/marketing authorization application/biologic license application • Real-world evidence (RWE)

DSUR, Development Safety Update Report; *PBRER*, Periodic Benefit-Risk Evaluation Report; *PROs*, Patient-Reported Outcomes; *PSUR*, Periodic Safety Update Report; *RMP*, Risk Management Plan.

The team will use various sources of information to aid their evaluation. Examples of the different types of information sources are shown in Table 13.2.

The Life Cycle Approach

The structured approach can be undertaken at select times during the product's life cycle, such as during early development, during late development, and when the product is on market (Fig. 13.7; Box 13.7).

Early development approach

During early development, typically after phase 1 or during phase 2, the structured approach can be used to construct the benefit-risk plan. This plan focuses on the product opportunity and product profile sections of the benefit-risk framework. The primary purpose of the benefit-risk plan is to inform preparation of the registration studies. The exact time to undertake this activity depends on the type of registration program being considered (i.e., a traditional, accelerated, or adaptive design program). The plan will also serve as a starting point for the benefit-risk assessment to be prepared later in the development life cycle.

In the benefit-risk plan, the product opportunity section provides the decision-makers with information about the analysis of condition, to enhance the team's understanding about the severity and consequences of the disease, and the current treatment options, to inform the team about the key benefits and risks of available treatments and the unmet medical need. The team can use the information about the product opportunity to provide the clinical context for planning out the product profile. An important early team activity is discussion about the product profile—the product's key benefits and risks. As there is limited data available during early development, the team can include aspirational benefits and potential risks. The team can gather information about potential risks by preparing a risk precedence analysis—an evaluation of the risks of products with a similar mechanism of action to their product and/or the risks associated with products indicated to treat the same condition as their product. The product profile can be displayed and recorded in a benefit-risk value tree (Figs. 13.11 and 13.12).

The benefit-risk plan prepared (Box 13.8) during early development can provide information and insights for other planning activities (Fig. 13.8). The team can use this information to inform pipeline milestone decisions and planning of the registration program, for example, to guide selection of the study population, comparator, doses, and endpoints (including the selection of PROs). The benefit-risk plan can also be used to support planning, preparation, or updating of key strategic documents, such as the developmental RMP Development

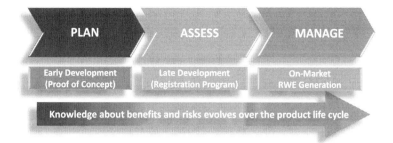

FIG. 13.7 Life cycle approach to benefit-risk.

Safety Update Report (DSUR), investigator brochure, and target product label.

Late development approach

During late development, typically after phase 2b or phase 3, the structured approach is used to conduct the full benefit-risk assessment (Box 13.9). The primary focus is on the product profile and product optimization sections of the benefit-risk framework, although the product opportunity section can be updated if needed (for example, if a new medication is on the market since the time the product opportunity evaluation was completed). The exact time to conduct the assessment depends on the type of registration program but should occur in time to support preparation of the marketing authorization application.

For the product profile section, the team returns to the product's benefit-risk value tree and updates it based on the information available from the registration studies. The team should include only the product's key benefits and key risks rather than a duplication of the various endpoints included in the studies.

Next the team focuses on product optimization, namely, risk management strategies, which are typically described in a product's risk management plan (RMP). An RMP is a document (prepared in accordance with EMA GVP Module V - Risk Management Systems [Rev 2][21]) that describes the current knowledge about the safety of the product. The RMP provides information on plans for pharmacovigilance studies and other activities to increase understanding of the product's safety profile, measures to prevent or minimize risks associated with use of the product, and plans to evaluate the effectiveness of these risk minimization measures (RMMs). Pharmaceutical companies are required to submit an RMP to regulatory agencies in many countries, including the EMA, at the time of the marketing authorization application.

One of the most important decisions the team will make is the types of RMMs needed to best manage the product's risks. RMMs are interventions that aim to prevent or reduce the *frequency* of a risk and/or to reduce the *severity* or impact (Box 13.10) on the patient should it occur. For most products, application of routine RMMs (Box 13.11) (product information/approved labeling, e.g., prescribing information [United States] or Summary of Product Characteristics [SmPC, European Union], and packaging [e.g., pack size and design plus information on the carton]) is usually sufficient to minimize the risk(s). However, some products have risks that require an extra level of risk minimization known as additional risk minimization measures (aRMMs).[22,23] In the United States, the FDA refers to aRMMs as Risk Evaluation and Mitigation Strategy (REMS).[24] These additional measures vary greatly depending on their purpose, design, complexity and the target stakeholder. (Table 13.3). RMMs are agreed between the marketing authorization holder and regulatory authorities at the time of product registration and may change during the life cycle of the product.

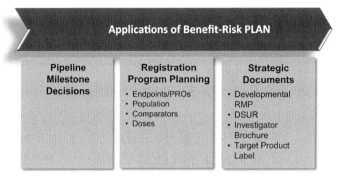

FIG. 13.8 *DSUR*, Development Safety Update Report; *PROs*, Patient-Reported Outcomes; *RMP*, Risk Management Plan.

BOX 13.9
Highlights of a Benefit-Risk Assessment in Late Development

A Benefit-Risk Assessment initially prepared during late development:
- Characterizes a product's key benefits and key risks based on evidence from the registration studies
- Describes measures to minimize the product's key risks
- Summarizes the product's benefit-risk profile in the context of its intended use and unmet medical need

---

BOX 13.10
Purpose of Risk Minimization Measures

Risk minimization measures are intended to prevent or reduce the frequency and/or severity of a risk.

BOX 13.11
Routine and Additional Risk Minimization Measures

Routine risk minimization measures, used for all prescription products, include
- product information (labeling)
- packaging

Additional risk minimization measures are used in select circumstances to achieve a favorable benefit-risk profile. These measures typically impact
- product distribution
- patient selection
- patient monitoring

To decide what types of RMMs are needed, the team can assess the effectiveness of risk minimization interventions used during the clinical trials, such as screening requirements, dose titration, prophylactic treatments, or patient-monitoring procedures. Additionally, the team can gather information about the types of RMMs used in healthcare settings for other products that have similar risks to the product undergoing the assessment. The team may also decide to conduct a failure modes and effects analysis (FMEA) to determine whether aRMMs are needed.[25] FMEA is used in a variety of settings, such as aeronautics, military, engineering, and manufacturing, to identify potential failures and mitigation options. With regard to the risk management of medicinal products, FMEA can identify failures in ideal behaviors or processes that could increase the likelihood of a patient experiencing the risk (e.g., product is prescribed to an inappropriate patient or prescriber writes a prescription at incorrect dose) and provide ways to minimize the failure, which ultimately would minimize occurrence of the risk and/or its severity should it occur.

Additional information about routine and aRMMs is provided in Appendix I.

The benefit-risk assessment prepared during late development (Box 13.12) can be used by the team to communicate the rationale for their decision to other key decision-makers. The assessment includes the most clinically relevant benefits and risks of the product and whether (and how) its risks can be managed. The assessment takes into account the context of the decision, which includes the patient population (e.g., chronically ill vs. acutely ill patients), the seriousness of the condition, and the relative benefits and risks of important alternative therapies available to patients. The assessment also denotes the limitations and uncertainties of the available evidence.

TABLE 13.3
Routine and Additional Risk Minimization

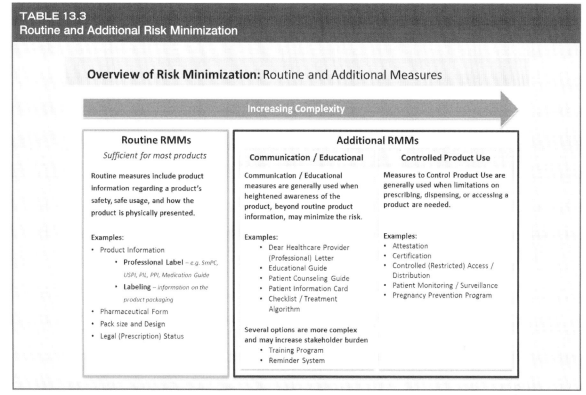

Overview of Risk Minimization: Routine and Additional Measures

Increasing Complexity

Routine RMMs	Additional RMMs	
Sufficient for most products	**Communication / Educational**	**Controlled Product Use**
Routine measures include product information regarding a product's safety, safe usage, and how the product is physically presented.	Communication / Educational measures are generally used when heightened awareness of the product, beyond routine product information, may minimize the risk.	Measures to Control Product Use are generally used when limitations on prescribing, dispensing, or accessing a product are needed.

Examples:
• Product Information
  • **Professional Label** – *e.g. SmPC, USPI, PIL, PPI, Medication Guide*
  • **Labeling** – *information on the product packaging*
• Pharmaceutical Form
• Pack size and Design
• Legal (Prescription) Status
	Examples:
	• Dear Healthcare Provider (Professional) Letter
	• Educational Guide
	• Patient Counseling Guide
	• Patient Information Card
	• Checklist / Treatment Algorithm
	
	Several options are more complex and may increase stakeholder burden
	• Training Program
	• Reminder System
		Examples:
		• Attestation
		• Certification
		• Controlled (Restricted) Access / Distribution
		• Patient Monitoring / Surveillance
		• Pregnancy Prevention Program

PIL, Patient information Leaflet; *PPI*, Patient Package Insert; *SmPC*, Summary of Product Characteristics; *USPI*, United States Prescribing Information.

BOX 13.12
Uses of a Benefit-Risk Assessment in Late Development

A Benefit-Risk Assessment prepared during late development can support:
• Preparation of submission documents and final product label
• Discussions with regulatory agencies
• Planning for product launch activities

The benefit-risk assessment can be reviewed by the company's safety governance board and pipeline decision-making board to support decision-making about a market authorization application and subsequent phase 3b and postmarket studies. Documentation of the assessment can be used to support preparation of key submission documents, such as the clinical overview and RMP.[20] Learnings from the assessment should also be used to guide preparation of the company's core product label (often referred to as the Company Core Data Sheet). The assessment can support interactions with the regulatory agencies, such as Pharmacovigilance Risk Assessment Committee (PRAC) and rapporteur meetings, and advisory meetings. Finally, the assessment can provide valuable information and insights for planning launch activities, including reimbursement strategies and product promotion campaigns (Fig. 13.9).

On-market approach

Once the product is on the market, efforts switch to managing the benefit-risk profile. Information (Box 13.13) about the product, especially about its risks, is readily available from a variety of sources. This information is based on use of the product in real-world conditions, typically from larger number of patients, using the product for longer durations, who are more heterogeneous than those who participated in the clinical trials. For example, rare or delayed adverse drug reactions would not be identified at the time of product approval. Industry and regulators have increasing access to real-world evidence (RWE)

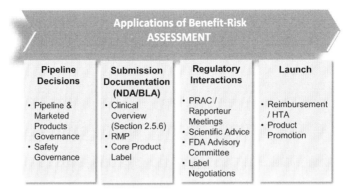

FIG. 13.9 *BLA*, Biologics License Application; *HTA*, Health Technology Assessment; *NDA*, New Drug Application; *PRAC*, Pharmacovigilance Risk Assessment Committee; *RMP*, Risk Management Plan

---

BOX 13.13
On-Market Benefit-Risk Assessment

Once on the market a product's Benefit-Risk Assessment is updated to address:
* Characterization of risks
* Effectiveness of risk minimization measures
* Optimization of product utilization

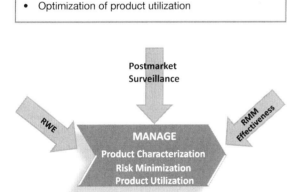

FIG. 13.10 On-market benefit-risk management. *RMM*, Risk Minimization Measure; *RWE*, Real-World Evidence.

from postapproval studies (such as phase 3b/4 studies, postauthorization safety and efficacy studies, and drug utilization studies), registries, electronic healthcare and claims databases, and even social media (Chapter 5). In addition, information about the product's risks is available from postmarketing pharmacovigilance surveillance efforts. Sometimes industry also gains information about their product from preapproval (early access) programs.

All this information can be used to manage the product's benefit-risk profile (Fig. 13.10). The risk profile should be reassessed, in an ongoing basis, to decide if new risks should be added or risks should be removed from the benefit-risk assessment. If the product was launched with aRMMs, then evaluation of the effectiveness of these measures can be used to modify the risk minimization strategies and specific tools. Most importantly, the ongoing assessment of the product's benefits and risks should guide the manner in which the product is used. For example, the target population, indication, and even duration of use may be modified during the product's life cycle to manage the product utilization in a manner that optimizes its benefit-risk profile. The ongoing benefit-risk assessment can be used to prepare either the Periodic Safety Update Report (PSUR) or the Periodic Benefit-Risk Evaluation Report (PBRER) which documents the integrated information about the product's benefits and risks throughout its life cycle.

Information gained about a product's risks while on market can further inform product decision-making. Updates to the product label are the primary form of risk communication. All other communication/educational efforts supported by the company must be "label consistent," otherwise the product may be found to be misbranded.[26] Patients and healthcare providers are increasingly requesting both the regulatory authorities and pharmaceutical companies to provide information about a product's benefits along with its risks to aid decision-making.

When developing risk communication materials, it is important to consider and test for health literacy. Health literacy is defined by the World Health Organization as "the cognitive and social skills which determine the motivation and ability of individuals to gain access to, understand and use information in ways which promote and maintain good health."[27] Many studies have examined comprehension of health-related materials and found that individuals with lower health literacy were significantly less able to navigate and retrieve risk-related information to support the safe and appropriate use of a medication.[28-31] Numeracy is an aspect of health literacy that refers to the ability to understand numbers.[32] Numeracy is especially relevant in drug information because risks and benefits may be expressed numerically as percentages or ratios.

VISUALIZATION OF BENEFIT-RISK ASSESSMENTS

Visual representations or displays of a product's benefits and risks can support the structured qualitative description of a benefit-risk assessment. Graphs (Box 13.14) and visual tools can facilitate comparison of the benefits and risks, by different treatment groups, and can display uncertainty. The visual display should integrate benefits and risks in a direct and understandable way, be practical and easy to generate, and ease cognitive workload. Sometimes specialized software is needed to generate the graphic displays.

BOX 13.14
Visualization of Benefit-Risk

Graphs and visual displays can be used to present a Benefit-Risk Assessment.

One useful display is the benefit-risk value tree (Figs. 13.11 and 13.12). Derived from decision analysis, a value tree is a visual map of the attributes or criteria of utmost importance to the decision-makers (Box 13.15). In the setting of benefit-risk assessment, a value tree is a hierarchical graphic depiction ("tree structure") of the key benefits and key risks that define the benefit-risk balance of the product.[33] Preparation of the value tree is an important initial effort undertaken by the team to capture their ideas about the product's key benefits and risks. The value tree can be updated throughout the phases of the development as data accumulate. A value tree generally has two branches, namely, benefits and risks. For each branch, multiple subbranches are created corresponding to one benefit or risk outcome (also referred to as an attribute). Creators of the value tree need to avoid "double counting," which can occur when one benefit or risk subbranch outcome overlaps with another subbranch outcome (e.g., reduction in hemorrhagic strokes [benefit outcome] and incidence of hemorrhagic strokes [risk outcome]). Another challenge in developing a value tree is to select only the outcomes that are critical to the assessment (which may require an exercise to "prune the tree," given the numerous endpoints usually included in clinical trials). Additionally, the team will need to distinguish between adverse drug reactions and the key risks (Chapter 4).

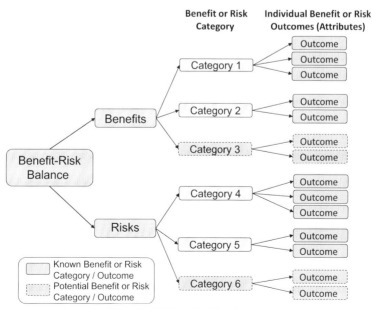

FIG. 13.11 Benefit-risk value tree.

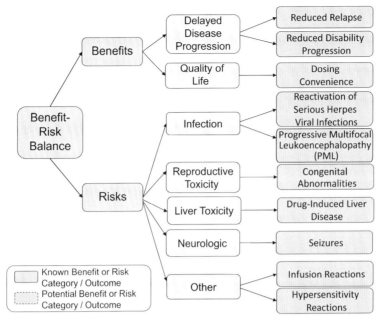

FIG. 13.12 Example of benefit-risk value tree for a hypothetical product to treat a chronic neurologic condition.

A variety of graphic displays can be used to illustrate the following features of a benefit-risk assessment:
• Magnitude—how large or small is the benefit or risk
• Comparison—relative magnitude of benefits and risks or weighting the importance of the different benefits and risks
• Cumulative—how benefit or risk changes over time; how magnitude may add up over time
• Uncertainty—variability or ranges related to the benefit or risk measurement.

The graphic displays can be generated using clinical trial data during development or RWE in the postmarket setting. Examples of some of the most frequently used graphic visualizations are (Fig. 13.13)[34,35]
• forest plot
• tornado plot
• heatmap
• waterfall plot
• stacked bar chart

Visualization of the benefit-risk assessment can provide a useful "snapshot" of the key information or data used by the decision-makers, along with its strengths, limitations, and uncertainties. In addition, the different graphic options can help "display" the qualitative assessment based on the benefit-risk framework.

QUANTITATIVE BENEFIT-RISK ASSESSMENTS

The field of quantitative methodology for benefit-risk decision-making is vast and evolving. For persons involved in assessing benefits and risks, it is important to know that quantitative assessments are available and can provide additional information to a qualitative assessment.

Quantitative assessments (Box 13.16) typically require a method to put benefits and risks on the same scale and calculate a benefit-risk score with associated uncertainty to numerically represent a benefit-risk balance. They usually involve an algorithm to combine metrics for specific benefit and risk attributes with measures that quantify the clinical impact or weight the importance of the attribute.

A key concern about quantitative methods is the use of a single value or number to represent the benefit-risk balance. A common criticism is that clinical judgment, which incorporates the subjectivity, complexities, and

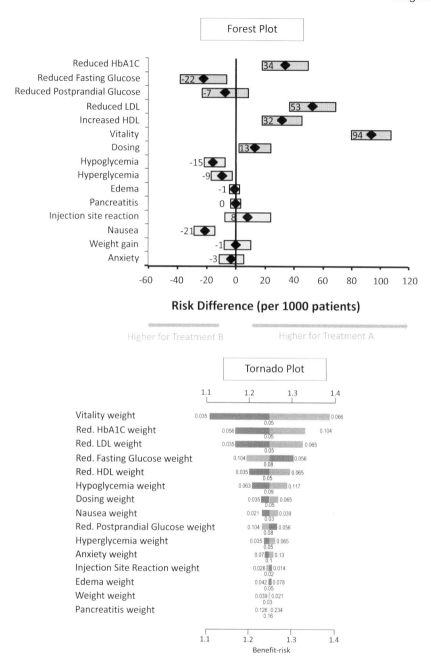

FIG. 13.13 Examples of benefit-risk graphic displays (forest plot and tornado plot). *HDL*, High-Density Lipoprotein; *LDL*, Low-Density Lipoprotein. (Berlin C, Nixon R. Presentation: An Example of Benefit-Risk Analysis Applying the BRAT Framework. DIA 2013 49th Annual Meeting)

BOX 13.16
Quantitative Benefit-Risk Assessment

A quantitative assessment can supplement a qualitative, structured benefit-risk assessment when the benefit-risk profile is complex.

nuances of conducting a benefit-risk assessment, is too complex to capture in a number. However, research has shown a strong correlation between clinical and statistical predictions.

An example of a quantitative methodology that is gaining popularity among academics, industries, and some regulators is the multicriteria decision analysis (MCDA).[36,37] MCDA is a useful methodology for integrating multiple benefit and risk attributes based on their perceived value (or weights), which can be used to make comparisons between alternative treatment options. All the attributes are weighted to create a common unit of preference value, or utility. Summing those common units of benefit and risk provides an overall benefit-risk preference value or utility for each treatment alternative, enabling calculation of the difference of the medicinal product of interest against the comparators. Stochastic multicriteria acceptability analysis (SMAA) is an extension of MCDA that uses probability distributions for data values instead of a point estimate and handles preferences expressed as ranking in the form of a distribution or range, or absent.

Examples of some of the most frequently used quantitative methodologies are listed in the following[38,39]; details about these methodologies are beyond the scope of this chapter but are summarized elsewhere:

- Bayesian statistics
- benefit-risk ratio
- incremental net health benefit
  MCDA
- SMAA
- Markov processes
- Kaplan-Meier estimators
- quality-adjusted life-years for modeling multiple health outcomes
- Conjoint analysis to elicit trade-off between effects, especially for patient preferences

The use of quantitative methodologies is not considered a routine part of benefit-risk assessment. However, in special situations, a quantitative assessment allows for specific probing of the data to obtain a clearer conclusion and enhance transparency in communicating the product's benefits and risks.

ROLE OF THE PATIENT IN BENEFIT-RISK ASSESSMENT

In the era of patient-centered healthcare, both the regulators and the developers have recognized the importance of capturing and incorporating patient input into benefit-risk decision-making. Patients (Box 13.17) who live with the disease are in a unique position to provide input on the product opportunity: the analysis of condition and the current treatment options (see Section 2). Patients can report how the disease impacts their lives, whether available treatments

---

BOX 13.17
The Patient Perspective and Benefit-Risk Assessment

Incorporation of the patient perspective is an important evolving aspect of benefit-risk assessment.
    Patient input can inform
- the product opportunity,
- the identification and weighting of a product's key benefits and key risks,
- the development of risk minimization measures.

---

are effective (or not), and what attributes they are looking for in a new product. Importantly, patients provide information about which benefits they prefer, which risks they are willing to tolerate, and their threshold of acceptable uncertainty about a product's benefit-risk profile.

Patients have taken actions to bring their voice to the forefront of benefit-risk decision-making. The outcry of HIV patients who demanded early access to experimental antiviral treatments has encouraged the formation of other patient groups to express their views, for example, by providing public testimony at the FDA advisory committee meetings. Patient advocacy organizations have been formed, such as the European Patients' Forum, PatientsLikeMe, and FasterCures, to actively bring the patient's perspective to the developers and the regulators.

The regulators are sponsoring initiatives (e.g., Patient-Focused Drug Development Initiative [FDA][40,41] and the Patients' and Consumers' Working Group [EMA][42,43]) to listen and learn from patients and then apply these learnings to their benefit-risk assessments. The FDA is including patients on advisory committee panels and the EMA is inviting patients to participate in the PRAC and the Committee for Medicinal Products for Human Use meetings.

The developers are realizing that patients enrolled in clinical trials can be a valuable resource to provide the patient perspective. In addition, developers are organizing meetings with patient groups to gather information about their weighing of a product's benefits and risks and their ideas about RMMs (for example, digital tools and innovative packaging). Finally, developers are inviting patients to participate in human factor testing of educational materials (assessing health literacy and numeracy), packaging designs, and other RMMs.

The developers and the regulators have started to conduct patient preference studies to obtain quantifiable evidence to reflect the views of patients about treatment options. In select cases, these studies have been part of marketing authorization decisions. One example of a patient preference study (Box 13.18) is a discrete choice experiment. In this study, patients are shown a series of hypothetical treatment pairs; each treatment has a unique benefit and risk profile. In each case the patients select their preferred treatment (Fig. 13.14). Analysis of the patients' choices provides information about which benefits and risks are most important to the patients and what maximal level of risk (known as the maximum acceptable risk) the patients are willing to accept for a given level of benefit.[44,45]

Patient preferences are critical to assess a product's benefits and risks but the process of evaluating patient-based information and accounting for variation within patient groups remains an emerging science.

BOX 13.18
Patient Preference Studies

Patient preference studies provide information about which benefits and risks are most important to patients and what maximal level of risk patients are willing to accept for a given level of benefit.

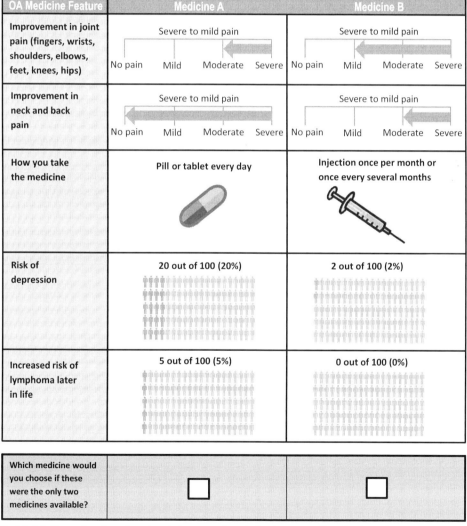

FIG. 13.14 Example of a discrete choice experiment: treatment profiles for hypothetical osteoarthritis products.

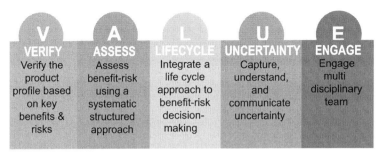

FIG. 13.15 The value concept for benefit-risk.

CONCLUSION

Formal benefit-risk assessments have been conducted since the introduction of the current regulatory systems following the thalidomide tragedy. Assessing the benefit-risk balance of medicinal products is an important challenge faced by all sectors of healthcare, from pharmaceutical developers and regulators seeking to provide patients with innovative treatment options to prescribers and patients seeking to make informed treatment decisions.

The critical appraisal of a product's benefits and risks is complex; it is thwart with uncertainty because of limited or conflicting data and heterogeneous effects across different patient populations. Additional uncertainty is expected as drug development pathways and regulatory approval processes accept conditional/accelerated approvals based on surrogate markers or interim analyses of pivotal trials. Importantly, different decision-makers can reach divergent conclusions based on the same benefit-risk information.

The regulators and developers have recognized the value and advantages of adapting a structured approach to their benefit-risk decision-making across the life cycle of the product (Fig. 13.15). A qualitative benefit-risk framework, supplemented with visual displays and quantitative methods, is being increasingly used to facilitate a structured approach to assess benefits and risks. Both regulators and developers are taking a more patient-centric approach by finding ways to incorporate the patient's perspective into their benefit-risk decision-making.

Sometimes a product's benefits are not worth its risks; other times, forgoing a product's benefits to avoid a risk can introduce other risks, such as prompting patients to use another treatment with significant risks, leaving a disease untreated, or deny some patients a potentially useful treatment. It is the responsibility of all participants in medicinal product development to ensure that products are developed, tested, manufactured, labeled, prescribed, dispensed, and used in a manner that maximizes benefits and minimizes risks.

APPENDIX I. REVIEW OF RISK MINIMIZATION

Routine Risk Minimization

Routine RMMs are used for all products. These measures usually include product information regarding safety, safe usage, and physical presentation of the product.

The types of routine risk minimization measures are:
1. Product Information
   a. Professional label (examples are shown for the European Union and the United States)

Professional Label	European Union	United States
Overall label	Summary of Product Characteristics	Prescribing information*
Patient-focused label	Patient information leaflet	Patient package insert, Medication guide

*May include a boxed warning, a concise summary of critical information for the prescriber, including restrictions on distribution or usage.

   b. Labeling - information that accompanies the product (i.e., on its container/wrapper)
      i. Outer: information on external packaging (e.g., carton)
      ii. Inner: information on package in contact with the product (e.g., vial, blister pack)

Manufacturer and regulatory authority must agree on the wording for product information. This is important because this information (particularly professional label) forms the basis for all other communications about the product.

2. Pharmaceutical form
   a. Size, shape, and color of the product to avoid medication error due to confusion with other medicines or other dosage strengths
   b. Low-dosage formulations
3. Pack size/design
   a. Limiting the quantity of doses in a pack
      i. Increases the frequency of interaction with the patient/caretaker or reduces the risk of overdose/abuse
   b. Restrictive packaging (e.g., childproof containers)
4. Legal (prescription) status
   a. Conditions or restrictions on supply or use of the product, such as controlling the conditions under which the product is prescribed, for example,
      i. specialist prescriber only,
      ii. treatment by physician experienced in the use of anticancer agents,
      iii. hospital use only (e.g., use in a setting where resuscitation equipment is available),
      iv. limiting prescription validity to a certain period (e.g., product must be dispensed within 7 days of prescription being written to ensure monitoring [such as pregnancy test result] is still valid at the time of dispensing),
      v. limit the number of automatic refills/repeat prescription,
      vi. subject to special medical prescription (e.g., due to abuse potential).

Legal status should be communicated in the professional label. Of note, measures to actively encourage or enforce the legal status are regarded as additional risk minimization measures (aRMMs).

Additional Risk Minimization Measures

Most risks can be effectively managed by routine measures, but in some cases, aRMMs may be needed to maintain a positive benefit-risk ratio. Several of these measures can be combined to address the risk minimization objective.

Additional risk measures (tools) can be grouped into two broad categories:
a. Communication/educational
b. Controlled product use

Communication/educational tools are generally used when a heightened awareness of the product, beyond routine product information, may minimize the risk. Messages should be nonpromotional, consistent with the professional label, and tailored to the stakeholder. These measures should utilize a variety of media and should be tested by the targeted users.

Purposes of Communication / Educational Tools
a. enhances understanding (knowledge), *for example,*
   i. patient selection criteria
   ii. complicated administrative procedures
   iii. recognition of signs and symptoms
   iv. treatment management (e.g., dosing, testing, monitoring, follow-up)
b. increases awareness about risk(s) and actions to minimize
c. provides reminders (what to do, what not to do)
d. provides counseling, information that needs to be discussed with the patient/caretakers before prescribing/starting treatment
e. influences/reinforces behaviors
f. informs on the specifics about the risk minimization program itself

Points to consider
a. Digital/Web-based versions should be utilized when possible
   i. download or online viewing
   ii. may provide options to evaluate effectiveness
b. Audiovisual options, such as DVDs, Webcasts, and smartphone applications
   i. video for procedural instructions
c. Interactive formats and computer simulations
d. Printable versions may be needed for certain patient populations or regions
e. Explore integration into Continuing Medical Education
f. Some of the communication/education tools can be linked to controlled product use options (e.g., a training program can be linked to certification [see below on controlled product use tools])
g. Disadvantages are
   i. dependent on health literacy
   ii. variable impact on behaviors
   iii. requires periodic updating (e.g., to align with product information)
   iv. patient versions may not be suitable for all countries
   v. can be burdensome

Examples of Communication / Educational Tools
1. Dear healthcare provider (professional) letter and dear professional society letter
2. Educational guide/brochure
3. Patient counseling guide

4. Patient information card (also referred to as "wallet" or "alert" card)
   a. used to alert other healthcare professionals (HCPs) about risk(s) and risk minimization actions
   b. instructs patients to show it to any HCP
   c. may include contact details of treating physician/center and dates or results of key tests
   d. designed to fit inside a wallet or handbag; electronic version for smartphone
5. Training programs
6. Prescribing guide
7. Checklist/treatment algorithm
8. Dosing guide/calculator
9. Reminder system
   a. Designed to enhance compliance with actions to minimize risk, such as monthly monitoring or testing (e.g., liver function testing or pregnancy testing).
   b. Reminders can be sent to the HCP and/or the patient via various means, such as e-mail, text, phone, or direct mail.
   c. Typically, the system is voluntary and customized to recipient's preferences.
   d. A variation to consider is call centers or integrated voice response systems to provide telephone-based support.
   e. Disadvantages are
      i. financial burden on the company
      ii. Patient privacy restrictions may complicate or restrict implementation

Controlled product use is generally used when limitations on prescribing, dispensing, or accessing a product are needed to ensure safe use of the product beyond routine risk minimization and communication/educational measures.

Purposes of Controlled Product Use
a. limits access to only appropriate patients,
b. limits prescribers and pharmacies that can prescribe and dispense the product,
c. minimizes off-label use.

Examples of Controlled Product Use
1. Attestation/informed consent/agreement
   a. Prescribers, other HCPs, or patients acknowledge (in writing) that they understand and accept the risk and agree to comply with actions to minimize the risk.
   b. Sometimes physician and patient cosign and commit to the minimization actions.
      i. For example, female patients of reproductive potential commit to monthly pregnancy testing.

2. Certification/registration
   a. Prescribers, other HCPs, or pharmacists become certified after they have met certain requirements or register for ongoing activities to gain access to a product.
      i. Certification can be mandatory or voluntary
   b. May involve maintaining a database of registered persons
   c. Examples:
      i. Physicians are certified after completing specialized training.
      ii. Pharmacists register into a restricted dispensing program that involves confirming laboratory test results or verifying counseling before dispensing each prescription.

Disadvantages (for 1 and 2):
a. Burdensome for prescribers/healthcare system
b. May discourage product use; limits product availability and accessibility
c. Unintended consequence of diversion to other treatment options

The controlled product use tool examples:
3. Controlled (restricted) access/distribution
   a. Requirements need to be met before the product is prescribed and/or dispensed, such as
      i. prescriber and/or patient certification (e.g., confirming receipt and understanding of information),
      ii. specific testing/evaluation results
         i. may necessitate using only certified or central laboratories to perform testing,
      iii. follow-up (e.g., inclusion in a data collection system such as a registry).
   b. Supply chain is restricted
      iv. A centralized/specialty pharmacy is used to distribute the product
         i. product can be traced through distribution stages,
         ii. enables verification,
         iii. eliminates wholesalers and large numbers of dispensing pharmacies.

Disadvantages (for 3):
a. Types of restriction allowed or available may vary between countries
   i. For example, access to specialist may be limited in certain areas or healthcare systems
b. May reduce prescribing or result in patient discontinuation
c. Burden on the healthcare system
d. Financial burden on the company

4. Patient monitoring/surveillance
   a. Monitoring could be required before initiating treatment or at specified time points during treatment.
      i. Purpose could be to check for adverse effects and laboratory/monitoring results (e.g., pregnancy test, blood cell counts, liver function tests, ECGs)
   Disadvantages:
   a. burdensome for prescribers/healthcare system,
   b. may require use of central or certified laboratory for testing,
   c. may reduce prescribing or result in patient discontinuation.
5. Registry
   a. A registry of patients who take the product can serve as a risk minimization tool by restricting access to the product; in this case, the registry would need to be mandatory.
   b. Typically, it is a pharmacovigilance activity used to capture additional safety information (on a voluntary basis).
   Challenges:
   a. Legal issues, such as confidentiality and data ownership (which varies between countries)
6. Pregnancy prevention program (PPP)
   a. A PPP is an example of a risk (e.g., known or potential teratogenicity) needing more than one additional risk minimization tool. A PPP groups together a combination of tools such as educational (with counseling), controlled (restricted) access based on pregnancy testing, and a mandatory pregnancy registry.
   Specialized purposes (typically for teratogenic product)
   a. prevents fetal exposure to the product,
   b. excludes pregnancy before and during therapy,
   c. educates and enables appropriate contraceptive use.
   Points to consider:
   a. Teratogenic risk identification—in humans or animal(s)
   b. Disease versus product-related risk (on fetus)
   c. Alternative therapies available
   d. Patient population treated (e.g., female patients with pulmonary arterial hypertension, obesity, or chronic pain)

REFERENCES

1. Bennett JW, Chung KT. Alexander Fleming and the discovery of penicillin. *Adv Appl Microbiol.* 2001;49:163—184.
2. US Food and Drug Administration. *Sulfanilamide Disaster. FDA Consumer Magazine;* June 1981. https://www.fda.gov/aboutfda/whatwedo/history/productregulation/sulfanilamidedisaster/.
3. Kelsey FO. Thalidomide update: regulatory aspects. *Teratology.* 1988;38:221—226.
4. Fintel B, Samaras AT, Carias E. *The Thalidomide Tragedy: Lessons for Drug Safety and Regulation.* Science in Society; July 28, 2009. http://scienceinsociety.northwestern.edu/content/articles/2009/research-digest/thalidomide/title-tba.
5. Franks ME, Macpherson GR, Figg WD. Thalidomide. *Lancet.* 2004;363:1802—1811.
6. Greene JA, Podolsky SH. Reform, regulation, and pharmaceuticals — the Kefauver— Harris Amendments at 50. *NEJM.* 2012;367:1481—1483.
7. Graham DJ, Campen D, Hui R, et al. Risk of acute myocardial infarction and sudden cardiac death in patients treated with cyclo-oxygenase 2 selective and non-selective non-steroidal anti-inflammatory drugs: nested case-control study. *Lancet.* 2005;365:475—481.
8. Karha J, Topol EJ. The sad story of Vioxx, and what we should learn from it. *Clevel Clin J Med.* 2004;71:933—939.
9. Mukherjee D, Nissen SE, Topol EJ. Risk of cardiovascular events associated with selective COX-2 inhibitors. *JAMA.* 2001;286:954—959.
10. Furberg CD, Pitt B. Withdrawal of cerivastatin from the world market. *Curr Control Trials Cardiovasc Med.* 2001;2:205—207.
11. Monahan BP, Ferguson CL, Killeavy ES, Lloyd BK, Troy J, Cantilena Jr LR. Torsades de pointes occurring in association with terfenadine use. *JAMA.* 1990;264:2788—2790.
12. Graham DJ, Green L, Senior JR, Nourjah P. Troglitazone-induced liver failure: a case study. *Am J Med.* 2003;(114):299—306.
13. Eichler HG, Pignatti F, Leufkens H, Breckenridge A. Balancing early market access to new drugs with the need for benefit/risk data: a mounting dilemma. *Nat Rev Drug Discov.* 2008;7:818—826.
14. Zafiropoulos N, Phillips L, Pignatti F, Luria X. Evaluating benefit—risk: an Agency perspective. *Regul Rapp.* 2012;9(6). https://embed.topra.org/sites/default/files/regrapart/1/4347/evaluating_benefit-risk._an_agency_perspective.pdf.
15. US Food and Drug Administration. *Structured Approach to Benefit-Risk Assessment in Drug Regulatory Decision-Making. Draft PDUFA V Implementation Plan. Fiscal Years 2013—2017.* 2013. Available online at: http://www.fda.gov/downloads/ForIndustry/UserFees/PrescriptionDrugUserFee/UCM329758.pdf.
16. EMEA/CHMP/15404/2007. *European Medicines Agency Reflection Paper on Benefit-Risk Assessment Methods in the Context of the Evaluation of Marketing Authorization Applications of Medicinal Products for Human Use.* March 19, 2008.
17. European Medicines Agency. *Benefit-Risk Methodology Project. Work Package 4 Report: Benefit-Risk Tools and Processes.* EMA/297405/2012-Revision 1. May 9, 2012.

18. ICH Final Concept Paper. *M4E(R2): Enhancing the Format and Structure of Benefit-Risk Information in ICH M4E(R1) Guideline*; 2017. http://www.ich.org/fileadmin/Public_Web_Site/ICH_Products/CTD/M4E_R2_Efficacy/M4E_R2__Final_Concept_Paper_27_March_2015.pdf.

19. ICH Harmonised Guideline. *Revision of M4E Guideline on Enhancing the Format and Structure of Benefit-Risk Information in ICH. Efficacy-M4E (R2). Current Step 4 Version*; 2017. http://www.ich.org/fileadmin/Public_Web_Site/ICH_Products/CTD/M4E_R2_Efficacy/M4E_R2__Step_4.pdf.

20. Wolka A, Warner M, Bullok K, Wang J, Radawski C, Noel R. Incorporation of a benefit-risk assessment framework into the clinical overview of marketing authorization applications. *Ther Innov Regul Sci*. 2016;50:130–134.

21. European Medicines Agency (EMA). *Guideline on Good Pharmacovigilance Practices (GVP): Module V — Risk Management Systems (Rev 2)* (EMA 838713/2011 Rev 2); 2017. http://www.ema.europa.eu/docs/en_GB/document_library/Scientific_guideline/2012/06/WC500129134.pdf.

22. Council for International Organizations of Medical Sciences [CIOMS]. *Report of CIOMS Working Group IX: Practical Approaches to Risk Minimisation for Medicinal Products*. Geneva: World Health Organization; 2014.

23. European Medicines Agency (EMA). *Guideline on Good Pharmacovigilance Practices (GVP): Module XVI —Risk Minimization Measures: Selection of Tools and Effectiveness Indicators (Rev 2)* (EMA 204715/2012 Rev 2). 2017. http://www.ema.europa.eu/docs/en_GB/document_library/Scientific_guideline/2017/03/WC500224576.pdf.

24. Food and Drug Administration. *Guidance for Industry. Format and Content of REMS Document. Guidance for Industry. Draft Guidance*; 2017. https://www.fda.gov/downloads/Drugs/Guidances/UCM184128.pdf.

25. Fetterman JE, Pines WL, Mickel WK, Slatko GH. *A Framework for Pharmaceutical Risk Management*. Washington, DC: Food and Law institute Press; 2003.

26. *Federal Food, Drug and Cosmetic Act*. 1938.

27. *World Health Organization*; 2011. http://www.who.int/healthpromotion/conferences/7gchp/track2/en/index.html.

28. Fiss T, Thyrian JR, Fendrich K, Van Den Berg N, Hoffmann W. Cognitive impairment in primary ambulatory health care: pharmacotherapy and the use of potentially inappropriate medicine. *Int J Geriatr Psychiatr*. 2013;28(2):173–181.

29. Wolf MS, Wilson EA, Rapp DN, et al. Literacy and learning in health care. *Pediatrics*. 2009;124(suppl 3):S275–S281.

30. Wolf MS, Gazmararian JA, Baker DW. Health literacy and health risk behaviors among older adults. *Am J Prev Med*. 2007;32(1):19–24.

31. O'Conor R, Wolf MS, Smith SG, et al. Health literacy, cognitive function, proper use, and adherence to inhaled asthma controller medications among older adults with asthma. *Chest*. 2015;147(5):1307–1315.

32. Peters E, Hibbard J, Slovic P, Dieckmann N. Numeracy skill and the communication, comprehension, and use of risk-benefit information. *Health Aff*. 2007;26(3):741–748.

33. Coplan P, Noel R, Levitan B, Ferguson J, Mussen F. Development of a framework for enhancing the transparency, reproducibility and communication of the benefit-risk balance of medicines. *Clin Pharmacol Ther*. 2011;89:312–315.

34. Hallgreen CE, Mt-Isa S, Liefucht A, et al. On behalf of PROTECT Benefit–Risk group. Literature review of visual representation of the results of benefit–risk assessments of medicinal products. *Pharmacoepi Drug Saf*. 2016;25:238–250.

35. IMI-PROTECT Benefit-Risk Group. *Recommendations Report: Recommendations for the Methodology and Visualisation Techniques to be Used in the Assessment of Benefit and Risk of Medicines. IMI-PROTECT Work Package 5*. http://www.imi-protect.eu/documents/HughesetalRecommendationsforthemethodologyandvisualisationtechniquestobeusedintheassessmento.pdf.

36. Mussen F, Salek S, Walker S. A quantitative approach of benefit-risk assessment of medicines. Part 1. The development of a new model using multi-criteria decision analysis. *Pharmacoepidemiol Drug Saf*. 2007;16:S2–S15.

37. Dodgson JS, Spackman M, Pearman A, Phillips LD. *Multi-Criteria Analysis: A Manual*. London: Department for Communities and Local Government; 2009.

38. Guo JJ, Pandey S, Doyle J, Bian B, Lis Y, Raisch DW. A review of quantitative risk-benefit methodologies for assessing drug safety and efficacy: report of the ISPOR risk-benefit management working group. *Value Health*. 2010;2010(13):657–666.

39. European Medicines Agency. *Work Package 2 Report: Applicability of Current Tools and Processes for Regulatory Benefit-risk Assessment, 33*. London; August 31, 2010 (Special topics, Benefit-risk methodology) www.ema.europa.eu.

40. Hoos A, Anderson J, Boutin M, Dewulf L, et al. Partnering with patients in the development and lifecycle of medicines: a call for action. *Ther Innov Regul Sci*. 2015;49:929–939.

41. Anderson M, McCleary KK. Patient Engagement. One the path to a science of patient input. *Sci Transl Med*. 2016;8(336):336ps11. https://doi.org/10.1126/scitranslmed.aaf6730.

42. European Medicines Agency (EMA). *The Role of Patients as Members of the EMA Human Scientific Committees* (EMA/351803/2010); 2017. http://www.ema.europa.eu/docs/en_GB/document_library/Other/2011/12/WC500119614.pdf.

43. European Medicines Agency (EMA). *Patients' and Consumers' Working Party (PCWP)/Healthcare Professionals' Working Party (HCPWP) Topic Groups. Consolidated Report on the Activities of Topic Groups Established in 2015* (EMA/225307/2017); 2017. http://www.ema.europa.eu/docs/en_GB/document_library/Annual_report/2017/05/WC500228518.pdf.

44. Johnson FR, Hauber AB, Zhang J. Quantifying patient preferences to inform benefit-risk evaluations. In: Sashegyi A, Felli J, Noel B, eds. *Benefit-risk Analysis in Pharmaceutical Research and Development*. New York: Chapman & Hall; 2013.

45. Johnson FR, Lancsar E, Marshall D, et al. Constructing experimental designs for discrete-choice experiments: report of the ISPOR Conjoint analysis experimental design good research practices task force. *Value Health*. 2013;16:3–13.

CHAPTER 14

Information Technology in Pharmacovigilance: Current State and Future Directions

SUNDEEP SETHI, MD, MBA • ROBERT HOGAN, PHD

INTRODUCTION TO PHARMACOVIGILANCE INFORMATION TECHNOLOGIES

Information technology (IT)—the use of electronic systems for the capture, storage, and manipulation of data—is a powerful and necessary enabler of all aspects of pharmacovigilance (PV). In the early years of regulated pharmacovigilance, relatively small volumes of data, the nascence of the scientific field, and limitations of early computing led to a predominance of analog, paper-driven processes for drug and device safety data management. The evolution of PVIT has been gradual, focused on incremental improvements in manual PV processes, and serviced by niche technology providers. Today, however, pharmacovigilance requires process automation and control, large dataset management, and complex analytics; as a result, robust PVIT is integral to modern drug and device safety.

The purpose of PVIT is to improve the efficiency and effectiveness of pharmacovigilance and risk minimization for all stakeholders. Patients and healthcare practitioners seek timely and transparent communication of product safety profiles. Health authorities expect robust and reproducible analyses and assurance of regulatory compliance. Biopharmaceutical companies desire improved productivity, insightful analyses, and effective risk minimization. This chapter focuses on the practical use of PVIT by biopharmaceutical companies, under regulations from the major foundational International Council for Harmonisation (ICH) health authorities (US Food and Drug Administration [FDA], European Union European Medicines Agency [EMA], Japan Pharmaceuticals and Medical Devices Agency (PMDA)).

Successful PVIT implementation must address industry-specific challenges. First, systems and data stores need sufficient interoperability to manage the multitude of data sources and integrate with other upstream/downstream PVIT applications. This is needed because manual data manipulation and transfer introduce inefficiencies and opportunities for error and loss of data integrity. Second, PVIT must be appropriately validated for reproducibility to ensure compliance to numerous regulations including those for pharmacovigilance, data privacy, and GxP compliance, which can be costly and time-consuming. Third, PVIT should be flexible and easy to update. Pharmacovigilance requirements and processes rapidly and, at times, significantly evolve, so PVIT must readily adapt. Such changes are catalyzed by a variety of sources, including regulatory (new or updated regulations, health authority commitments), product (specific data or techniques utilized as a product's benefit-risk profile evolves), partners (co-development or co-marketing relationships with other companies), and internal (continuous improvement efforts or other business factors).

Current and emerging technologies offer tremendous opportunities for pharmacovigilance. Large-scale data capture and analysis opens the door to surveillance of exponentially growing information. Enabling technologies, such as robotic automation and cognitive computing, increase process efficiency and

---

General Points to Consider

- Information technology improves efficiency, effectiveness, and regulatory compliance of all PV activities
- Much more important than in the past due to increased data volume, scientific complexity, and regulatory expectations
- Implementation challenges include ensuring interoperability, appropriate technical validation, and flexibility for often-changing requirements

reproducibility. Finally, digital trends in mobility, social media, and Internet connectivity create new patient information pathways.

Taking heed of *Amara's Law* that the effect of technology tends to be overestimated in the short run and underestimated in the long run, this chapter focuses on current and near-term PVIT, yet invites its readers to imagine the long-term possibilities.

PHARMACOVIGILANCE DATA AND DATA FLOW

Much of the day-to-day work of pharmacovigilance revolves around the acquisition, curation, analysis, and interpretation of data regarding patient experiences with medications and medical devices. Therefore, to best understand the use of technologies that support pharmacovigilance, it is helpful to first examine the sources and nature of safety data and explain how it is used.

Safety Data Sources

Fig. 14.1 provides an overview of the safety data ecosystem. Almost all information relevant to patient safety is produced directly or indirectly as a result of an interaction between a healthcare provider (HCP) and patient. This information is available for pharmacovigilance via three major ways: direct reporting, indirect reporting, and through the healthcare system.

Direct Reporting: When an HCP or patient suspects an adverse event (AE) is associated with a therapy, either may directly report such information into the pharmacovigilance system. Such a report, often called "spontaneous reporting," follows international standards and contains a minimum of four data elements (reporter, patient, therapy, and clinical event). The HCP or patient may directly report to a biopharmaceutical company or their health authority (e.g., the FDA MedWatch system). In both scenarios, those recipients

follow specific regulations to process such adverse reactions and record them in a safety database.

Indirect Reporting: Information about AEs is available from sources other than spontaneous reports. HCPs may publish case studies in scientific literature. Clinical research, including registries, also capture and report adverse experiences in association with patient therapy. Patients also create information about AEs when they post a comment on social media or a patient support website. These alternative data sources are surveyed by biopharmaceutical companies and health authorities to varying degrees.

The special case of a "solicited" AEs report is a hybrid of direct and indirect reporting. It occurs when outreach from a biopharmaceutical company that is not intended for safety data collection (e.g., a patient support program) incidentally identifies a potential AE. In such cases, the biopharmaceutical company typically creates an AE report (AER).

Health Care System: When a doctor, nurse, or other provider interacts with a patient, information is captured within the healthcare system, often as a medical record entry, a prescription, or an insurance claim. Statistical analysis of this real-world data (RWD) can derive safety insights. Data aggregators (see Fig. 14.1) are companies and organizations that collect data from multiple hospital systems, insurance companies and pharmacy benefit managers to create very large datasets for such analyses. Aggregate data may be distributed (e.g., FDA's Sentinel system or Patient-Centric Outcomes Research Institute's PCORNet) or be consolidated into a single database by commercial firms or health authorities (e.g., the UK Medicines and Healthcare Products Regulatory Agency's Clinical Practice Research Datalink). Note that even if a safety issue is not identified from healthcare system information, it is still important and utilized in pharmacovigilance to develop comparison background rates of adverse experiences in relevant populations.

Biopharma Safety Data Flows

Fig. 14.2 is a high-level depiction of the major PV value chain elements and associated safety data ecosystem within a biopharmaceutical company.

Adverse Event Report Capture: The acquisition and entry into a database of AEs from all sources, including spontaneous reporting, literature, and clinical trials (see Chapter 4).

Surveillance: Review of safety information from multiple data sources to identify and confirm potential safety signals using standard analytical data reports and visualizations (see Chapter 2).

> **PV Data and Data Flow**
>
> - Most safety data arise from a patient's interaction with an health care provider
> - Safety data can be directly reported, indirectly reported, or aggregated from healthcare system data
> - Biopharmaceutical companies will bring in safety data, evaluate it, and take action to optimize product benefit-risk
> - Throughout the various stages of biopharmaceutical pharmacovigilance, different databases and applications are utilized

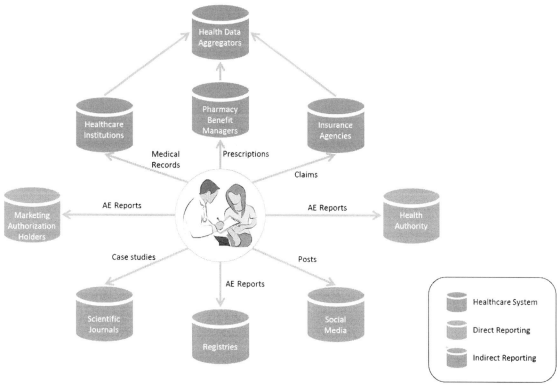

FIG. 14.1 Safety data ecosystem. *AE*, adverse event. (Image: Robert Hogan, Sundeep Sethi. Patient-physician icon licensed from © Can Stock Photo Inc.)

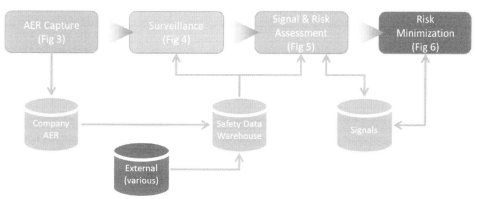

FIG. 14.2 Overview of safety data flows for a biopharmaceutical company. *AER*, adverse event report. (Image: Robert Hogan, Sundeep Sethi)

Signal and Risk Assessment: Comprehensive evaluation of a safety signal using further data sources to assess criticality and causality including measures of patient exposure and background event incidence as well as benefit-risk assessment (see Chapter 2).

Risk Minimization: Actions to minimize a risk including risk communications (such as product labeling and Dear Health Care Provider letters), product approval status changes, HCP training, and distribution restrictions (see Chapter 13).

Major pharmacovigilance data repositories that biopharmaceutical companies maintain include:

Adverse Event Report Database: A transactional database of all AERs for a company's products used to capture, curate, and transmit individual case safety reports (ICSRs) to marketing partners, health authorities, and other designated recipients. Clinical studies likely have independent databases with information from participating subjects including serious and nonserious AEs.

Safety Data Warehouse: An analytical data store containing multiple datasets, including the company's AER data and data imported from other sources in an optimized form suitable for routine surveillance, signal, and risk assessment.

Signal Database: A database containing an audit trail of all signal management activities throughout a product's lifetime, including information used, analyses performed, and decisions made.

PHARMACOVIGILANCE INFORMATION TECHNOLOGIES FOR ADVERSE EVENT REPORT CAPTURE

The basic building block for pharmacovigilance today is an AER. It is a primary (though not exclusive) source of information for much of downstream pharmacovigilance and risk management, and as such, a significant portion of pharmacovigilance human and technological resources are dedicated to AE data management. The objective of AE capture is to take raw safety data from the environment and structure it for analysis. It entails four major steps: intake (acquisition of AE source data), processing (transforming into a structured AER), reporting (transmitting AER to health authorities, partner companies, and internal stakeholders), and archiving (store and enable access/reporting of AER data for surveillance, as well as processing audit trails).

The multiple PVIT associated with AER capture are often collectively referred to as the "AE safety database."

> **Special Considerations for AER Capture**
>
> - Adverse event reports (AER) are the fundamental source of safety data for pharmacovigilance
> - Significant technology emphasis is placed on rapid processing and regulatory submission of AER to comply with health authority regulations
> - International conventions and regulations ensure standardization of AERs worldwide, enabling reproducibility and data sharing

It is often a complex set of interrelated systems and can manage data on multiple products.

Special Considerations for Adverse Event Report Capture

There are specific processing requirements that provide helpful context on the design and use of AER technologies.

Regulatory Reporting: Certain AERs are required by law to be submitted to oversight bodies and stakeholders (e.g., health authorities, clinical trial ethics committees, and investigators, and co-marketing/co-development partner companies) in an expedited fashion. As a result, the processes and systems surrounding AE data management emphasize not only quality but also speed of data management.

International Council for Harmonisation Standards: The ICH guidelines E2A and E2D (https://www.ich.org) define the minimum criteria for a complete AER: identifiable patient, identifiable reporter, a clinical event, and a medicinal product. In addition, the ICH E2B provides a global standard for electronic exchange of AERs. This is the de facto data protocol for AER transmission with health authorities and co-development/co-marketing partners.

Coding Dictionaries: The Medical Dictionary for Regulatory Activities (MedDRA) is the recognized international standard for clinical terms and is used extensively in AER management. Chartered and maintained under ICH, MedDRA is a hierarchical ontology that allows for assigning ("coding") a clinical concept (e.g., symptom, test, procedure, diagnosis) to a specific term. This enables standardization across languages and variable reporting terms in order to support repeatable categorization and analysis. Similarly, WHODrug (chartered under the World Health Organization and maintained by the Uppsala Monitoring Committee) is

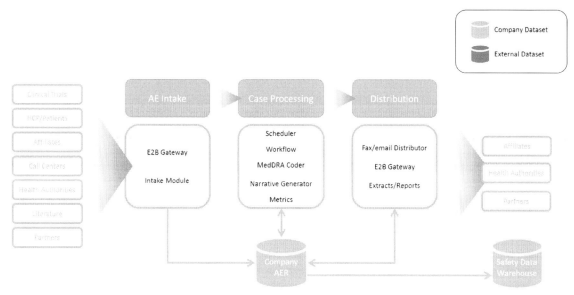

FIG. 14.3 Pharmacovigilance information technologies for adverse event report capture. *AE*, Adverse Event; *E2B*, International Council for Harmonisation Guideline E2B for Transmission of Individual Case Safety Reports; *HCP*, healthcare provider. (Image: Robert Hogan, Sundeep Sethi.)

a broadly recognized hierarchical dictionary for medications.

Current State of Pharmacovigilance Information Technologies for Adverse Event Report Capture

Fig. 14.3 shows the relationship of a modern AE safety database and related applications.

Data sources

Clinical Research: Clinical research captures AEs and serves as a source of safety data for investigational compounds as well as new investigational uses of marketed products. All safety data for a study should reside in the clinical trial database, but a subset of AER, specifically serious AER, may be replicated into the AE safety database to allow for expedited reporting (i.e., 7- or 15-calendar days after awareness) to health authorities, ethics committees, and/or investigators. In such cases, periodic reconciliation is required to assure consistency of the safety data between the two databases.

Postmarket: AEs that are directly or indirectly reported (see Safety Data Sources section) in the approved marketing stage of a product are considered "post-market" reports. AE data may be routinely acquired from other databases internal to a biopharmaceutical company. This includes databases of medical information queries, product quality complaints, and patient support programs. Biopharmaceutical companies must evaluate and transfer AE data from within these databases to the AE safety database.

Co-development/Co-marketing Partners: Biopharmaceutical companies will often collaborate in development and/or marketing of the same product. In such cases, and usually defined in a specific contract, AER will need to be exchanged between companies to support their respective pharmacovigilance efforts and regulatory obligations. Often one partner's AE safety database is defined as the definitive database for all safety information and referred to as the "global safety database" for the product.

PVIT for AER Capture - Current State

- Adverse event report (AER) technology commonly includes a large-scale database and related applications for AER data management
- Unstructured AER data must be processed into a standard report file; structured AER data can be brought in via standard electronic data exchange protocols ("ICH E2B")
- Pharmacovigilance information technologies for AER generally include intake modules, a processing interface, process automators, workflow managers, and distribution tools

Applications

A company's AER technology will include a database and many supportive applications.

Database: The AER safety database should provide terabyte-scale storage for AERs and associated information (as a large biopharmaceutical company may have millions of AERs). Information within an AER can include hundreds of fields with both structured and unstructured data, the former being well organized and defined (and therefore easily searchable) and the latter being variable in format and consistency (and therefore more difficult to search and analyze). In parallel to each AER, which may have multiple historic versions, audit trail and workflow data for the processing history of that AER will be maintained. In addition, the AER record needs to contain (or be linked to a document management system that contains) the source documentation for the AER, such as the initial email from the reporter. At the administration level, database tables define roles and permission levels, control user access, and establish code lists for structured fields.

Intake: AEs may be reported by a variety of means, including unstructured phone and handwritten source documents, semi-structured email and facsimiles, and structured ICH E2B transmissions and local data entry applications. Unstructured and semi-structured data must be manually entered into the AER database. Optical character recognition technologies are useful when large volumes of AEs are received in predictable, machine-readable forms (such as facsimile, PDF, or email forms from other databases). An ICH E2B file meets international standards and so can be transmitted between compliant databases by means of an established transmission gateway. This is rapid, is cost-efficient, and given the electronic handshake between the systems, eliminates the need for manual reconciliation of the transmission. Finally, commercial safety database applications may have an "affiliate" module that allows a call center, local operating company, or vendor to conduct data entry of an AE. If this module is field-mapped to the AER database, it can be seamlessly transmitted into it.

Workflow: AE processing, especially at large volumes, often adopts an assembly line approach. Electronic workflows provide process assurance and monitoring by specifying the steps in production of an AER with associated user groups assignments, such as by geography, product, or skill level (or permutations of all three). Different workflows can be developed for different AE types. As an AER moves through the workflow steps, it is incrementally processed until it emerges as a completed file. Major steps include data entry (input of reported information about the patient, drug, and event), event assessment (determining seriousness, expectedness, causality, and medical terminology coding), and narrative generation (creating a free-text summary of the AER).

A valuable feature of AER workflows is the ability to add alerts and validations to the processing steps. In an alert, if an in-process AER meets certain criteria, then notification can be provided to relevant individuals; an example of this would be a reminder that this specific event requires special follow-up questions to the reporter. A validation is a signal to a human processor that something needs to be done in order to progress the case to the next step (such as completing a missed required field).

Within the transactional database, analytic capabilities are typically kept to operational metrics. Monitoring (such as intake/output volumes, workflow queues, and processor productivity) can be accomplished by business intelligence queries and visualizations or metric reports.

Automation: AER workflows may include applications that automate certain processing steps. Current-state technologies use deterministic automations (i.e., they do not employ any system cognition) that read a specific input field and, based on predetermined rules, populate a fixed value in an output field. Examples of this include the following:

- Autocoding: common verbatim terms are assigned to corresponding MedDRA codes
- Autolabeling: common MedDRA events are assigned a value of "yes" or "no" for presence in product reference safety information
- Autoseriousness: common MedDRA events are assigned to "yes" or "no" for whether they meet AER seriousness criteria
- Autonarrative: a template for the unstructured AER narrative field is partially or fully populated with specific field values from the rest of the AERs.

Such automations can add efficiency but require continued manual maintenance of tables and rules, typically only have simple rule systems, and do not return values if a perfect match is not found.

Distribution: The final step is identification and transmission of reportable AERs to appropriate recipients. Distribution engines can, at the completion of AER processing, identify specific report characteristics and automatically transmit the AERs in appropriate format to the appropriate recipient (e.g., all AERs of a certain product to be emailed to a co-marketing partner). Just as with intake, the ICH E2B protocol enables electronic transmission of completed reports to health authorities and co-marketing/co-development partners.

Other distribution mechanisms include sending to affiliate modules for local operating company review and reporting, and facsimile or email transmissions. Web portals are gaining in popularity for distribution of expedited clinical trial reports to investigators as more rapid, cost-effective, and traceable than traditional email, fax, or physical distribution.

It is not a best practice to conduct analysis directly in the transactional database as the information is dynamic and not optimized for rapid searching or output manipulation. Therefore, another routine distribution method is frequent (i.e., nightly) transfer of AER data from the transactional database where the processing occurs to the safety data warehouse from which surveillance occurs (the latter being optimized for rapid search and analysis).

Emerging Technologies for Adverse Event Report Capture

Given the significant resources allocated to AER capture and processing, the ability of emerging technologies to improve the efficiency and quality of AE capture has the potential to unlock tremendous value that can be reallocated to downstream pharmacovigilance (surveillance, signal assessment, and risk minimization).

Infrastructure hosting

At this writing, many large companies continue to maintain on-premise and individually configured instances of an AE safety database. Doing so, however, results in significant costs and management effort to maintain such systems. Advances in cloud infrastructure and security, along with continued regulatory standardization, are improving feasibility and provider options for hosted AE safety databases, including Software-as-a-service and multitenant models. Such a trend has the potential to not only reduce overall industry costs for AER systems but also facilitate standardization and commoditization of AER management, with fewer, larger networked databases.

Intake

Existing AE intake technologies only address a portion of sources, specifically those that are routine and structured. Natural language processing (NLP) is being developed as a means to facilitate and potentially automate the identification and intake of AE from unstructured sources in order to increase efficiency and consistency of capture.

Two areas of interest as safety data sources are mobile applications and social media. Mobile applications designed for AE reporting have been developed, notably MedWatcher in the United States and WEB-RADR from Europe. Social media is being explored by multiple entities for possible utility in pharmacovigilance. Neither has yet become a primary source of AERs, and further research is needed on both to identify best use cases for safety data capture. Importantly, new surveillance methods may be needed given their differences from traditional pharmacovigilance data sources.

Processing

Several emerging technologies have the potential to significantly increase automation of the AER production process. Robotic process automation can allow programs to conduct many of the simple, rote tasks that human processors are currently conducting, such as transcription and reconciliation. Natural language generation can come to replace the algorithmic templates for current generation autonarrative capabilities, leading to more readable AERs. Finally, cognitive computing holds the promise of replacing the limited deterministic automations, such as those for autocoding and autolabeling, with probabilistic techniques and machine learning.

SURVEILLANCE PROCESS TECHNOLOGY

Marketing authorization holders are required by regulation to conduct periodic reviews of AERs for each product to determine whether there is evidence of an emerging safety issue. That evidence may include new AEs associated with a product or changes in the frequency, duration, severity, or outcome of a known AE. For biopharmaceutical companies with very few AERS, these processes may be performed manually. However, some companies receive thousands of AER monthly (or even daily!). With such high volumes of AERs and increasing expectations from health authorities for more sophisticated analytical approaches to surveillance, many companies seek to automate surveillance to varying degrees. Biopharmaceutical companies and health authorities conduct separate surveillance on medical therapies; an example of the latter is the European Medicines Agency's (EMA) Pharmacovigilance Risk Assessment Committee. Regulations (e.g., EMA Guideline on Good Pharmacovigilance Practices Module X) are accelerating the need for advanced analytical methods and expanding sources of data, causing a trend of increasing use of technology for surveillance.

Current State of Pharmacovigilance Information Technologies for Surveillance

Fig. 14.4 depicts the major activities and data sources in the surveillance process.

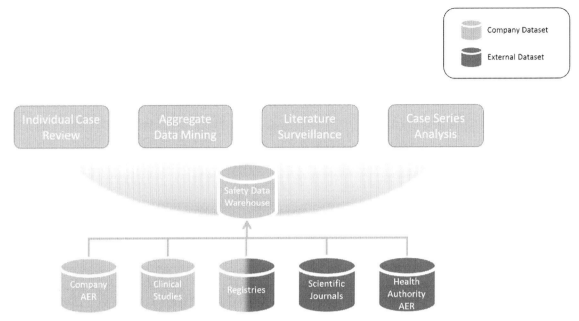

FIG. 14.4 Pharmacovigilance information technologies for surveillance. *AER*, adverse event report. (Image: Robert Hogan, Sundeep Sethi.)

PVIT for Surveillance

- Surveillance technologies support scanning and signal identification across various datasets
- Data warehouses are helpful in managing the various internal and external datasets
- Advanced reporting, visualization, and analytical technologies enable signaling in large and diverse data types

Data sources

The primary data sources for surveillance are generally the company's own AER data (postmarket and clinical) and health authority databases such as the FDA's Adverse Event Reporting System (FAERS) and the EMA's EudraVigilance database. These data sources are on the order of gigabytes and can be easily managed using traditional relational database technology. They can be brought into an analytical safety data warehouse. In addition, the scientific literature must also be screened. Finally, other safety-related datasets (e.g., poison control center data, registry reports) may be evaluated as part of surveillance.

Processes and applications

Each of the subprocesses in Fig. 14.4 uses software applications to automate the process to a greater or lesser degree.

Individual Case Review: Review of individual AERs may identify new associations between medications and events. The workflow component of the AE safety database can be used to route ICSRs to the appropriate medical professionals for assessment (during and/or after AER processing). Different companies have different policies regarding which cases should be reviewed immediately upon receipt based on seriousness, expectedness, occurrence of designated medical events, or other events of interest.

Aggregate Data Mining: This part of surveillance involves conducting statistical analyses and graphical data visualizations to identify patterns and trends in aggregated ICSR data that may predict an adverse reaction. Automated algorithms are used to help identify potential new AEs and changing trends in frequency, duration, severity, or outcome, such as disproportionality statistics including Proportional Reporting Rate and the Empirical Bayesian Geometric Mean (see Chapter 2). Commercial software is readily available that can automatically flag results above a preset threshold level for further review, provide additional reports to evaluate suspected trends, and allow users to drill down to lists of similar cases, even individual case details.

Literature Surveillance: Biopharma companies are required by regulation to conduct periodic reviews of the medical and scientific literature; this can be accomplished through weekly or biweekly searches of multiple literature databases (e.g., Medline, Embase), for which the level of automation may vary. A company with a limited product portfolio may conduct manual searches using online access tools and manual searches. For large portfolios, literature search tools may be employed that store search queries, execute them automatically, present them for review, and track the review and disposition process. It is critical for companies to develop (and maintain) optimal search queries that find important articles and eliminate those that are irrelevant.

Case Series Analysis: This surveillance activity involves in-depth analysis of a group of similar AERs in order to confirm signals. Commercial aggregate data mining tools provide some simple capabilities for case series analysis such as searching, sorting, filtering, and generating simple breakdown statistics for a case series. More sophisticated analysis is often required where cases are annotated with new variables derived from medical review of the case and more sophisticated analyses performed with the derived data. At the time of this writing, there are no commercial products that provide full case series analysis capabilities, so the predominant model is to download and analyze data in spreadsheet applications.

Surveillance Tracking: A biopharmaceutical company must track its surveillance processes and document them in a form that supports internal and health authority audits. Current commercial surveillance tools do not provide automated workflow and tracking tools fit for this purpose. As a result, this is often a manual process with schedules stored in standard business productivity software or simple database. Business process management (BPM) technology is increasingly being configured by companies for this pharmacovigilance purpose, as it not only supports process compliance with controlled and consistent workflows, process alerts and reminders to users, and monitoring reports but can also provide audit trails of surveillance activities.

Emerging Surveillance Pharmacovigilance Information Technologies

The next generation of surveillance technology will be characterized by:

- expanded data sources for aggregate data mining,
- more sophisticated predictive analytical methods,

- integrated software applications with enhanced data visualization and support for the end-to-end surveillance process, and
- validated "signals" databases that capture a comprehensive history of all surveillance, signal evaluation, and benefit-risk assessment activities over the life cycle of a product.

Expanded Data Sources: Review of company internal AE data will remain a cornerstone of surveillance. However, there will be expanded use of health authority data beyond FAERS. EMA regulations (Good Pharmacovigilance Practices Module IX) require surveillance of EudraVigilance data. Although not required, companies can use World Health Organization VigiBase data as well to provide a more globally diverse source of AE data.

One of the limitations of health authority data is the relatively long refresh periods. As the industry and regulatory authorities move toward faster approvals with more sophisticated perilaunch risk management strategies, there will be increasing use of data from electronic health record systems as a means for near real-time surveillance of safety issues.

Sophisticated Predictive Analytics: Although disproportionality scores are useful for prioritizing drug-event combinations for review, they have limitations (see Chapter 2). Most notably, disproportionality scores are only meaningful if the data source is sufficiently diverse to enable calculation of background rates for events. That works well for health authority databases spanning all marketed products but not so well for company databases based on a limited product portfolio that may be dominated by one or two high-volume products. Research is underway to identify new methods that do not depend on background rates. Jokinen et al.,[1] for example, developed a "sieve analysis" algorithm that simulates the approach expert reviewers use to evaluate event frequency trends. They found sieve analysis to be consistent with, and complementary to, disproportionality scores. This kind of research is expected to accelerate using advanced predictive statistics and machine learning algorithms to identify specific cases of interest and patterns of suspicious events in aggregate data. Next generation surveillance systems will need to be flexible enough to support such experimentation and rapidly implement effective analytical methods in production use.

Integrated Surveillance Software: Expanded data sources, more sophisticated analytical methods, increasing regulatory scrutiny, and the limited availability of experienced safety data scientists are some of the factors driving development of the next generation of surveillance software, characterized by:

- seamless integration of application functionality
- end-to-end workflow automation
- plug-and-play data sources
- research sandboxes for new surveillance algorithm development
- graphical visualization of individual cases and aggregate data trends
- NLP/machine learning algorithms for literature and unstructured data surveillance
- full function case series analysis tools.

Several commercial vendors are currently developing cloud-based web applications to fully automate the surveillance process and facilitate compliance with rising regulatory expectations. Many of these systems will use BPM technology as a foundational tool to automate surveillance workflow and tracking. BPM tools will scan online surveillance schedules, generate analyses/reports/graphics in the background, route them to safety analysts for review, and capture assessment results in a signal database to document compliance. The user interface for these surveillance applications will be seamlessly integrated across the business process, enforcing process consistency, and optimizing the productivity of safety analysts.

There is a tremendous opportunity to improve productivity and effectiveness in literature surveillance and evaluation of unstructured (even internal) datasets using NLP and machine learning technology. Today, static searches must be very broad to ensure that nothing important is missed. As a result, human review of large numbers of irrelevant articles or records is required to identify any "needles in the haystack." Advanced technologies can have early value by filtering search results for human reviewers to focus analysis on only the most relevant articles.

Future systems are also expected to provide significant improvements for case series analysis. New technology is not required but application software must be developed that provides the flexibility of a spreadsheet with automated support for case annotation, statistics, and visualization.

Signals Database: Demonstrating compliance with regulations will require maintaining a database of all surveillance activities over the life cycle of a product. The BPM tools used for surveillance tracking can do much of the work by automatically recording surveillance activities as they occur. It will also be necessary, however, to maintain links to the actual data that was used, the analyses that were performed, and documentation of the thought process that went into

determining whether a signal did or did not exist. The signals database will capture this information for surveillance and extend downstream through the signal evaluation, risk and benefit-risk assessment, and risk management to provide a comprehensive safety history for each product.

SIGNAL AND RISK ASSESSMENT TECHNOLOGY

Following signal confirmation, in-depth signal assessment determines whether there is an adverse drug reaction (i.e., causal relationship with therapy) and, if so, the magnitude of the risk to public health. If it is determined that there is a risk, further analysis takes place to determine whether a new adverse drug reaction impacts the overall balance between the benefit and risk of the medication (i.e., benefit-risk assessment [see Chapter 13]).

Surveillance and signal/risk assessment are on a continuous spectrum. Though surveillance involves routine evaluations of a limited data source using standardized analyses, signal/risk assessment, in contrast, involves design of issue-specific analysis strategies, data from multiple sources, and more sophisticated analytical methods. Safety Management Team members collaborate to develop an assessment strategy, acquire the appropriate data, analyze and interpret it, and prepare an assessment report.

PVIT for Signal and Risk Assessment

- Signal and risk assessment often require validation with additional external datasets, including large real-world datasets
- "Big data" challenges arise in these circumstances, including sufficient repository scale, sophisticated analytical methods and applications, and satisfactory system performance

---

Current State of Pharmacovigilance Information Technologies for Signal and Risk Assessment

The technology used for signal and risk assessment (see Fig. 14.5) tends to be an extension of surveillance technology with a few key differences.

Patient Exposure Estimation: The assessment of risk requires the normalization of AE data using estimates of population exposure. Patient exposure estimates often use sales or distribution data as a surrogate of exposure. However, these commercially oriented data may not

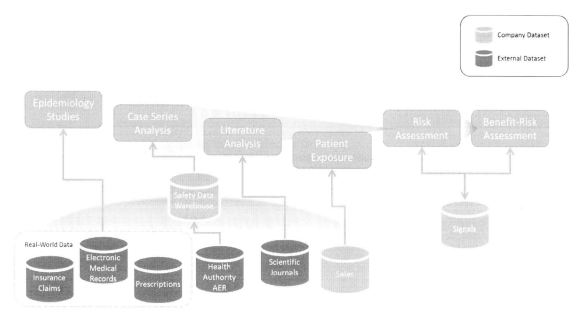

FIG. 14.5 Pharmacovigilance information technologies for signal and risk assessment. *AER*, adverse event report. (Image: Robert Hogan, Sundeep Sethi.)

readily provide the clinical exposure needed, so complex calculations may be required, which can be facilitated and even automated by PVIT.

Real-World Safety Data: One of the goals at this stage is to use additional data sources to assess signals and risk. RWD such as insurance claims, prescriptions, and electronic health records provide alternative ways to answer safety hypotheses. However, pharmacoepidemiologic analysis of these "big data" sources faces several challenges, the most fundamental being data volume (i.e., managing enormous datasets).

At this writing, at least one well-regarded claims database contains ∼3.6 TB of insurance claims data, approximately 1000 times the size of FDA's entire 2017 safety database. Working with terabyte-scale databases is problematic because of the performance limitations of network and hard disk technology. With standard data transfer speeds of networks, it still takes several hours to run a single pass through such a large dataset, and often several passes are needed in pharmacoepidemiologic cohort development. Radically different technology is needed to enable high-speed cohort generation and facilitate sophisticated analyses using real-world evidence as described below.

Benefit/Risk Assessment: Although signal and risk assessment are highly analytical and quantitative, the assessment of benefit-risk is currently more subjective. Frameworks and graphical visualizations of the benefit-risk balance (e.g., forest plots, value trees) provide support for what is fundamentally a medical judgment (see Chapter 13).

Emerging Pharmacovigilance Information Technologies for Signal and Risk Assessment

Technology advancement for signal and risk assessment is anticipated to progress in two dimensions simultaneously:

Integrated Safety Assessment Platform: Most commercial development is focused currently on integrated surveillance systems as described in the Emerging Surveillance Pharmacovigilance Information Technologies section. In the future, the distinction between surveillance and assessment will be blurred and a single integrated safety assessment platform supporting the full-signal life cycle will emerge. Analysts will have direct access to all data sources and a rich set of analytic and visualization tools with which to rapidly explore safety issues. The platform of the future will also provide "sandboxes" for the development and evaluation of new analytical tools. This will be particularly useful for benefit-risk assessment where multiple qualitative and quantitative methods exist, and new ones are being evaluated (see Chapter 2).

High-Performance Safety Real-World Data Analytics: Near-future safety RWD analytics platforms will be characterized by speed, visualizations, and tracking. Massively parallel databases deployed in a cloud will be capable of storing hundreds of terabytes of data. High-speed computing and search tools will need to accelerate pharmacoepidemiologic cohort generation by one to two orders of magnitude to create an environment in which hypotheses can be rapidly explored using RWE. This may be achieved by splitting RWD databases across many servers and executing parallel searches on the database "shards". Open source technologies like Hadoop, and the many tools built upon it, have been developed for this purpose and are used in current RWD analytics platforms. Once the fundamental performance problem is solved, it is relatively straightforward to create a data science analytics environment that integrates access to cohort data, code development with various statistical analysis languages, data visualization, and audit trail.

PHARMACOVIGILANCE INFORMATION TECHNOLOGIES FOR RISK MINIMIZATION

In contrast to the earlier parts of the pharmacovigilance data flow, which focus on *intake* and internal analysis, risk minimization places an emphasis on information *outflow* to patients, HCPs, and other stakeholders. This includes both routine risk minimization (e.g., product labeling) and additional risk minimization measures (e.g., a formal Risk Evaluation and Mitigation Strategy [see Chapter 13]).

Technology Goals for Risk Minimization

The goals for PVIT in support of risk minimization efforts (see also Chapter 13) are to:
- streamline development of risk minimization programs and materials
- ensure robust implementation of risk minimization programs
- enable evaluation of risk minimization program effectiveness.

PVIT for Risk Minimization

- Routine risk minimization does not require specialized pharmacovigilance information technologies (PVIT)
- Additional risk minimization measures rely on data and PVIT for program design, implementation, and evaluation
- Future risk minimization may utilize mobile applications, connected devices, and cognitive computing for improved interventions

---

Beyond routine measures, risk minimization programs vary greatly (e.g., patient/HCP education, additional laboratory monitoring, restricted distribution) and therefore employ a wide variety of supportive technologies specific to the nature of each program. These are often general applications used for PVIT, rather than pharmacovigilance-specialized applications.

Current State of Pharmacovigilance Information Technologies for Routine Risk Minimization

Routine risk minimization measures (typically product labeling, pack size and packaging, and prescription status) are part of standard activities in product approval and ongoing management, so specialized PVIT are not routinely employed. However, the parent activities of product labeling, packaging, and approvals are often managed by cross-functional teams and involve regulatory interactions and submissions, so workflow technologies and document repositories are used for process adherence, communication, and documentation.

Current State of Pharmacovigilance Information Technologies for Additional Risk Minimization

Fig. 14.6 illustrates the data sources and applications frequently used in additional risk minimization program management.

Program Design: Various source data are utilized in risk minimization program creation. Signal assessment data outlines the nature of the product risk. Prescription and/or electronic health record data provide insight into practice patterns and likelihood of the risk. For programs with communication components (e.g., Dear Health Care Provider letters), databases of prescribers can be used to target communications to the most appropriate audience.

Design and materials development for additional risk minimization measures often involve large, cross-functional teams which utilize coordinating technologies for process workflow and document management. Program materials can also be tested for potential effectiveness prior to implementation by software assessment of readability or other relevant human factors.

Program Implementation: Within a biopharmaceutical company, workflow and document repositories are utilized to manage distribution of program information and materials to local operating companies (i.e., affiliates) or partners who implement in their respective territories. These systems can facilitate two-way communication, including negotiation/approval of local program variations.

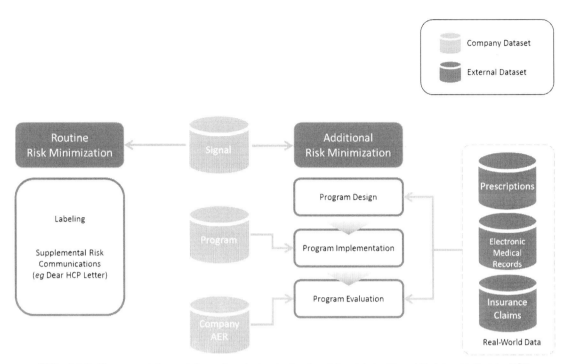

FIG. 14.6 Pharmacovigilance information technologies for risk minimization. *AE*, Adverse Event; *HCP*, healthcare provider. (Image: Robert Hogan, Sundeep Sethi)

For programs with a one-way education component, websites or mobile applications may be used to distribute materials in addition to traditional means, and a database is necessary to record materials distribution. If registration, certification, or attestation is needed from HCPs, pharmacies, or patients, then a system, such as a web-based portal, can be used to facilitate and track these two-way transactions. With highly complex programs that restrict distribution (e.g., to certified providers or pharmacies) and/or require additional monitoring (e.g., negative pregnancy test), sophisticated program-specific systems and databases are established along with channels to various third-parties to exchange and store patient, prescriber, pharmacy, and product information.

Program Evaluation: Evaluation of additional risk minimization programs is divided into process and outcome measures (EMA Good Pharmacovigilance Practices Module XVI). Process measures evaluate the reliability of the program operations. For programs with distribution and enrollment requirements, reports from the implementation systems noted above are critical and should be considered in the design of the database and applications. Some programs require evaluation of comprehension of educational and program materials

and so frequently use electronic surveys. Clinical practice patterns can be evaluated by statistical analytical tools applied to electronic health records, prescription, and claims databases (i.e., utilization studies). Outcome measures evaluate the actual occurrence of AEs and, depending on the nature of the risk, may be assessed from the core safety database (spontaneous AEs).

Emerging Technologies for Risk Minimization

Emerging technologies have the opportunity to improve the options and effectiveness of risk minimization programs. Mobile applications are already being used in some programs but greater penetration, security, and sophistication in mobile applications will increase reach, especially in countries with limited traditional infrastructure, and may enhance learning effectiveness with users. Additionally, the rise of Internet-connected devices and wearables may improve management of risks where patient behavior is a factor and may allow for real-time patient monitoring and early detection of AEs when on therapy. Finally, improved availability and curation of healthcare data sources along with increased use of electronic health records can improve timeliness and confidence in outcome effectiveness measurement (vs. the current approach of lengthy and costly utilization and epidemiologic studies).

ADDITIONAL INFORMATION TECHNOLOGIES FOR PATIENT SAFETY

IT is used in various ways throughout healthcare ecosystems to ensure patient safety. Two significant areas outside of a biopharmaceutical company's purview are the patient care setting and health authorities.

Pharmacovigilance Information Technologies in the Patient Care Setting

A considerable focus of patient safety in the care delivery setting is the avoidance of medication errors. Clinical decision support systems may be utilized by hospitals and pharmacies; on electronic order entry, such systems can advise users of potential drug allergies, drug-drug interactions, and dosing parameters. At the point of delivery, both drug and patient identification can be scanned to ensure the correct product is being administered to the correct patient.

Pharmacovigilance Information Technologies and Health Authorities

Health authorities carry the mandate to ensure the safety and well-being of their citizens. This not only entails establishing and enforcing regulations on biopharmaceutical developers, manufacturers, and marketers but also involves conducting their own pharmacovigilance and risk minimization efforts. To that end, they use similar technologies previously described in this chapter to directly capture AEs, analyze safety data, and assess and manage risk.

Health authorities are also in unique positions to sponsor large-scale technology initiatives. One example is the WEB-RADR project, funded by the European Union's public-private partnership for health research, the Innovative Medicines Initiative. The project "seeks to utilise the powers of social media and new technologies for pharmacovigilance purposes" including development of a mobile application for AER capture and tools for mining social media data (https://web-radr.eu). Another example is the FDA's Sentinel Initiative. Designed to complement their traditional AER program, Sentinel enables the FDA to "rapidly and securely access information from large amounts of electronic health care data, such as electronic health records (EHR), insurance claims data and registries, from a diverse group of data partners" (https://www.fda.gov/Safety/FDAsSentinelInitiative).

CONCLUSION

Sophisticated technology applications are a de facto requirement for a modern pharmacovigilance system, from the databases and processing workflows that capture essential safety data to the analytical and reporting tools that enable scientists to elucidate a product's clinical risk profile. A wide range of commercial and in-house tools are currently in use by pharmacovigilance units of biopharmaceutical companies and health authorities, with more developed each year.

The evolution of biopharmaceutical product safety surveillance capabilities from the low volume, highly subjective practice of years past to the high volume, systematic science of today is intrinsically tied to the advancement of the ITs that support it. This pattern will undoubtedly continue. Stakeholders—patients, HCPs, health authorities, and biopharmaceutical manufacturers—will develop more complex clinical treatments, create higher standards of information transparency and public health protection, and demand greater efficiency in healthcare systems. As a result, the expectations of pharmacovigilance insight and risk management will correspondingly increase, and it will be the newer, emerging technologies—novel data sources, improved computing capabilities, process enabling applications, and human networks—that will provide the solutions.

APPENDIX I: GENERAL PV TECHNOLOGY FRAMEWORK

Table 14.1 below provides a framework of the categories and specific types of technologies utilized in pharmacovigilance.

Patient Safety IT Outside Biopharma

- While this chapter focused on pharmacovigilance information technologies from the perspective of a biopharmaceutical company, there are other important players
- Healthcare systems can use technologies at point-of-care to minimize medication errors
- Heath authorities also conduct surveillance and are actively exploring new data models and technologies to support pharmacovigilance and the public health

TABLE 14.1
Technologies with current or potential utility in pharmacovigilance

Category	Technology	Description
Enabling software	Databases	Data stores that house multiple types of structured and unstructured data for transactional (curation), analytic (manipulation), and archival (recording) purposes. Can be linked and aggregated into larger data stores (e.g., "data warehouses" and "data lakes")
	Workflows	Software that manages work through different preset steps in a process, potentially for different users at each stage. Used for assurance of process compliance and also records activities for audit and reporting purposes
	Robotic process automation	Rules-based tools that mirror rote human tasks, such as transcribing (copying) or transforming (looking up value) data within/between systems
	Reporting	Output tools that pull data from systems and databases into structured forms for end-user consumption. Includes visualization tools with graphic displays/outputs
Hardware and infrastructure	Distributed computing	Networks of physical or virtual computers operating in parallel to enhance the speed of large computational tasks
	Hosting/cloud computing	Applications and data stores that are managed centrally, typically by third-parties and in large data centers, and are accessible via the Internet without the need for local copies
	Mobile applications	Applications designed for networked personal devices such as smart phones and tablets
	Internet of things	General term for Internet (Bluetooth, WiFi, cellular) connectivity by devices other than computers; connections can send and/or receive data
	Augmented/virtual reality	Digitally driven sensory experiences that either merge (augmented) or replace (virtual) a person's environment
Artificial intelligence	Natural language processing	Semantic technologies that can accurately assess content of complex human speech or text as an instruction or data
	Natural language generation	Semantic technologies that can output data as syntactically correct complex speech or text
	Predictive analytics	Statistical techniques that evaluate data in order to detect trends and patterns
	Machine learning	Facilitated or automated method of improving system accuracy via feedback on accuracy of prior outputs
Human networks	Crowdsourcing	Harnessing the capabilities of large groups to solve complex problems by breaking them down into smaller fragments, distributing for evaluation, and aggregating results
	Social media	Any of a number of information platforms that allow users to rapidly and easily transmit (one-way) or exchange (multiway) user-generated content
	Patient portals	Websites where patients contribute their experiences directly to data repositories with intent of user sharing

REFERENCE

1. Jokinen JD, Lievano F, Scarazzini L, Truffa M. An Alternative to Disproportionality: A Frequency-Based Method for Pharmacovigilance Data Mining. *Therapeutic Innovation & Regulatory Science.* 2017;52(3).

CHAPTER 15

The Future of Safety Science

MONDIRA BHATTACHARYA, MD • LINDA SCARAZZINI, MD • FABIO LIEVANO, MD • SUNDEEP SETHI, MD, MBA

BACKGROUND

As drug development evolves with the latest approaches in technology, data analytics, and patient engagement, so does safety science. In the most general sense, safety science is "knowledge about safety related issues and the development of concepts, theories, principles, and methods to understand, assess, communicate, and manage (in a broad sense) safety."[1] To succeed in this rapidly evolving era of safety science, pharmaceutical companies and regulatory authorities need to use integrated approaches, timely evaluation of data, and detailed analysis of safety signals. The three building blocks for the future of safety science, cognitive and behavioral systems, medical assessment, and data sciences (see Fig. 15.1) complement each other in quantitative and qualitative approaches.

Novel quantitative approaches to data and the expertise to transform information into insights will drive the value of safety science organizations. Quantitative departments, such as epidemiology and safety statistics, will analyze big data to identify target patient populations most likely to benefit from new therapies and those whose risk is decreased. Cognitive and behavioral expertise will yield patient-centric guidance allowing patients to make informed decisions regarding medications. Medical assessment applied continuously throughout a product life cycle, accomplished through creation of safety assessment committees, will emphasize life-cycle safety monitoring. Organizational design and processes implemented with these building blocks, and their intersections, in mind will yield a life-cycle approach to benefit-risk assessment that will significantly impact public health (Box 15.1).

> **BOX 15.1**
> **Future Safety Science Practice**
>
> • Integrated strategies and processes across multiple scientific disciplines (medical, pharmacologic, statistics, behavioral health, information technology) will be required for successful deployment of safety science capabilities.

Before these approaches can be implemented, safety science departments at pharmaceutical companies and regulatory agencies must overcome certain limitations. First, safety science departments traditionally suffer from a disjointed structure, making collaboration across groups and functions difficult. Second, safety science operations were transactional and process focused, which led to data generation, yet failed to provide elucidation of findings. Finally, safety science was constrained by the available technology and lack of resources.

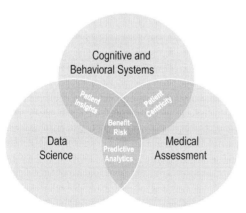

FIG. 15.1 Intelligent pharmacovigilance.

The future of safety science is monitoring risk throughout the drug development cycle to inform benefit-risk management. An intelligently resourced and high-functioning safety science organization not only enables risk management but also prescribes guidance, continuous safety monitoring, and identification of target patient populations, such that benefit-risk for a product is optimized.[2–5] The following sections explore the three building blocks of safety science in the context of optimizing benefit-risk profiles and risk management.

COGNITIVE AND BEHAVIORAL SYSTEMS

Cognitive and behavioral systems describe a field of study dedicated to the communication, comprehension, adherence, and performance of the actions needed to optimize patient outcomes. Cognitive behavioral sciences are an increasingly important contributor to pharmacovigilance (PV). Although PV scientists endeavor to understand, generate, detect, and/or validate signals, cognitive behavioral science examines this same information through a different lens. Their expertise is focused on the determination of the root cause of patient safety issues and is applied through approaches such as Human Factors Engineering and user-centered design. These issues then can be addressed through systemic changes—design changes in the product, care delivery, or intervention. The combination of cognitive behavioral science and pharmacovigilance results in a cognitive and behavioral system with the goal of continuous learning resulting in incremental improvements in patient safety outcomes.

Since 2011, updated regulations and guidance from global health authorities required makers of new products to provide information on how patients and healthcare providers interact with these products in the real world.[6–12] In an effort to improve patient outcomes and reduce the harm caused by medication errors, application of human-factors engineering, i.e., usability engineering or user-centered design, has been encouraged.

The expanding scope of cognitive behavioral work will initially focus on those areas that are most likely to benefit. Telemedicine, medical devices, mobile applications, text message reminders, remote nurse follow-up, and medication guides, for example, are approaches in healthcare that would benefit from user-centered design and development.[13,14] Regulators want sponsors to identify tools that are useful in real-world practice and support by evidence generated from human factors and health literacy research that impact prescribing behavior and the safe use of drugs on market[14] (Box 15.2).

> **BOX 15.2**
> **Importance of Cognitive Behavioral Science in Pharmacovigilance**
>
> - Cognitive behavioral science principles are increasingly important in pharmacovigilance activities
> - The discipline's expertise is critical to understanding of patient safety issues, design of products and packaging, and in transparent communication of risks and benefits to patients.

Patient Centricity: Cognitive and Behavioral Systems and Medical Assessment

A cognitive behavioral approach shifts patient engagement from a best practice to an expected standard and creates an integrated model focusing on producing usable tools that facilitate patients' and providers' understanding of risks, benefits, and required actions for safe and effective product use.[3–5,15] Through questionnaire design and development (e.g., patient reported outcomes), patient advocacy group interactions, and patient-centered data sources, safety science is positioned to advance the patient perspective throughout the entire product development life cycle. The use of terms like patient engagement and patient centeredness are now ubiquitous throughout healthcare and increased focus on the patient's experience is driving patient-centered guidance for benefit-risk and the safe use of new drugs.[16,17]

MEDICAL ASSESSMENT

Drug discovery medical assessment teams bring together the study of toxicity and toxicogenomics, biomarkers, and special populations to personalize the benefit-risk profile. To achieve this end, however, safety assessment must occur simultaneously with the assessment of product efficacy to ensure the benefit-risk profile is considered throughout drug development. In recent years, medical assessment teams have expanded to include personnel with substantive clinical expertise, as well as leadership skills (e.g., communication and decision-making). As medical assessment teams get involved earlier in the drug discovery process, they can provide unique perspectives and interpretation of potential adverse events (AEs) in the clinic.

Predictive Analytics: Medical Assessment and Data Science

Medical assessment applied in drug discovery has the potential to identify and predict AEs and toxicities throughout the drug development pipeline; in *silico* modeling provides insights into AEs like QT prolongation or hepatotoxicity.[18,19] Identifying toxicities of potential drug candidates in the development pipeline is beneficial for understanding which toxicities are tolerable relative to potential benefit and how those toxicities may change with changing dose and treatment regimens.[20] Drug development teams collaborating with medical safety should be empowered to predict, diagnose, and manage these toxicities.[21] Efficient and validated models in other lower animal species, such as zebrafish, have the potential to replace mammalian prescreening experiments to detect AEs not detected in in vitro experiments.[22] Toxicogenomics will use genomic technology to predict, identify, and extrapolate pathways leading to drug toxicity.[23,24] Medical assessment teams will be able to drive the early identification of drugs with a positive or negative benefit-risk profile.

Additionally, the combination of medical assessment and data science contributes to biomarker research to aid determinations of benefit-risk. The safety profile of each drug product may have a biomarker profile unique to a subset or cluster of patients, as some patients may be more prone to certain events than others, based on genetic predisposition, and future products may be individualized.[25,26] Biomarkers are currently limited by a lack of specificity and limited sensitivity in determining disease state, difficulty in correlating disease development with new markers, and intensive qualification required to validate clinical biomarkers.[25,26] Despite these current limitations, the potential is tremendous. For example, injury response biomarkers may be developed that help diagnose toxicity and have the specificity to distinguish injury from benign events.[24] These new biomarkers can grade progressive injury and fibrosis to determine if the injury can be reversed and to detect the injury earlier.[27] Biomarkers may be used to classify subpopulations of patients into groups that are more prone to certain drug-drug interactions (DDIs) and predict DDIs in others (Box 15.3).

BOX 15.3
Integrated Data Usage for Product Characterization

- The integration of scientific data from multiple sources (clinical, toxicology, biomarkers, genomics, etc.) to support sound decision-making and product characterization relies on team-based medical assessments.

One of the most interesting outcomes of "big data" efforts is the impact on individuals and small groups.

Medical assessment science will contribute to drug development through the design of studies for special populations, including the elderly or children, or individuals unable to take certain drugs due to a history of AEs or drug ineffectiveness. Studies of various forms (e.g., observational studies, registries, and pragmatic clinical trials) may be co-developed with clinical research personnel early in the product life cycle for special populations, providing early identification and prevention of potential DDIs.[28] In fact, as modeling becomes more predictive, the need for certain clinical trials will be obviated (Box 15.4).

BOX 15.4
Life-cycle Real World Data Analysis for Benefit-Risk Assessments

- Traditional scientific data emerging from clinical development programs will be supplemented by real world data using electronic datasets, registries, etc. early in product life cycle to identify benefit-risk profiles in subpopulations historically excluded from clinical trials.

A key competency of data science is database integration. Surveillance in the future requires the seamless integration of data from spontaneous report databases, health records, and social media. Data sources will be integrated and analysis-ready, enabling predictive analytics and providing real-time monitoring.[29] Safety alerts may then be generated from monitoring postmarket situations, as well as blinded and unblinded reviews of clinical trial data. The Sentinel Initiative at the Food and Drug Administration is intended to achieve this goal—compiling multiple data sources into a single interface that enables proactive safety monitoring.[30] Additionally, pharmacogenomics with genome-wide association searches can help to predict the predisposition of adverse drug reactions from multiethnic populations.[31]

DATA SCIENCE

Data science in a safety organization encompasses statistical expertise and computer hardware and software designed to address the rapidly changing requirements for evidence generation. Software advancements for medical analytics allow for easy access, analysis, and visualization of safety trends in clinical trials, epidemiological studies, postmarketing events, and publications.[29,32] Future software tools will connect with different structured and unstructured databases and allow simple visualization of outputs from complex statistical modeling or simulation routines. Safety experts will be able to document all scientific work in this single application, simplifying the process for reporting to regulatory officials and developing a safety profile for each product specific to patient populations or global regions.[33]

High-performance computing will enable analytic approaches to electronic health records (EHRs), claims, and spontaneous report data to identify potential safety issues.[34,35] Clinical development safety monitoring will include earlier and more-frequent examination of safety data from products in development.[29] In addition, there will be an evolution of algorithms for improved signal detection and medical and scientific review of potential safety issues in newly created databases. Machine learning will be employed to refine algorithms to increase sensitivity and specificity of data-mining methods. With these advances in data access and analysis, clinical trial safety assessment committees will review unblinded data with prespecified analyses on a periodic basis, providing quicker feedback to ensure rapid detection of potential safety signals[36] (Box 15.5).

BOX 15.5
Role of Data Science in Pharmacovigilance

- Data science within safety will allow for
  - Better and faster evidence generation
  - Employment of varied data sources such as EHRs, spontaneous and clinical trial data, patient preference, quality-of-life measures
  - Integration of data from disparate sources to create patient insights
  - Employ scientists from many disciplines including biostatistics and epidemiology

---

Computing power and advanced software do not replace the need for data science expertise. Most databases, such as EHR databases, are not constructed for the purpose of conducting research. Additionally, idiosyncrasies of each database, such as geographic distributions, patient populations contained therein, under- or overrepresentation of disease states require data scientists. Their knowledge is requisite to accessing and transforming data and insuring appropriate questions are posed to appropriate data.

Patient Insights: Data Science and Cognitive and Behavioral Science

An integrated safety data science and statistics organization will evolve from more traditional biostatistics and epidemiology departments to a field incorporating statistical techniques more common in psychometrics, marketing analytics, and forecasting.[29] This transition will facilitate a move from reactive, safety analytics to predictive modeling designed to generate insights regarding a patient's care or disease state to refine the benefit-risk profile of products. For example, patient preferences gleaned from quality of life or other psychometric instruments may serve as inputs to statistical models comparing drug candidates or dose levels of the same drug candidate. In the same manner that consumer goods manufacturers select new products for the market, new drug candidates may be selected that maximize patient's preferences for outcomes or potential adverse effects. Patient insights enable regulators and the industry to focus development and postmarketing pharmacovigilance surveillance on safety issues of most concern to the patient.[37] Safety statistics organizations, including industry and regulatory agencies, will require diverse expertise in data and cognitive and behavioral science to gather patient perspectives, leverage atypical real-world data sources, and bring correct data and analysis to safety scientists and physicians.[38]

Special populations have unique issues to consider when physicians develop treatment plans and make prescribing decisions. Patient registries designed to collect data from special populations are likely to become more common and easier to access, creating a resource to which physicians may refer. Pregnant women have their responses and AEs related to different drugs tracked in registries.[39] In elderly populations, because of the concern about polypharmacy, EHR data help track outcomes and DDIs.[40] Another special population is children, who pose a unique challenge to physicians and caretakers due to their limited ability to express symptoms of adverse reactions to drugs and vaccines. To counter this concern, the Center for Disease Control and Prevention has implemented the Vaccine Safety Datalink initiative to track reactions to vaccines.[41] In the future, patient registries will need to be transparent, cost-effective, and designed in plain language to be health-literacy friendly, with increased patient access.[42] Also, patient registries will evolve to contain all medical records so that physicians are fully informed of other prescriptions and potential DDIs.[34] The ultimate goal of efforts to synthesize disparate sources of data is to make all available data readily accessible to physicians, patients, and payers across the healthcare ecosystem.

A recent study by the Massachusetts Institute of Technology and SAS Institute, Inc. demonstrates that while the amount of data available is rapidly increasing, the ability to generate insights from the data is decreasing.[43] The major causes are an organization's inability to integrate disparate sources of data and the lack of appropriate analytical skills.[43] Safety statistics is central to the organization with cooperation from safety science and other quantitative departments. The result of this collaboration will be earlier and better characterization of benefit-risk profiles.

Epidemiology is becoming essential for all phases of clinical trials. Epidemiology estimates disease background rates and describes patient burden and unmet patient needs, which identifies target population preapproval. Epidemiological research provides input to clinical growth, such as identifying or developing patient-reported outcome tools. Early in drug development, the process of building epidemiologic real-world data capabilities begins by establishing collaborative networks, leveraging existing data, or expanding strategies for data collection through registries. The outcomes of this early development work are disease state and comorbidity insights, and postmarketing patterns of already approved treatments, which provide the foundation for later-phase studies (e.g., cost-effectiveness and comparative effectiveness). Additionally, epidemiologists can contribute to creation of different data sources that encompass the full spectrum of healthcare from patient to payer to healthcare professional.[38] Three types of databases are useful for epidemiology and the future of safety science: disease specific, innovative platforms (social media), and treatment type combined with patient molecular profiles.[44] These databases will provide the platform for more detailed information and population-level medical needs (Box 15.6).

BOX 15.6
Role of Epidemiology in Pharmacovigilance

- Epidemiologic research supports all stages of clinical development. In early development, it contributes to disease characterization. Later more extensive research allows for linkage of data sources including those with patient molecular profiles allowing for recreation of personalized medicine paradigms in real-world datasets.

Epidemiology groups have traditionally defined the disease state (i.e., background rates of events in the population) based on published data on historical control arms of clinical trials. A similar methodology is now evolving where control subjects from multiple trials are being aggregated to serve as a synthetic control for small phases 1 and 2 clinical trials, after matching for baseline covariates to the trial participants. This approach allows for assessment of key outcomes for investigational therapies where either due to ethical issues or scarcity of available trial participants, trials are conducted in an uncontrolled fashion.

The importance of incorporating high-quality data into assessment of a drug's effectiveness and safety is even more relevant today due to the use of accelerated pathways in the US (fast track, break-through designation, etc.) and Europe (Priority Medicine initiative) to gain marketing authorization for diseases in which there is a high unmet medical need (frequently oncology and infectious diseases). These programs are often very small, use open-label design, lack comparator arms, and are conducted in patients with advanced disease where patient comorbidities further confound safety assessments.[45] These postmarketing requirements that are becoming standard at the time of approval will need to be conducted expeditiously to communicate effectively the evolving benefit-risk profile of these critically needed therapies (Box 15.7).

BOX 15.7
Changes in Regulatory Science Driving Greater Evidence Generation after Approval

- New regulatory pathways that allow for accelerated approval require the generation of new evidence after approval.

BENEFIT RISK: BRINGING IT ALL TOGETHER

Fig. 15.1, intelligent pharmacovigilance, is not a process map or a flow chart. Rather, it depicts the overlapping and interacting disciplines required to drive safety science forward. Effective collaborations among these pharmaceutical industry departments propel companies away from the historic and all-to-common approach where one department (or group of departments) is responsible for efficacy and a separate portion of the organization responsible for collecting evidence pertinent to the safety. Those of us who have participated in drug development for many years also realize that these departments are not only physically separate but they also seem to exist in different time epochs. The present-day drug development process is dominated by the generation of evidence required to establish efficacy sufficient to receive regulatory approval. Postapproval is when safety science takes shape and plays a prominent role. Efficacy, however, has largely been established by the time the drug is marketed so the responsible departments move resources to other projects and are partners with safety only in a perfunctory sense. This approach is satisfactory when the pharmaceutical company's view regulatory authorities as their primary audience and safety science as an activity that scrutinizes data sources to identify new safety concerns.

Alternatively, if the goal is to develop a drug-life-cycle approach to benefit-risk; an approach which results in critical information for not only regulatory authorities but also for patients, payers, and providers; an approach which continually assesses evidence to identify both efficacious and safe use; an approach which combines medical, data, and cognitive and behavioral science disciplines, then a fully integrated organization and process is required. We started this article by offering a definition of safety science. But safety science is, in the words of Hollnagel, an umbrella term for many disciplines.[46] In this paper, we discuss three building blocks and their overlapping segments, but even within the building blocks, there are certainly multiple disciplines that come together to insure a drug's benefits and risks are appropriately considered for the intended patient population. In an integrated approach to benefit risk, the intended patient population also has a voice in the process, contributing critical data through patient reported outcomes, for example. When safety sciences shifts our mind-set from one of reacting to AEs and signals of disproportionate reporting to an organizational mentality dedicated to the identification of the right drug for the right patient at the right time, the value of these building blocks will be fully realized.

Patients, payers, and providers of healthcare are demanding for more transparency and guidance regarding the safe use of medicinal products. In an era when virtually any information can be found on the web, the paucity of information available to allow stakeholders to weigh benefits and risks for themselves is disappointing. The stakeholders in the best position to provide this information are pharmaceutical companies. To do this—to truly respond to the demands of the changing market—pharmaceutical companies need to realize that the primary audience for information is no longer regulatory authorities (Box 15.8). Then, companies additionally need to realize that this isn't an exercise with a defined start and stop conducted within segregated departments. As new evidence emerges through literature, clinical studies, real-world evidence, and spontaneous report data, the evidence is weighed by experts from these disparate disciplines and benefit-risk determinations reevaluated as appropriate. Additionally, this evidence is made available to

---

BOX 15.8
Life-cycle Benefit-Risk Assessments Linked to Evolving Prescriber and Patient Knowledge

- The safety science discipline requires a commitment by pharmaceutical companies to always reevaluate the benefit-risk profile of their products, focused not only on regulators but also more significantly on prescribers and patients to provide them with the best evidence for decision-making in the era of personalized medicine.

---

all stakeholders, as soon as practical, allowing them to think through uncertainties and to make the right choices for the patients. This is only achievable through a fully integrated organization receptive to insights from patients and whose patient-centric values compel the organization to act upon these insights throughout the life cycle of pharmaceutical development.

CONCLUSION

The future of safety science is happening now. Advances in cognitive behavioral systems, medical assessment, and data science are modernizing the benefit-risk paradigm and will continue to do so as each approach is incorporated into the larger PV structure and processes. Assessing evidence that impacts the benefit-risk profile of a product as it is developed and delivered into the population informs drug development and, ultimately, improves patient outcomes.

REFERENCES

1. Aven T. What is safety science? *Saf Sci.* 2014;67:15−20.
2. Pronovost PJ, Holzmueller CG, Molello NE, et al. The Armstrong Institute: an academic institute for patient safety and quality improvement, research, training, and practice. *Acad Med.* 2015;90(10):1331−1339.
3. Pleasant A, Rudd RE, O'Leary C, et al. *Considerations for a New Definition of Health Literacy.* National Academy of Medicine; 2016.
4. National Patient Safety Foundation. *Free from Harm: Accelerating Patient Safety Improvement Fifteen Years after To Err Is Human.* Boston, MA: National Patient Safety Foundation; 2015.
5. Pronovost PJ, Ravitz AD, Stoll RA, Kennedy SB. *Transforming Patient Safety: A Sector-Wide Systems Approach.* Report of the WISH Patient Safety Forum. 2015.
6. Food and Drug Administration, Center for Drug Evaluation and Research. *Safety Considerations for Container Labels and Carton Labeling Design to Minimize Medication Errors Draft Guidance.* Silver Spring, Maryland: Food and Drug Administration; 2013.

7. Food and Drug Administration, Center for Drug Evaluation and Research, Center for Biologics Evaluation and
Research, Center for Veterinary Medicine. *Brief Summary
and Adequate Directions for Use: Disclosing Risk Information
in Consumer-Directed Print Advertisements and Promotional
Labeling for Prescription Drugs*. Maryland: FDA; 2015.

8. Health Canada Health Products and Food Branch. *Questions and Answers: Plain Language Labelling Regulations*. Canada: Minister of Public Works and Government Services;
2015.

9. European Medicines Agency Pharmacovigilance Risk
Assessment Committee. *Good Practice Guide on Risk Minimisation and Prevention of Medication Errors*. European Medicines Agency; 2015.

10. Food and Drug Administration Center for Devices and
Radiological Health. *Design Considerations for Devices
Intended for Home Use*. Maryland: FDA; 2014.

11. Food and Drug Administration Center for Devices and
Radiological Health. *Applying Human Factors and Usability
Engineering to Medical Devices*. Maryland: FDA; 2016.

12. Food and Drug Administration Center for Drug Evaluation
Research. *Safety Considerations for Product Design to Mini-
mize Medication Errors Guidance for Industry*. Maryland:
FDA; 2016.

13. Wolf MS, King J, Wilson EA, et al. Usability of FDA-
approved medication guides. *J Gen Intern Med*. 2012;
27(12):1714–1720.

14. Bailey SC, Navaratnam P, Black H, Russell AL, Wolf MS.
Advancing best practices for prescription drug labeling.
Ann Pharmacother. 2015;49(11):1222–1236.

15. Rosen MA, Goeschel CA, Che XX, et al. Simulation in the
executive suite: lessons learned for building patient safety
leadership. *Simul Healthc*. 2015;10(6):372–377.

16. Stegemann S, Ternik RL, Onder G, Khan MA, van Riet-
Nales DA. Defining patient centric pharmaceutical drug
product design. *AAPS J*. 2016:1–9.

17. Parker RM, Wolf MS. Health literate equates to patient-
centered. *J Health Commun*. 2015;20(12):1367–1368.

18. Davies MR, Wang K, Mirams GR, et al. Recent develop-
ments in using mechanistic cardiac modelling for drug
safety evaluation. *Drug Discov Today*. 2016;21(6):
924–938.

19. Raunio H. In silico toxicology - non-testing methods. *Front
Pharmacol*. 2011;2:33.

20. Relling MV, Dervieux T. Pharmacogenetics and cancer
therapy. *Nat Rev Cancer*. 2001;1(2):99–108.

21. Weng L, Zhang L, Peng Y, Huang RS. Pharmacogenetics
and pharmacogenomics: a bridge to individualized cancer
therapy. *Pharmacogenomics*. 2013;14(3):315–324.

22. Barriuso J, Nagaraju R, Hurlstone A. Zebrafish: a new companion for translational research in oncology. *Clin Cancer
Res*. 2015;21(5):969–975.

23. Foster WR, Chen SJ, He A, et al. A retrospective analysis of
toxicogenomics in the safety assessment of drug
candidates. *Toxicol Pathol*. 2007;35(5):621–635.

24. Qin C, Tanis KQ, Podtelezhnikov AA, Glaab WE,
Sistare FD, DeGeorge JJ. Toxicogenomics in drug develop-
ment: a match made in heaven? *Expert Opin Drug Metab
Toxicol*. 2016;12(8):847–849.

25. Olson S, Robinson S, Griffin R. *Accelerating the Development
of Biomarkers for Drug Safety: Workshop Summary*. Washington, DC: National Academic Press; 2009. p. 100.

26. Harrill AH, Ross PK, Gatti DM, Threadgill DW, Rusyn I.
Population-based discovery of toxicogenomics biomarkers
for hepatotoxicity using a laboratory strain diversity panel.
Toxicol Sci. 2009;110(1):235–243.

27. Motola DL, Caravan P, Chung RT, Fuchs BC. Noninvasive
biomarkers of liver fibrosis: clinical applications and
future directions. *Curr Pathobiol Rep*. 2014;2(4):245–256.

28. Workman TA. *Engaging Patients in Information Sharing and
Data Collection: The Role of Patient-Powered Registries and
Research Networks [Internet]*. Rockville, MD: Agency for
Healthcare Research and Quality; 2013.

29. Chuang-Stein C, Xia HA. The practice of pre-marketing
safety assessment in drug development. *J Biopharm Stat*.
2013;23(1):3–25.

30. Food and Drug Administration. *FDA's Sentinel Initiative*.
2016 [Updated 10/05/2016; cited 2016 24 October].

31. Chan SL, Jin S, Loh M, Brunham LR. Progress in understanding the genomic basis for adverse drug reactions: a
comprehensive review and focus on the role of ethnicity.
Pharmacogenomics. 2015;16(10):1161–1178.

32. Duke SP, Bancken F, Crowe B, Soukup M, Botsis T,
Forshee R. Seeing is believing: good graphic design principles for medical research. *Stat Med*. 2015;34:3040–3059.

33. European Medicines Agency. *Guideline on Good Pharmacoviligance Practices (GVP) Module V- Risk Management Systems*.
European Medicines Agency; 2014:1–60.

34. Kelly BJ. In: Colquitt J, ed. *The Registry of the Future: Leveraging EHR and Patient Data to Drive Better Outcomes*. Quin-
tiles; 2016:27.

35. Center for Innovation in Regulatory Science, ed. *RWD
Collection, Analysis and Reporting: How Do We Maximise its
Use to Optimise the Effectiveness of Medicines Post-approval?
Real World Data to Real World Evidence for Assessing Efficacy
and Effectiveness: Opportunities and Challenges for New Med-
icines Development, Regulatory Review and Health Technology
Assessment; 2016 June 23 and 24*. Tysons Corner, USA: Hyatt
Regency Hotel; 2016.

36. Leaf C. *Here's the Surprising Reason IBM is Partnering with
Celgene*. Time; November 1, 2016.

37. Center for Innovation in Regulatory Science, ed. *How Could
RWD and Alternate Data Source Shape a More Predictable Pro-
cess of "efficacy to Effectiveness Assessment" Using Evidence
Generated Both in and outside the Clinical Drug Development
Process? Real World Data to Real World Evidence for Assessing
Efficacy and Effectiveness: Opportunities and Challenges for
New Medicines Development, Regulatory Review and Health
Technology Assessment; 2016 June 23 and 24*. Tysons Corner,
USA: Hyatt Regency Hotel; 2016.

38. Center for Innovation in Regulatory Science. In: *What Framework(s) Needs to Be in Place to Overcome Barriers to the Implementation of RWD? Real World Data to Real World Evidence for Assessing Efficacy and Effectiveness: Opportunities and Challenges for New Medicines Development, Regulatory Review and Health Technology Assessment; 2016 June 23 and 24.* Tysons Corner, USA: Hyatt Regency Hotel; 2016.

39. Food and Drug Administration. *Pregnancy Registries.* 2016 [Updated 03/31/2016; August 03, 2016].

40. Institute of Medicine. In: Baciu A, Stratton K, Burke SP, eds. *The Future of Drug Safety: Promoting and Protecting the Health of the Public. Committee on the Assessment of the US Drug Safety System.* 500 Fifth Street, N.W., Washington, DC, 20001: The National Academies Press; 2007, 332 p.

41. Centers for Disease Control and Prevention. *Vaccine Safety Datalink (VSD) Centers for Disease Control and Prevention.* 2016 [Updated May 13, 2016; August 03, 2016].

42. Firth S. *Patient Registries See Promise and Challenges Ahead-Physician-Driven Registries Adapt to a Changing Health System. Practice Management [Internet];* 2015. Access date: August 03, 2016. Available from: http://www.medpagetoday.com/practicemanagement/practicemanagement/53516.

43. Ransbotham S, Kiron D, Prentice PK. *Why Competitive Advantage from Analytics Is Declining and What to Do about it. Beyond the Hype: The Hard Work behind Analytics Success [Internet];* August 02, 2016. Available from: http://sloanreview.mit.edu/projects/the-hard-work-behind-data-analytics-strategy/.

44. Berlin JA, Glasser SC, Ellenberg SS. Adverse event detection in drug development: recommendations and obligations beyond phase 3. *Am J Public Health.* 2008;98(8): 1366−1371.

45. Naci H, Smalley KR, Kesselheim AS. Characteristics of preapproval and postapproval studies for drugs granted accelerated approval by the US Food and Drug Administration. http://jama.jamanetwork.com/article.aspx?doi=10.1001/jama.2017.9415&utm_campaign=articlePDF%26utm_medium=articlePDFlink%26utm_source=articlePDF%26utm_content=jama.2017.94154.

46. Hollnagel E. Is safety a subject for science? *Saf Sci.* 2014;67: 21−24.

Index

Note: Page numbers followed by "f" indicate figures, "t" indicate tables and "b" indicate boxes.

Printed in the United States
By Bookmasters